Kettlebell Rx

A More Excellent Way

Jeff Martone

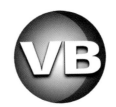

Victory Belt Publishing Inc.

Las Vegas

ISBN: 978-1-936608-99-7

This book is for educational purposes. The publisher and author of this instructional book are not responsible in any manner whatsoever for any adverse effects arising directly or indirectly as a result of the information provided in this book. If not practiced safely and with caution, kettlebell training can be dangerous to you and to others. It is important to consult with a qualified kettlebell coach before training. It is also very important to consult with a physician prior to performing the techniques in this book.

RRD1211

TABLE OF CONTENTS

Section 3: Turkish Get-Up Series

Section 4: Clean Series

Section 5: Overhead Series

Section 6: Kettlebell Rx Program Design

Part II: Rotational Power Development

H2H Program Design

Part III: Introduction to Kettlebell Sport

About the Author

Jeff Martone, founder and CEO of Tactical Athlete Training Systems, Inc., is considered a pioneer and one of the "founding fathers" of the modern kettlebell movement in the United States.

— First to implement kettlebell program into a federal law enforcement academy, 2001.

— Creator of H2H Kettlebell Drills (i.e., kettlebell juggling), 2002.

— Creator of TAPS (Tactical Athlete Pull-up System) & Tactical Rings, 2003.

— Senior instructor for the RKC (Russian Kettlebell Challenge), 2001–2005.

— CrossFit Level-1 Coach, 2004.

— CrossFit Level-2 Coach, 2006.

— Kettlebell SME (subject matter expert) for CrossFit, 2006–present.

— Creator of CrossFit Kettlebell Trainers Course.

— Creator of S.H.O.T. (Super High Output Training), 2006.

— American Kettlebell Club Coach, 2006.

— Kettlebell Sport Lifting Coach, IKSFA, St. Petersburg, Russia, 2010 and 2011.

— First Place New York Open Kettlebell Championship, achieved Rank 1 in Long Cycle, 100 kg weight class (IKSFA Ranking Table), June 2011.

— Presenter at national and international conferences, seminars, and workshops.

— Clients include multiple federal, state, and local law enforcement agencies, special operations personnel, and professional athletes, including top MMA coaches and fighters.

Jeff served seventeen years as a full-time defensive tactics, firearms, and special response team instructor, providing low-profile operator development training for the Nuclear National Security Administration (NNSA).

Jeff is a lifelong martial artist. He achieved the rank of black belt in two styles of kung fu by age eighteen. He boxed in the amateurs and served two years with 19th SFG, RI Army National Guard while in college. He's currently a Gracie Barra BJJ blue belt, under Samuel Braga.

He resides in East Tennessee with the wife of his youth and their two children.

Dedication

Soli Deo Gloria

(for God's glory alone)

"Yet those who wait for the LORD will gain new strength; They will mount up with wings like eagles, They will run and not get tired, They will walk and not become weary."
Isaiah 40:31

And He has said to me, "My grace is sufficient for you, for power is perfected in weakness." Most gladly, therefore, I will rather boast about my weaknesses, so that the power of Christ may dwell in me.
2 Corinthians 12:9

"I can do all things through Him who strengthens me."
Philippians 4:13

"And I show you a still more excellent way."
I Corinthians 12:31

OVERVIEW

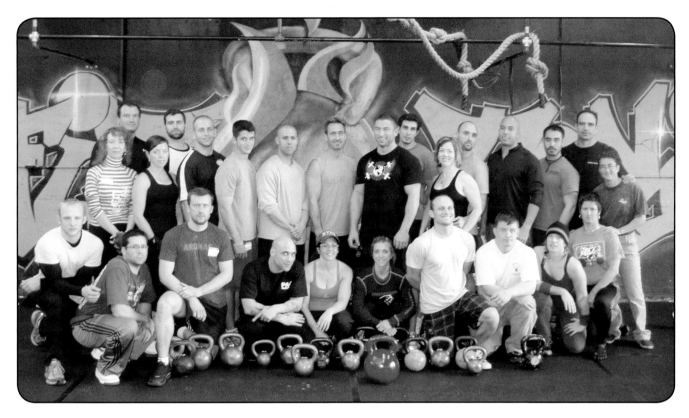

The objective of this book is to share a tested, systematic approach to kettlebell lifting that will maximize your ability to learn, improve, and master fundamental kettlebell exercises in minimum time. This book has three distinct parts. Part 1 and 2 are complete, stand-alone training programs, and part 3 is a primer to kettlebell sport. Essentially, you are holding three separate, yet complimentary, books bound together in one comprehensive training system.

Part I:
Kettlebells for CrossFitters

This is the complete, updated level-one trainer's curriculum that I developed and that I teach all over the world for CrossFit and my company Tactical Athlete Training Systems, Inc. This program will benefit athletes of all disciplines, and even non-athletes. You don't have to be a CrossFitter or a Tactical Athlete to experience the benefits from this general physical preparation (GPP) kettlebell program.

Part II:
Rotational Power Development

This is a unique series of simple hand-to-hand (H2H) KB drills designed to dynamically strengthen core muscles and develop exceptional rotational strength and power. The drills are applicable to any sport or vocation.

Part III:
Introduction to
Kettlebell Sport Technique

This is an introduction to the sport of kettlebell lifting and the unique benefits of practicing the sport technique and specialized physical preparation (SPP) training methods.

This book is written from a coach's perspective. Attention to detail and mastery of the fundamentals are key to minimizing risk of injury and maximizing athletic potential. The difference is always in the details. This is what separates world-class performers from the rest of the pack.

As you begin to learn and apply the training principles outlined in this manual, your athleticism, general well-being, and ability to optimize the full potential of your kettlebells will be significantly enhanced.

A properly implemented kettlebell training program will effectively build functional strength, endurance, and flexibility to your major muscle groups and dramatically increase your anaerobic capacity without running. In addition, it will increase the tensile strength of your connective tissue and strengthen all the stabilizer muscles surrounding your joints. These are just a few of the reasons why the kettlebell has become known as an amazingly effective pre-habilitation and rehabilitation tool for the lower back, knees, and shoulders.

On the other hand, an improperly implemented kettlebell training program will quickly aggravate old injuries or create new ones. Our goal is to train, not to maim anyone in the process. All movements must be performed correctly.

"Learn it right, and you will do it right the rest of your life. Learn it wrong, and you'll spend the rest of your life trying to get it right... and in battle, you meatheads that get it wrong—the rest of your life will be very short."
—Sgt. Steve Prazenka, WWII veteran, 28th (Bloody Bucket) Division

The key to avoiding injuries is to practice correct technique. We've all heard the saying "practice makes perfect." Vince Lombardi clarified and raised the bar by stating that it's not practice that makes perfect; rather, it's perfect practice that makes perfect. Perfect practice—right on! However, I believe Olympian Tommy Kono's statement concerning practice is the most accurate: "Practice makes permanent." Whatever you practice, whether good, bad, or ugly, will be permanently ingrained into your being. This only reinforces the importance to "learn it right the first time."

How to Accelerate the Learning Process

This book is a resource for coaches, trainers, parents, and athletes. To "learn it right the first time," it is critical that you clearly understand the principles behind the teaching methods used throughout this book. This knowledge will aid you in your ability to model the basic skills, evaluate progress, individualize instruction, and accelerate the learning process.

Let's begin by looking at the definition of a motor skill. A motor skill is any act or task that has a goal to achieve and that requires voluntary body or limb movement to be properly performed. Life is one big motor skill. Motor skills can be categorized as either fine or gross. Fine motor skills involve the smaller muscles of the fingers in coordination with the eyes where accuracy is very important (e.g., handwriting, typing, sewing). Gross motor skills, on the other hand, involve movements of the large muscles of the body (e.g., arms, legs, and torso). Running, jumping, throwing, squatting, and kettlebell lifting are examples of Gross motor skills.

Five Steps to Developing Competence

Effective coaches, instructors, and educators follow the five simple steps to develop competence in their students.

1. Tell—Clearly explains the task and its relevance.

2. Show—Demonstrates the skill to be performed.

3. Do—Allows athletes to practice the skill.

4. Observe performance—It is essential that all practice sessions during the first stages of learning are under the coach's supervision.

5. Reward, redirect, and reinforce—Constant feedback is a critical component for learners to correct, modify, and overcome technical deficiencies.

Let's take a closer look:

Steps 1–2: If you are reading this book and I did my job correctly, the steps of explaining and demonstrating have already been done for you. You can look at the pictures, read the captions and exercise descriptions as many times as necessary.

Step 3: The quality and length of your practice sessions are critical for improving skill ability. Follow the teaching progressions as outlined in this book. Repetition establishes habit. In order for you to achieve maximum benefit, I have broken complex skills down into easily digestible parts. Practice the individual parts, then piece them back together and practice the whole skill. This simple strategy will save you a lot of time and unnecessary frustration.

Steps 4–5: There is no substitute for a coach. Because "practice makes permanent," it is ideal to have a coach observe your practice sessions and give you immediate feedback. Technical deficiencies need to be immediately identified and corrected before they become permanent. If you don't have a coach, then find a training partner. For optimal results, you should really find both. The importance of this will become more evident as you finish reading the rest of this chapter.

Three Stages of Skill Development

Awareness and proper understanding of the three stages of skill development (i.e., cognitive, associative, and autonomous stages) are critical for efficient progress from novice to expert. Anytime you learn a new skill, you will go through these same three stages of learning. Exceptional coaches know how to (1) identify which stage of learning his student is in, (2) how to best structure his practice sessions based on that stage of skill development, and (3) give the right coaching cue at the appropriate time to maximize the training results and advance his athlete to the next level.

The Cognitive Stage is the first stage of learning and is the first experience the learner has with the new skill. Learners at this stage have a lot of questions, make lots of mistakes, and are unable to detect and correct errors. They are usually one of two things: (1) unconsciously incompetent—ignorant of the subject or unaware the skill exists—or (2) consciously incompetent—aware the skill exists but with no realistic idea how to perform it.

They need several demonstrations of the correct skill, one or two simple instructions to concentrate on, and short practice sessions with plenty of rest periods in between. Fatigue can hinder correct movement. At this stage, keep your practice sessions short and happy! Repetition establishes habit. As Coach Tommy Kono said: "Practice makes permanent. Practice correct technique!"

The Associative Stage is the second stage of learning. The basic skills are to some extent learned. The learner is attempting to refine the skills they have developed and have some ability to detect errors. Errors have become less frequent and the skill more refined. The learner is now consciously competent—aware and performing the skill, as long as he has time to think, decide, and take action.

Continue to keep practice sessions short and happy. Think quality not quantity. The key to progressing to the next stage is to find an analogy or make a link from an existing skill and apply it to the new skill you are practicing (e.g., vertical jump for hip drive). This facilitates learning because you aren't really "learning" a new skill, only adapting one you mastered in the past to a different task.

The Autonomous Stage is the final stage of learning. It is at this stage that the skill appears to be automatic. The learner does not have to attend to every phase of the skill, and is able to detect and correct his own errors. This is referred to as unconscious competence (mastery). The autonomous stage is only accomplished with correct practice. How many reps does it take to reach the autonomous stage? Some research says thousands of reps, others suggest 100 percent more repetitions than it took the student to accomplish the skill one time correctly without help. Other studies have shown that the higher the motivation and importance, the fewer repetitions are needed to become skillful.

Note: It is only in this stage that skills should be practiced in a fatigued state. It is imperative that you always terminate practice just before proper form begins to deteriorate. Work out smart and focus on quality training. Practice sessions should be challenging and enjoyable. It's best to leave with the knowledge that you learned something and achieved the best possible performance for that day.

Find a Training Partner

The goal when training is to move through the above stages of skill acquisition as quickly and efficiently as possible. There is no substitute for a good coach. If you don't have a qualified coach in your area, then I strongly recommend that you find a training partner. A like-minded training partner is an essential ingredient for your success

"Two are better than one because they have a good return for their labor."

—Ecclesiastes 4:9

As we just discussed, during the first stages of learning, you will make lots of errors and have no ability to detect and correct common errors. A good coach provides constant feedback while the student is performing the skill and after the skill is practiced. Feedback is information given to learners that helps them learn, modify, and correct their performance. This allows learners to think about what they did right or wrong. It's all about efficiency—streamlining and facilitating the learning process. The one major limitation when it comes to learning motor skill from books and DVDs—they can't provide feedback during your practice sessions! This is why everyone needs a coach or training partner.

A good training partner also serves as a good spotter. A spotter is essential to maximizing training safety. A good spotter gives you the confidence to try something new and the freedom to fail by minimizing the consequences for failure.

"For if either of them fall, the one will lift up his companion, but woe to the one who falls when there is not another to lift him up."

—Ecclesiastes 4:10

Teaching others accelerates our learning. It's been said that if you really want to master a subject, then try to teach it to someone else. The teaching process forces you to examine what you are doing and why. Pay close attention to teaching sequences in this book. They are designed to be self-correcting. Common errors will be addressed and eliminated as you practice and progress through the different drills and skills. The difference is in the details.

"Iron sharpens iron, so one man sharpens another."

—Proverbs 27:17

If your circumstances are such that you don't have a coach and can't or won't find a training partner, then the next best step would be to videotape your practice sessions, then compare them to the examples in the book. Recording your training sessions can be a powerful learning tool. Many times what we think we're doing and what we're actually doing are two totally different things. It can be quite the eye opener.

If you're really technologically challenged, then I guess you can use a mirror. I'm not a big advocate of training in front of mirrors. Use them sparingly, just quickly check your form and move on before you get mesmerized into an "I'm so wonderful" self-love-fest.

Learning Styles

As a coach, training partner, or athlete, it is important to understand that there are three primary styles of learning: visual, kinesthetic, and auditory. Adult learners generally have their preferred method of learning, even though they use a variety of all three styles. Understanding this information will enable you to adjust your teaching style to better fit the needs of the person you are training.

Visual Learners focus on the visual part of the instruction. Demonstrations (live, video, or pictures) are vital to these learners because if they can "see it," they can "do it." Visual learners have a need to "see" everything. In a classroom or group setting they tend to sit/stand toward the front of the class. They want to be close but not too close because they want to take in the "entire picture." If you listen closely, visual learners will use "visual references" in their speech like "I don't see the big picture" or "I just can't imagine that" or "yes, I see what you are saying."

Kinesthetic Learners are the "touchy-feely" folks in the group. They need to touch and feel everything, physically or emotionally. Practice sessions are key to this type of learner. The practice sessions allow the learner time to get the "feel of the motor skills they are attempting to learn." In a classroom environment, this type of learner must be comfortable in order to learn. They also look like they have ADD (attention deficit disorder) because they will be anxious to get to the practice session so they can check themselves out on the skill. Kinesthetic learners tend to use "physical/emotional" references, saying things like: "I can't get a handle on this" or "I don't feel like I'm getting this."

Auditory Learners tend to take in their information through the hearing process. These learners like a good verbal description of the task required of them. The most common type of auditory learner is the digital. Digital learners like to learn the task in a logical, sequential order. They prefer to have the task broken down into numbered steps and in the correct order. These learners tend to have their ear toward the speaker and will be greatly distracted by noise outside the learning environment. They will use references like "there is a piece missing" or "this doesn't make sense."

Taking It Full Circle

All learners use all three styles of learning. They just tend to favor one and will use it as often as they can. Oddly enough, by following the "Five Steps to Developing Competence" you will address all three learning styles in one fell swoop.

1. Tell—(Auditory): Clearly explains the task (logical, sequential order) and its relevance.

2. Show—(Visual): Demonstrates the skill to be performed. Sets the standard of performance, provides a mental template of the example to be followed.

3. Do—(Kinesthetic): Allows athletes to practice the skill. When in doubt, break the skill down into easily digestible parts, and then piece it back together.

4. Observe performance—It is essential that all practice sessions during the first stages of learning are under a coach's supervision. Coaches need to assess the situation: actually see and analyze what's happening. Fatigue in the early stages of learning is counterproductive. Practice sessions need to be short and happy!

5. Reward, redirect, and reinforce—Constant feedback is a critical component for learners to correct, modify, and overcome technical deficiencies. Focus on correcting one or two errors at a time. Try to link the new skill to a skill they already mastered in the past. Be creative and be patient. They will eventually transition into the Autonomous Stage.

Conclusion

Coaching can be challenging and very rewarding. It has been said that there is no such thing as a bad student, just bad teachers. It is important to take the time to understand the reasons behind the teaching methods we use and to use the appropriate method or technique at the right time. If you do not understand the "why" behind the teaching methods, it is difficult to become an effective coach.

This book is designed so that you can easily follow the pictures, read the explanations, practice the drills, observe and compare the results to a standard, make corrections, and then continue onward making forward progress. Stay the course, enjoy the process, and finish strong!

The mediocre teacher tells.
The good teacher explains.
The superior teacher demonstrates.
The great teacher inspires

—William Arthur Ward

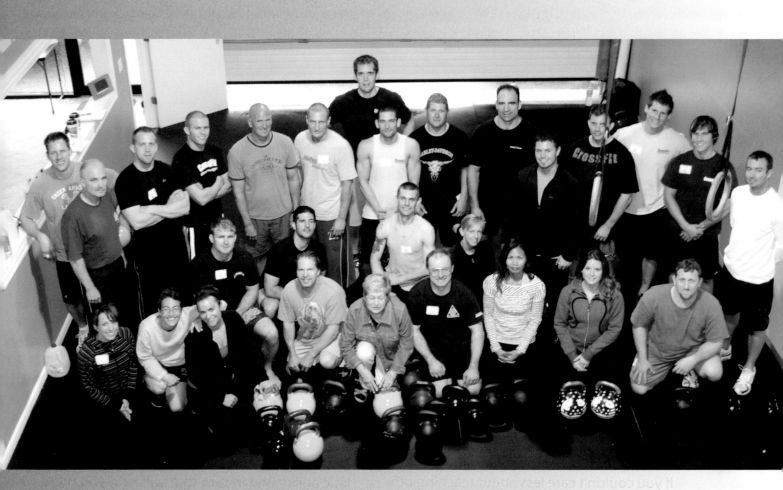

If you couldn't care less about a healthier lifestyle but just want to learn how to stretch, then

Part I

Kettlebells for CrossFitters

Part One consists of the Level-1 Kettlebell Trainers Course curriculum that I developed and teach all over the world for CrossFit and for my company Tactical Athlete Training Systems, Inc. This is a General Physical Preparedness (GPP) Kettlebell fitness program that's applicable to any sport or vocation.

If you have already attended and passed either the CrossFit or Tactical Athlete Kettlebell Trainer courses, then Part One will serve as an updated training resource with many new training insights and teaching progressions.

If you are considering attending a Level-1 Kettlebell Trainers Course in the near future, then this information will give you a solid foundation and help you to properly prepare for that event.

If you couldn't care less about teaching others but just want to learn how to safely train with kettlebells and implement them into your existing routines or CrossFit WODs (Workout of the Day), then Part One will serve you well.

If, on the other hand, you don't do CrossFit, you never heard of CrossFit, or maybe you don't even like CrossFit, but want to learn how to properly use a kettlebell and get into the best shape of your life with minimal time, then this is the program for you.

The kettlebell is probably still one of the most misunderstood and under-utilized tools within the fitness community. Regardless of your kettlebell experience, this curriculum is designed to adeptly take you from a kettlebell zero to hero. Part One of this book and the accompanying DVD set "Beyond the American Swing" are resources that will help expand your ability as an athlete and a coach to unlock the full potential of your kettlebells.

What Is GPP?

General Physical Preparation (GPP) is defined as any non-sport-specific workout that develops a set of general athletic qualities or physical skills. This includes: cardiovascular and respiratory endurance, strength, stamina, flexibility, power, speed, coordination, accuracy, agility, and balance. By Improving GPP, you increase your athletic ability and in turn that will help you more effectively train for sport-specific or job-specific activities in other workouts.

Part One is comprehensive and systematic GPP kettlebell training program. It is broken down into the following six sections:

Section 1: Joint Mobility/Flexibility
Section 2: Swing Series
Section 3: Turkish Get-Up Series
Section 4: Clean Series
Section 5: Overhead Series
Section 6: Program Design

GPP vs. Sport

You can train with kettlebells for general fitness to enhance your sport, or you can train with kettlebells as a sport. In a similar fashion, you can practice the Olympic weighting style movements as a means to increase power output for your sport, or you can train specifically to compete in the sport of Olympic weightlifting. Just as you can do CrossFit to improve general athletic qualities for your sport or you can do CrossFit as a sport. There are technical and programming differences based on the goals you are trying to achieve. Part Three of this manual will specifically address the techniques, goals, and objectives used within the sport of kettlebell lifting.

What Is CrossFit?

CrossFit, founded by coach Greg Glassman, is a strength and conditioning program built upon constantly varied, functional movement, executed at high intensity. Functional movements are safe, common, multijoint movements utilizing universal motor recruitment patterns. They are efficient and effective movements you see and use all the time. The CrossFit "movement pool" is derived from movements used in Olympic weightlifting, power lifting, kettlebell lifting, gymnastics, running, biking, rowing, swimming, striking, jumping rope, and so on.

Functional Movement Is Functional Movement

Kinesiology is the study of the principles of mechanics and anatomy in relation to human movement. It is not only important to understand how certain movements are executed, but also why they are executed in such a way. Throughout this book we will discuss and clarify basic body mechanics as it relates to efficient movement and effective lifting style.

Years ago, I was invited to present at the July 2006 CrossFit Training Seminar, hosted at CrossFit San Diego. In between my kettlebell training sessions, I would watch, listen, and learn from the other presenters. Most of those coaches now teach their own discipline for what is now known as the CrossFit Specialty Courses. I found the whole event inspiring for three reasons. First, the level of athleticism and motivation of the participants was phenomenal. Second, it was an awesome opportunity to get personal instruction from a diverse group of truly great teachers. Third, I was struck by observing the pervasiveness of a common thread of movement mechanics—specifically hip flexion to extension—that weaves through the disciplines that make up CrossFit.

During his presentation, Tony Blauer made the statement that "good information doesn't displace other good information." The seminar was practical evidence of this assertion, as it seemed that the more different coaches offered information, the more it all came together, and the more they reinforced each other's points and methods. Mark Rippetoe's detailed analysis of the deadlift is a perfect example. The mechanics of the deadlift and the importance of achieving and maintaining lumbar and thoracic back extension during the deadlift are also essential when performing Olympic lifts or kettlebell swings, cleans, and snatches. The same holds true for Coach Burgener's definition of the Olympic lifts as "a vicious extension of the ankles, knees, and hips that creates momentum and elevation of the barbell." This same "vicious extension" also takes place in the jumping movements of gymnastics and parkour. One movement, many applications—now, that's inspiring.

That also makes perfect sense. In sports, we adopt postures that give us stability, mobility, and strength. We can enhance our efficiency by co-opting existing body positions that have proven successful and adapting them to a different task. The benefits of co-opting existing body motions are threefold:

- They are easier to learn because you aren't really "learning" them (i.e., only adapting them).

- They are easier to master rapidly and consistently.

- They are easier to execute on demand under stress.

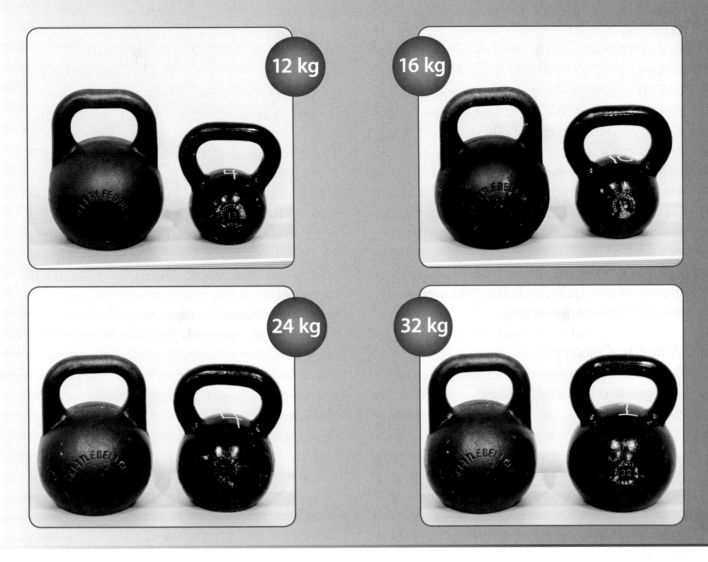

These are critical but rarely acknowledged concepts and are a great way to explain to athletes of all levels why certain techniques work best. Get in the habit of thinking about and analyzing every movement you practice and why it is the best solution. This is something my training partner and I do on a consistent basis. My training partner, Richie Carter, summed it up best one day when he said, "If a something works, you'll see it in multiple disciplines."

Kettlebell Selection

Kettlebells come in a variety of shapes and sizes. Prices vary depending on perceived quality and country of manufacture. It is amazing to see how many manufacturers have jumped on the kettlebell bandwagon over the last few years. I honestly don't even try to keep track of whose making what version anymore. Listed below are some basic criteria to consider before purchasing a kettlebell.

There are basically two main styles of kettlebells: The Dragon Door style kettlebells (aka Russian Kettlebells) and Competition Style kettlebells, which are considered the "standard" in Russia for the sport of kettlebell lifting (aka kettlebell sport). There are pros and cons to training with each style. A lot of it depends on your training goals.

Dragon Door was the first company to manufacture and sell kettlebells in the USA. In 2001, the very first "Russian Kettlebells" hit the market. The Dragon Door style kettlebells are distinguished by a handle that resembles the outline of a Mickey Mouse ear, and the bell (i.e., the sphere or ball portion of the Kettlebell) is cast solid. The handle thickness and bell size varies depending on the weight of the kettlebell. As the weight of the kettlebell increases, so does the size of the bell and thickness of the handle. A benefit to this style KB is that you can usually fit both hands rather comfortably on to the handle for a variety of two-handed swings. These kettlebells are also great for juggling or H2H KB drills because they tend to rotate quicker and are a little easier to handle than the competition style. The down side to this style kettlebell is that as the kettlebell gets lighter, the handle and bell (i.e., sphere) gets smaller. This leads to inconsistent trajectory patterns and constant minor adjustments in technique when changing weights. Smaller kettlebells have less surface area and tend to land like a ball-peen hammer on the back of your arms, especially when you are trying to learn how to clean and snatch.

The competition style kettlebells are considered the standard in the sport of kettlebell lifting. The shape and diameter of the handle as well as the dimensions of the bell are consistent, regardless of the weight. The benefit is that every size kettlebell has the same feel and trajectory. It's also great for beginners, youths, and females because of the size of the bell—it has more points of contact in the rack position (clean) and a bigger surface area on the back of your forearm (snatch). It's similar to the advantages of training with Olympic bumper plates, where all bumpers are the same diameter. Whether it is 10-pound or 45-pound plates, your height of the bar and your pull starts from the exact same height every time. It's all about consistency.

I personally own and train with both styles. Most CrossFit Gyms use some variation of the Dragon Door Style KBs. That's fine for general fitness. If you aspire to compete in the sport of kettlebell lifting, then I would strongly recommend the competition-style kettlebells. If I were going to open a gym tomorrow, the bulk of my kettlebells would be the competition style. Unless I'm specifically practicing H2H drills, I find myself training more and more with the competition-style kettlebells.

All other kettlebells are some variation on the theme. Some handles are taller, shorter, wider, etc. Never purchase a kettlebell without first physically getting hold of one to try it out and see how it feels.

Which size should I start with?

Generally speaking, 8 kilograms (kg) is a great beginning weight for women and young teens. Sixteen kilograms is a good starting weight for men. The traditional standard weights lifted in competition are 16 kg, 24 kg, and 32 kg. You get the most mileage out of kettlebells of 8, 12, 16, 20, and 24 kg.

How many should I purchase?

A lot depends on your budget. For a home gym, ultimately, you want to get at least two of each size.

Safety 101

Safety is the name of the game if you're looking for longevity as a coach or an athlete. The following guidelines cannot cover all training contingencies and there's no substitute for common sense.

General Guidelines:

- Consult your physician before attempting any new conditioning program.

- Use only high-quality kettlebells. They will last you a lifetime.

- Keep your training area clutter free

- Always have a first aid kit available

- Stay hydrated

- No horse play

Basic Safety Rules to Consider before Training with Kettlebells

- Train where there is no concern about property damage or injury to anyone in your vicinity.

- Practice proper lifting techniques at all times, even with very light kettlebells. Remember, repetition establishes habit.

- Don't try to recover a questionable rep. When in doubt—drop the kettlebell(s). Guide the falling KB, if necessary, but don't fight it. Keep in mind, "Quick feet are happy feet."

- Wear flat-sole shoes for GPP (i.e., wrestling shoes, Chuck Taylors, Inov-8s, Vibram 5-Fingers, etc.) Avoid training in running shoes with big cushy heels.

- Work within your current flexibility limits.

- Build up your training load gradually, using common sense.

- When in doubt, consult a sports doctor when dealing with preexisting injuries.

"Life is hard; it's harder if you're stupid."

—John Wayne

The Keys to Learning It Right

The "Rules of Engagement" are proven teaching strategies that will enhance your ability to learn it right the first time, avoid common pitfalls, and address common errors before they become habit.

Rules of Engagement:

- Begin each training session with a simple warm-up; refer to Section 1 Joint Mobility/Flexibility.

- Master the Russian swing first! Establish a solid, unshakable foundation by wisely investing your time and getting this exercise correct.

- Master the exercises in the sequence presented! This can be a tough for some people. A lot of us want to learn everything all at once. Stay focused. Each exercise builds upon the previous one. This is by design to accelerate your learning process.

- Master each section in the order presented: swings, cleans, then the overhead series; in that order. The Turkish get-up (TGU) series stands alone. You can practice that section anytime before, during, or after the swings.

- Limit the number of reps in your learning sets to 10 repetitions or less for all swings, cleans, and snatches. Strive for perfect form—not a workout. It's better to do multiple sets of low reps to perfect your form.

- Give yourself plenty of rest in between sets. Stay as fresh as possible to maintain precise form. The irony is that you will get a good "workout" while you are practicing.

- Focus your attention on the mechanics and nuances of generating maximum power from your hips.

- Limit the number of reps of strength exercises from three to five when practicing and refining your skill. These exercises would include pressing movements and TGU series.

- Get a training partner and commit to excellence.

- As a learner, focus on the pictures that show you how to do it right. The teaching sequences are designed to be "self-correcting." Common errors are minimized through good practice.

- As a training partner, compare your partner's movement with the standard. If something doesn't look right, search through the common error pictures until you find one that matches. Actually see and analyze what's happening. Identify errors, and then apply the corrective action.

- Have fun, enjoy the learning process, and savor every victory!

Conclusion

There are many kettlebell exercise variations. Master the basic lifts (virtuosity) and the principles of power generation. When training, use liberal amounts of common sense. Finish your sets before your form starts to deteriorate. Never go to failure! Treat each workout as a practice session and constantly try to improve your form, striving to make each exercise effortless.

It is your choice whether to follow the simplicity of the kettlebell-only routines, or turn your current fitness routines into a killer package of all-around strength and conditioning by simply adding a few new kettlebell exercises. The choices are many and the benefits are plenty.

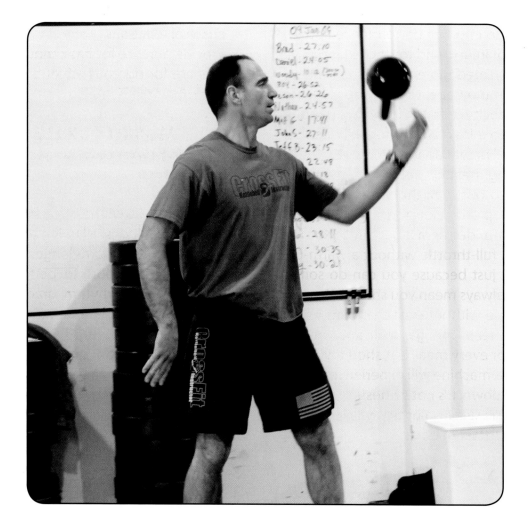

Section 1
Joint Mobility/Flexibility

"Blessed are the flexible, for they will not be broken."
—Pastor Chuck Smith

INTRODUCTION

A proper warm-up is critical for optimum performance, and it becomes more important as we age. It is an absolutely essential part of our daily routines to improve performance and reduce the risk of injury. And for those who have already accumulated more "miles" then that of a person twice their age, there's hope; proper warm-ups, mobility drills, and paying attention to detail will go a long way in rehabilitation of old injuries and prevention of new ones.

Most young, healthy people have a natural tendency to overlook the importance of a proper warm-up and cool-down. I know I did. Some athletes pride themselves on their ability to perform full-throttle without a warm-up. Keep in mind; just because you can do something doesn't always mean you should. You can run your vehicle without ever changing its oil; you can put water in your gas tank; and you can eat Twinkies for every meal, but should you? At some point the machine will experience a catastrophic breakdown. It's not a question of if, but rather when. The same holds true with our bodies. It's only a matter of time.

Warm-up Criteria:
- Increase body temperature and heart rate
- Provide some stretching
- Stimulate the entire body and major biomechanical functions
- Provide practice for basic movements
- Prepare for rigorous athletic training [(CrossFit Journal, issue 8, April 2003)]

I. JOINT MOBILITY DRILLS
—Maintain proper form longer and with less discomfort.

The following drills will help you smoothly move into athletic positions, allowing you to achieve and maintain proper form longer and with less discomfort. It is import to perform mobility drills in a controlled rhythm, gradually increasing to maximum range of motion. Note: these drills are not static stretches. Neither are they bouncy ballistic movements! The emphasis should be on smooth movement, staying within a comfortable range of motion (ROM), gradually increasing ROM as your muscles and joints warm up (i.e., increase blood flow to muscles, synovial fluid to the joints, body temperature, etc.). Think of it as "oiling" the joints. Be patient and consistent, and gradually you begin to regain your God-given freedom of movement.

Ideally, the repetitions should match the age of the participant. Realistically, 20–30 repetitions will be sufficient to achieve desired results. If you have an injury, you may need to increase your reps to 50–100. Initially you may have to break the drills down into multiple sets of lower reps. Gradually work toward fewer and fewer sets until you're performing one set of the total number of reps.

According to Pavel Tsatsouline's book *Super Joints,* "Rotating a joint through its anatomically complete range of motion—or trying to approach that ROM if the joint is damaged—smoothes out the joint surfaces and lubricates them. This contributes greatly to the joint's health. A full range of motion is gained or maintained."

Therefore, a few minutes of daily practice first thing in the morning, prior to a workout, is ideal. If necessary, repeat before retiring. Habitual practice will put you on the right road to enhancing your joint health, economy of motion, and painless movement.

Joint mobility drills can serve as a total body warm-up, a form of active recovery, and a means to regain normal range of motion that was lost through injury or inactivity. The body is designed to move. Range of motion (ROM) is a "use it or lose it" proposition. If you don't use a ROM, you will lose it. Find a toddler and carefully watch how he moves. Toddlers have amazing flexibility and full range of motion in all their joints. They perform effortless rock bottom squats and maintain perfect posture when sitting on the floor playing with their toys. If you perform a few mobility drills before you go to bed at night, it will make getting out of bed much easier the next morning. For years, I crept out of bed feeling like the Tin Man from the Wizard of Oz before Dorothy applied the oil. I remember thinking to myself; man, I shouldn't hurt this bad (i.e., crippled) at this young of an age (early to mid-thirties). Now that I'm in my mid-forties, I have better range of motion than when I was in my twenties. It didn't happen overnight. It took a little determination and consistent effort. That's a small price to pay for pain-free movement and mobility.

General Guidelines:

- Perform first thing in the morning or prior to a workout.

- Keep good posture (i.e., chest up, shoulders back and down).

- Perform movements in a controlled, smooth rhythm.

- Always stay within a comfortable ROM.

- Never force a range of motion. Let your body warm up naturally.

- Gradually increase speed of movement.

- Gradually increase ROM.

- Never use bouncy ballistic movements.

- Do as many reps as your age. Realistically, 20–30 repetitions should be more than sufficient to achieve the desired results.

- Perform mobility drills before retiring makes getting out of bed much easier in the morning.

- For best results, practice mobility drills from head to toe (i.e., top to bottom).

a. Tilting—Forward/Back

Gently move your chin down toward your chest and up toward the ceiling.

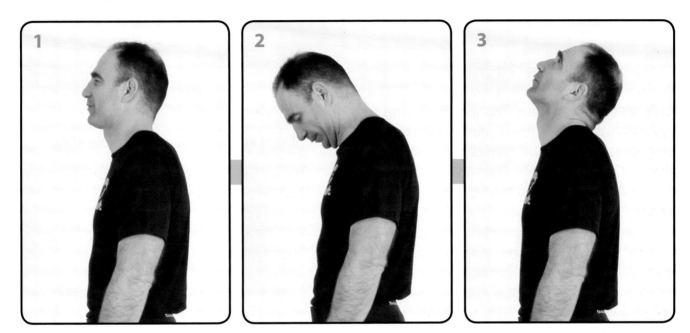

b. Rotating—Left/Right

Keeping your head in good alignment, turn your head to the left and right. Every couple of reps, try to turn your head a little further. Look in the direction you are turning your head and gradually pick up your speed of movement.

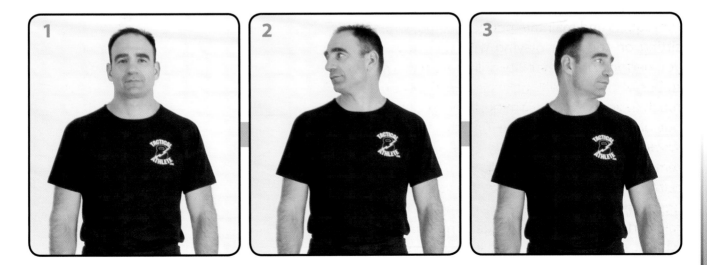

c. Tilting—Left/Right

Try to move your left ear toward your left shoulder, then your right ear toward your right shoulder. After a few reps and your neck is feeling loose, try lifting the side of your jaw toward the ceiling instead. You should feel a distinct stretch and a noticeable increase in your ROM.

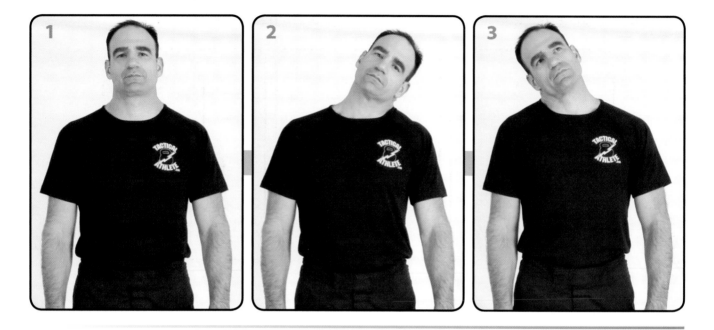

d. Sliding head—Forward/Back

Begin by sliding your head forward, until your chin is directly over your toes, and then reverse the direction. As your head moves back towards the neutral position, lift the crown of your head towards the ceiling. Sometimes it's helpful to imagine you have strings attached to the crown of your head like a marionette puppet, and someone is pulling up on the string. This will also cause your chest to open (i.e., lift) up.

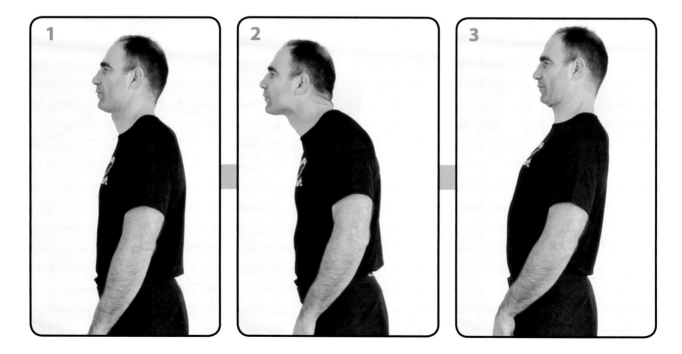

e. Sliding Head to Left/Right

Keeping your head vertically oriented, slide it to the left then right. The easiest way to get the motion of this exercise is to extend your arms over your head and interlock your fingers. Keeping your head upright, slide it over (without tilting) until your left ear touches your left biceps, and then slide your head in the opposite direction until your right ear touches your right biceps. Initially, it may be helpful to practice this exercise in front of the mirror until you get the movement correct.

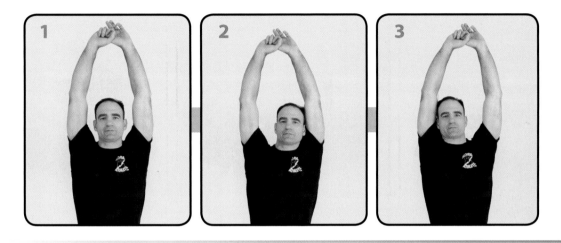

2. SHOULDERS

a. Arm Circles Overhead

Extend your arms straight overhead (i.e., elbows locked, wrists straight, biceps close to ears) and rotate your arms in small circles. Be sure to keep your chest open throughout the entire drill. Be sure to work both directions.

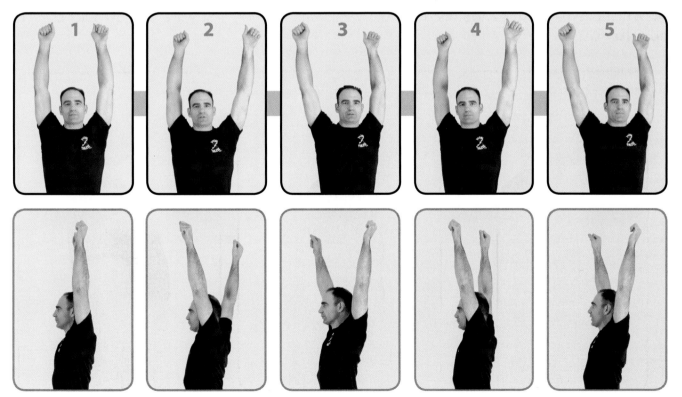

b. Shoulder Rolls Forward & Back

— Begin in a neutral stance, arms by your sides.
— Move your shoulders in a circular motion (i.e., back, up, front, and back to start point). Every few reps, gradually try to increase the entire ROM.
— Reverse direction and repeat.

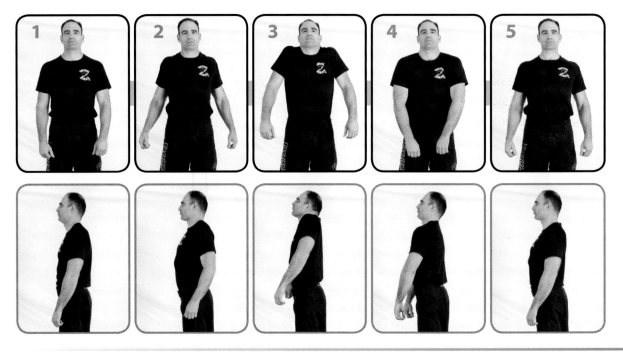

c. Scarecrow

— This is a great exercise to loosen up the rotator cuff.
— Begin by lifting your elbows to shoulder height, pinch your shoulder blades (i.e., scapulae) toward each other and open your chest.
— Maintain a 90-degree bend in your elbows then slowly rotate your forearms up (palms facing away) and down (palms facing behind you). Be sure to keep your shoulder blades pinched through the entire exercise!
— Go slow, be smooth, and always stay within a comfortable range of motion.

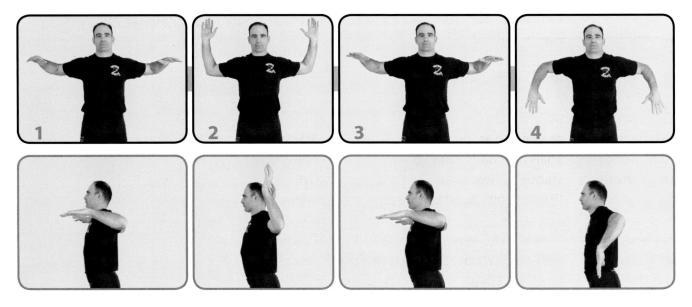

d. Egyptian

— Begin with your arms outstretched to the sides. Imagine someone tied thick bungee cords around your wrists, stretching your arms apart.
— Initiate movement with the right shoulder and hip, pivoting on the ball of your right foot. The shoulder moves up toward your ear then rotates over.
— Reverse the movement until you're back in the neutral position.
— Repeat same movement on the left side.

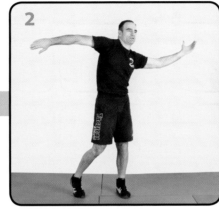
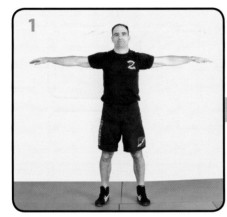
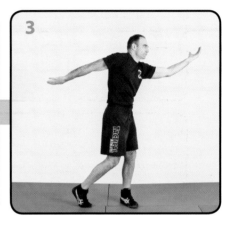
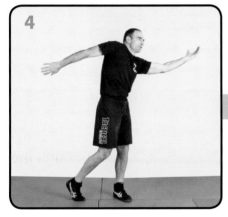
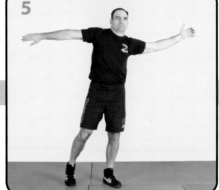
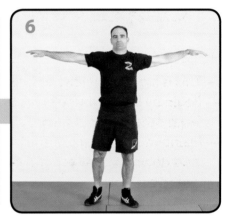
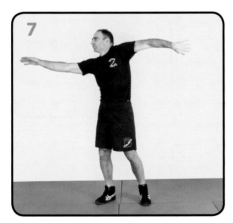

a. Side Circles

— Begin with arms extended out to the side, hands clenched as if holding a piece of chalk.

— Keep elbows at shoulder height and simultaneously draw two big circles. Both hands move up toward the head then down away from the body, in a circular motion. Be sure your elbows fully flex and extend with each rotation for the desired number of reps.

— Change directions & repeat.

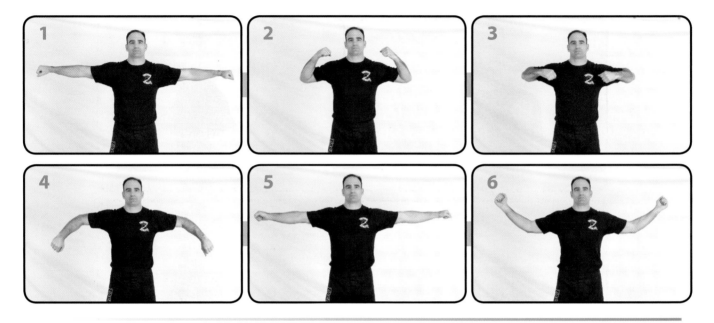

b. Speed Bag

— Loosely clenching your hands, lift them in front of your chest and face. Your right hand should be above the left, elbows slightly flared toward the outside.

— Extend your top hand, similar to a boxer extending to strike a speed bag. Alternate extending and flexing each arm in a circular manner.

— Change directions and repeat for desired number of reps.

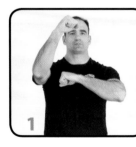
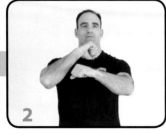
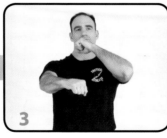
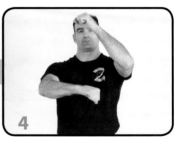
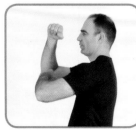
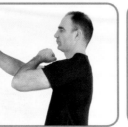
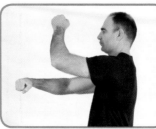
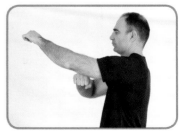

c. Wrist Circles

— Begin by clenching your fists and placing them in front of your chest, elbows down, knuckles out, and wrists slightly flexed.
— Flex your wrists and rotate your knuckles toward each other.
— Continue the rotation until your wrists are straight, knuckles up, thumbs outboard.
— Rotate thumbs inboard, flexing wrists, palms down.
— Repeat circles for desired reps.
— Change direction and repeat.

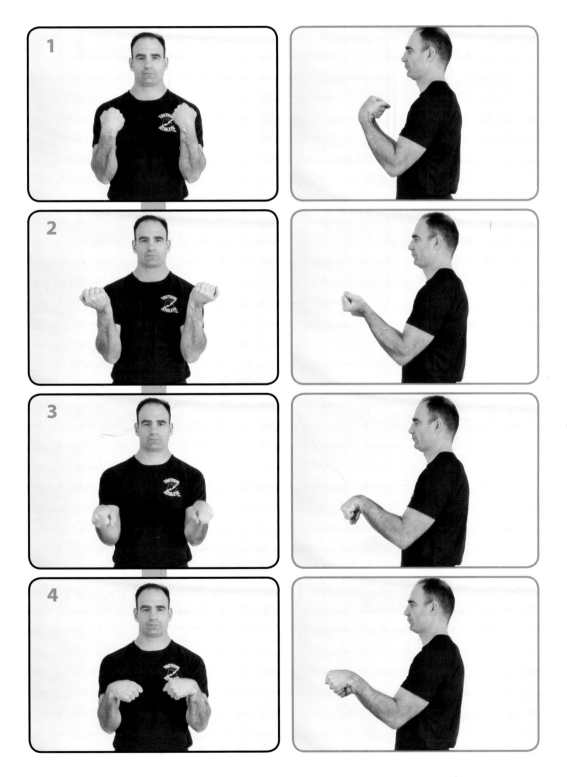

Joint Mobility/Flexibility

d. Finger Waves

— Begin with loosely clenched fists in front of your chest.
— Simultaneously extend your thumbs and rotate your thumbs to the outside, palms up.
— Extend each finger sequentially, starting with the index finger until all your fingers are totally extended.
— Rotate your hands palms down.
— Flex all your fingers, one at a time, starting with the index finger until your fists are clenched.
— Repeat for desired reps.

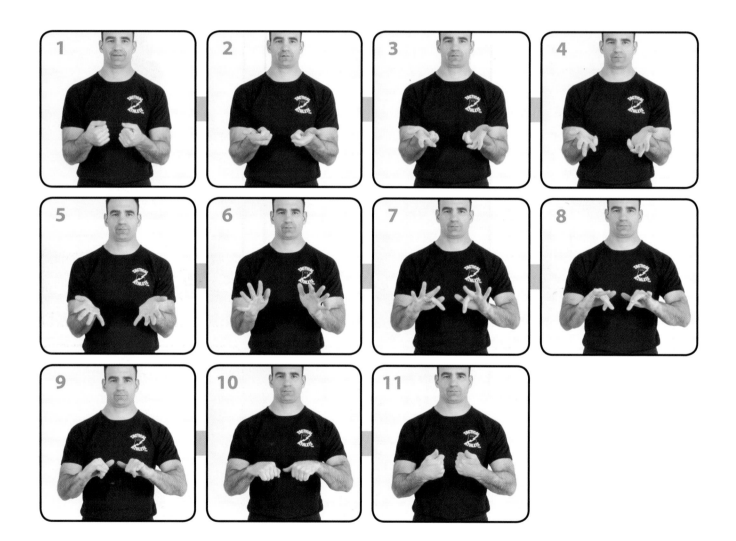

a. Spinal Rotation

— Begin in a neutral stance, toes forward.
— Initiate movement with your eyes by looking at a point behind you. Where the eyes go, the body will follow.
— Rotate your head and shoulders to the right and left keeping your arms relaxed.
— Attempt to go a little farther every few reps.

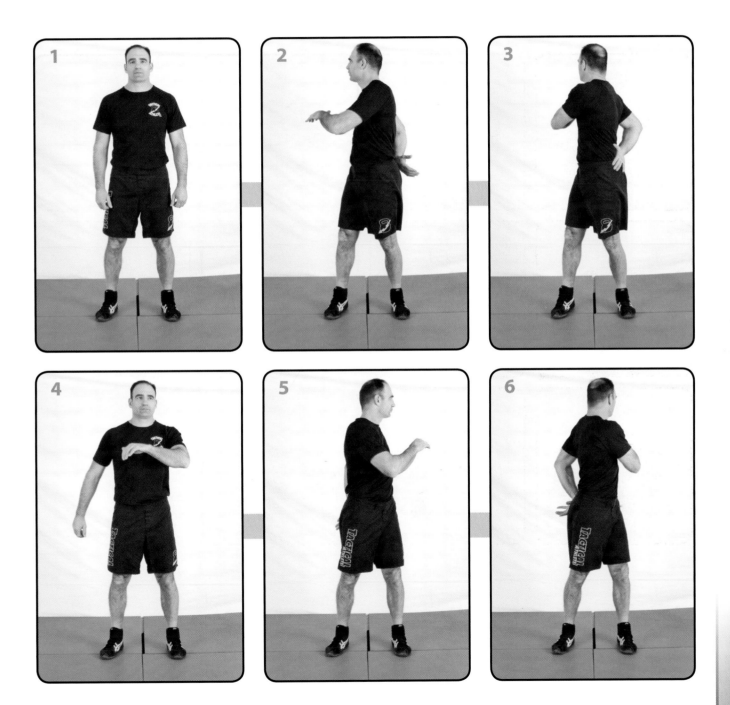

b. Lateral Spinal Flexion

— From a neutral stance, perform a side bend by extending your left arm up and over your head while leaning toward your right.

— Reverse directions by extending your right arm over your head and leaning toward your left.

— Keep your hips square and avoid any type of twisting of your torso.

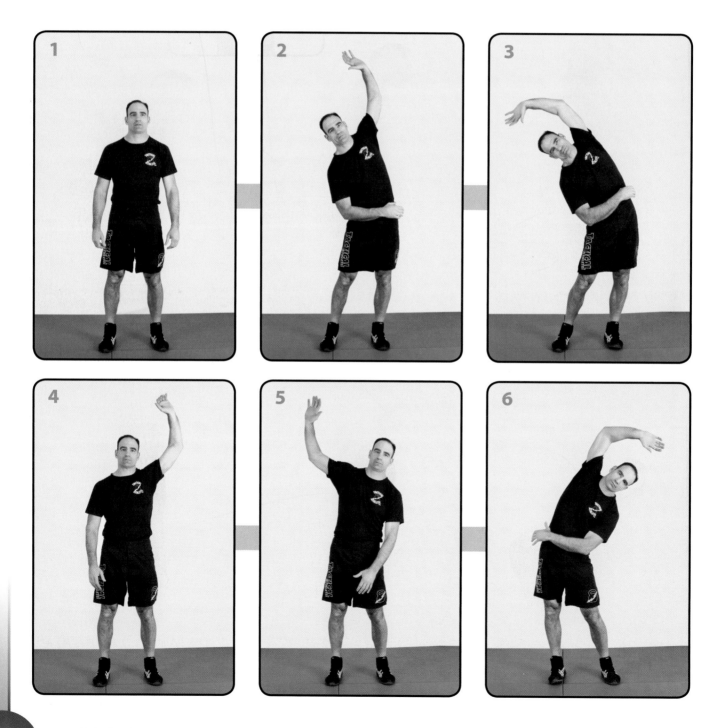

c. Good Mornings

— Begin in a neutral stance, feet hip width apart.
— Interlock your fingers behind your head and pull your shoulder blades together, opening your chest.
— Move your hips backwards, knees slightly bent. Your shins stay vertical; weight transfers to your heels.
— Once you feel a little tightness in your hamstring, return to the starting position.
— Repeat for desired number of reps, attempt to increase ROM every couple of reps.

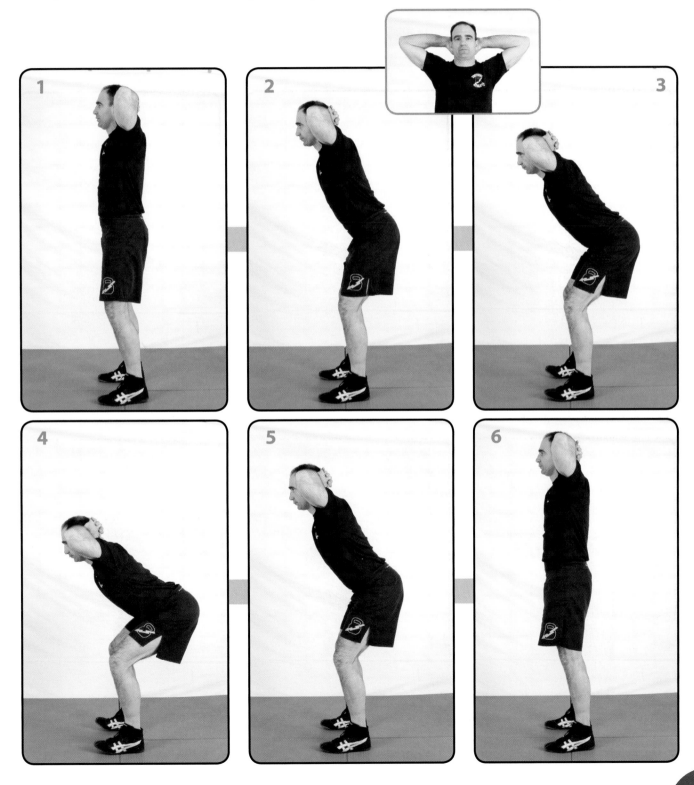

d. Spinal Flexion/Extension

— Begin in a neutral stance, feet shoulder width apart.

— Bend over by folding at the hip, hands move through center of legs. It's important to exhale through your mouth as you bend over. This will help relax your hamstring muscles and increase your ROM.

— Once you reach your bottom position, reverse direction.

— Inhale through your nose on the way up, packing air into your diaphragm (i.e., lower abs).

— As your body straightens, extend your arms over your head, tighten your glutes, and lean backward as if you were attempting to wrap yourself around a very big ball.

— Return to neutral position and repeat.

— Try to gradually increase your ROM during both the flexion and extension phases of movement.

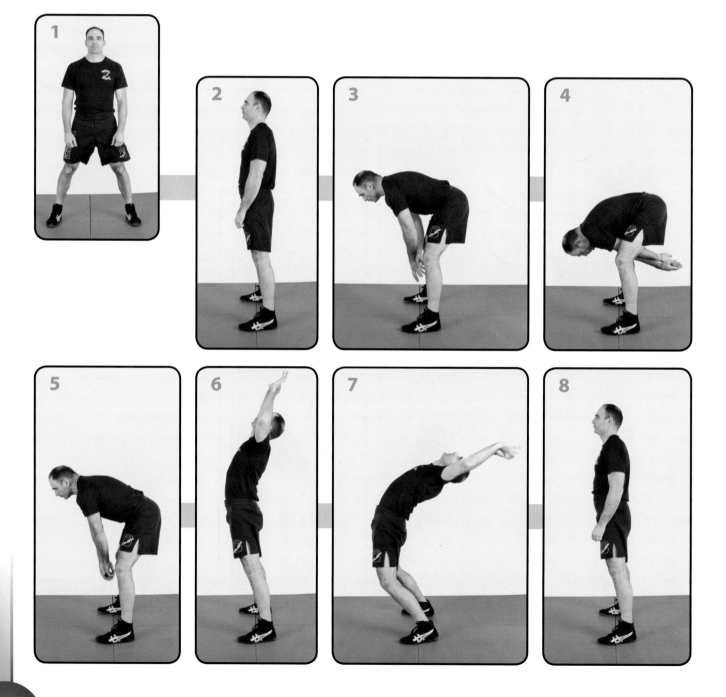

e. Spinal Flexion—Rotation/Extension

— Begin in a neutral stance, feet together.
— Bend over by folding at the hip, extend your right hand toward the outside of your left ankle. Exhale through your mouth as you bend over.
— Once you reach the bottom position, return to neutral, extending your arms straight overhead. Contract your glutes and lean backward as if attempting to wrap yourself around a very big ball.
— Return to neutral and then fold at the hip, reaching your left hand toward the outside of your right ankle.
— Repeat alternating sides for desired number of reps.

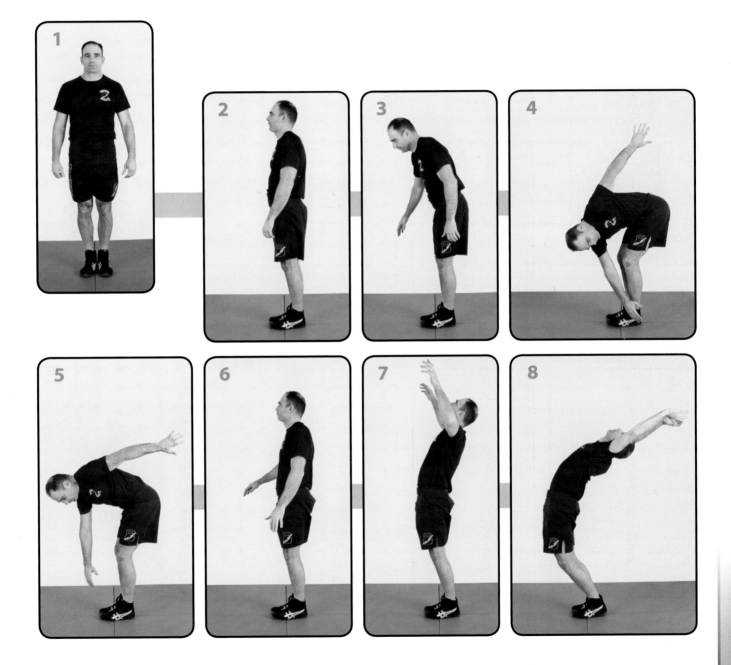

a. Hip Circles

— Begin in a neutral stance, feet hip width apart.

— Place your hands on your hips and slowly move your hips in a circular motion to the left, front, right, and back. The motion is similar to using a hula-hoop.

— Shoulders stay directly over your feet. Move only your hips.

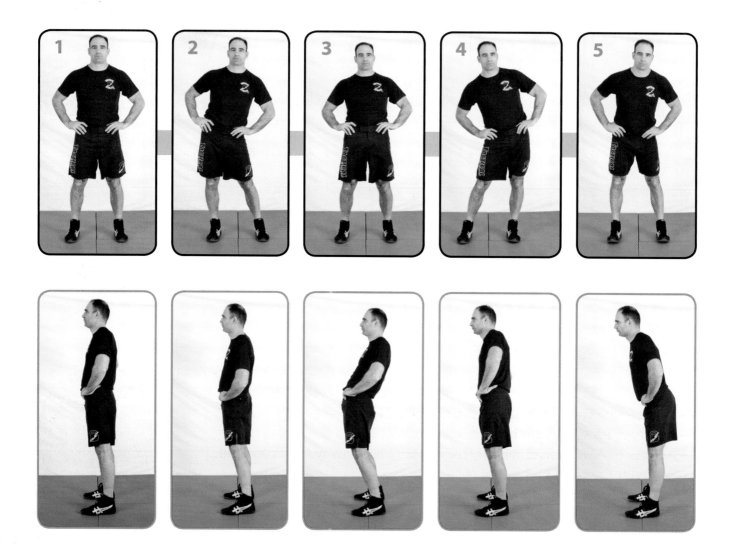

6. KNEES & ANKLES

a. Rotation

— Begin in a neutral stance, feet together.
— Keeping your back straight and chest open, move your hips back, bend your knees, and place your hands on your knees.
— Rotate your knees in a clockwise direction (i.e., left, center, right, back).
— Be sure to keep your ankles relaxed and allow them to loosen up also.
— Continue for desired number of reps.
— Reverse direction and repeat.

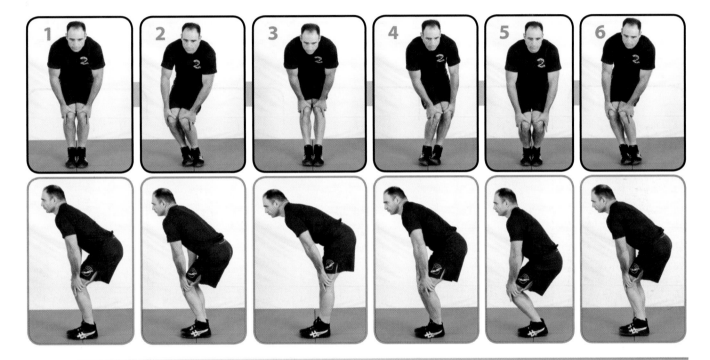

b. Ankle Flexion

— Begin in a neutral stance, feet together.
— Bend over and place your palms on the ground. Walk your feet back until your legs are straight and you feel a slight stretch in your calf.
— Your weight is on your hands and the balls of your feet.
— Alternate pressing your heels into the mat.
— As your ROM increases, slightly move your hands away from your feet.
— Repeat for desired number of reps.

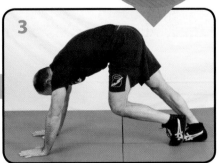

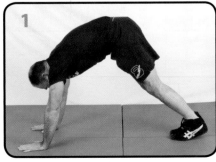
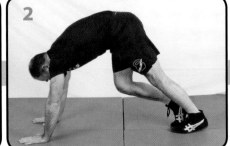

Joint Mobility/Flexibility

c. Ankle Extension

— Begin on your hands and knees. Be sure your ankles are extended and your toes are straight.
— Fully straighten your legs, pressing the top of your foot/base of your toes into the mat.
— Fully flex your knees and repeat.

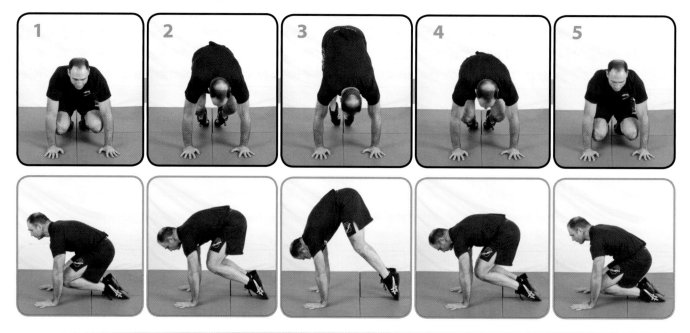

d. Knee Extension/Flexion (feet together)

— Begin in a neutral stance, feet together.
— Bend over and place your hands on the floor in front of your feet, knees flexed, weight on the balls of your feet.
— Fully extend your legs until your knees are straight. If you can't straighten your legs, move your hands away from your toes until you can.
— Rebend your knees (full flexion), then back to full extension.
— Repeat for desired number of reps.

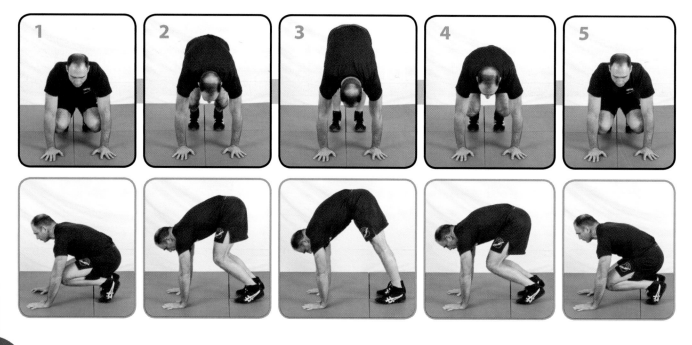

e. Knee Extension/Flexion (feet apart)

— Begin in a neutral stance, feet between hip and shoulder width apart, toes pointing slightly out.
— Keeping your chest open and back straight, squat down, placing the palms of your hands on the ground between your feet.
— As you squat be sure to open your hips and shift your weight to your heels. Ensure your knees track in the same direction as your toes. Do not let your knees collapse inward; instead, press them slightly outward when you squat.
— Keeping your hands on the ground, fully extend your legs, and then return to the squat (full flexion).
— Repeat.

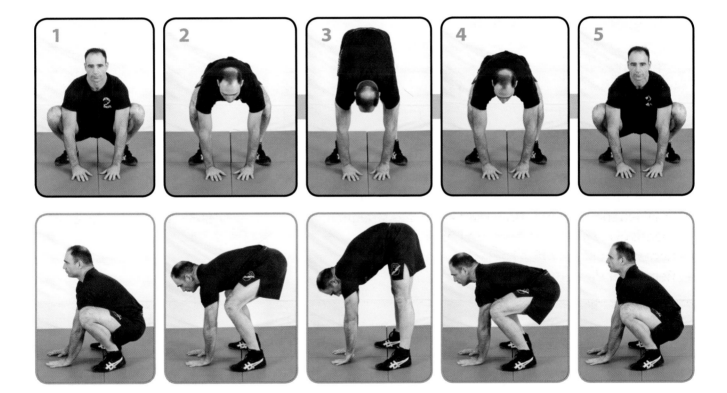

f. Side Lunge (foot flat)

— Begin in a neutral stance, feet wider than shoulder width.
— Keeping your chest open and back straight, move your hips back and to the right.
— Bend your right leg as you extend your left leg; weight transfers to your right heel.
— Drive off your right heel, extending your right leg. Body shifts to neutral position, hips back, chest open, weight equally distributed on heels.
— Flex your left leg as you continue to extend your right; weight transfers to left heel. Be sure the toe of the extended leg stays on the ground.
— Repeat alternating left and right for desired number of reps.

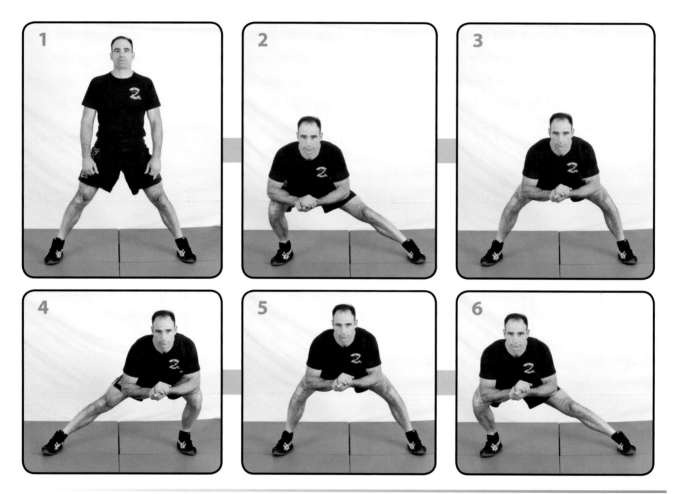

g. Side Lunge (toe up)

— Follow the exact procedure above, except allow the toe of your extended leg to rotate off the ground and point toward the ceiling. This will allow your hip to open up to a greater ROM.

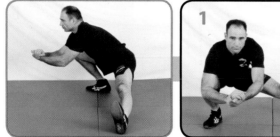 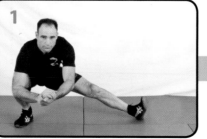 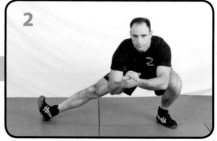

II. DYNAMIC FLEXIBILITY

Dynamic flexibility drills are best performed immediately after mobility drills. The purpose of the dynamic flexibility drills is to "reset" the stretch reflex. This allows for even greater range of motion and dramatically decreases the chance of "muscle strains." The key is to move your limbs while staying as loose as possible. Always move within a comfortable range of motion. Never allow the stretch reflex to activate. Gradually increase the range of motion and speed of movement. Perform drills in the morning or prior to a training session. Some research claims that if you perform dynamic flexibility drills in the morning, you'll be good to go for the rest of the day. I know from experience that it will keep you loose for a couple of hours. If at some point during the day you are starting to feel a little stiff, just do another set.

Leg Swings—Front

— Begin in a neutral stance.
— Keep your shoulders, hips, knees, and feet square.
— Gently swing your leg forward and back in a comfortable ROM. Keep your swinging leg as loose as possible.
— After a few reps, slightly increase your ROM.
— Passively exhale through your mouth each time your leg swings up in front of you. This will help keep your muscles relaxed.
— If at any time your leg muscles become tight, stop and shake out the tension. When it feels loose, pick back up where you left off.

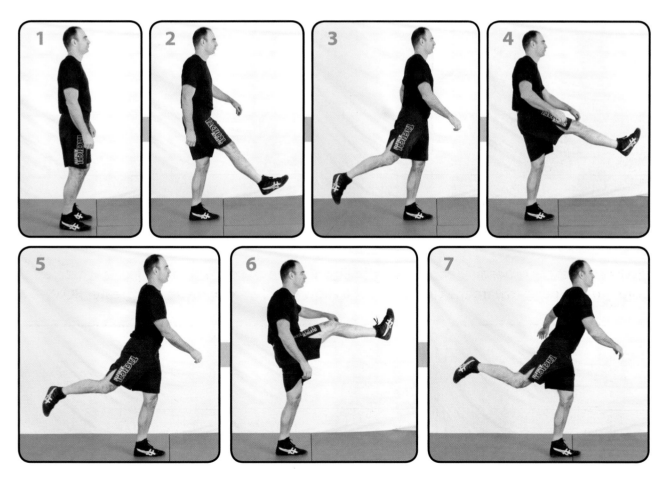

a. Leg Swings—Side

— Follow the same procedures above, except this time swing your leg side to side in front of your support leg.

— Be sure to keep swings low and controlled. Be patient with this exercise. The ROM won't come as quickly or as easily as in the front-leg swing. Feel free to experiment and vary the foot angle of the swinging leg from time to time.

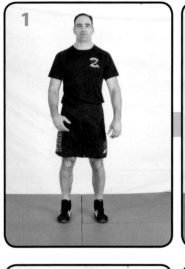

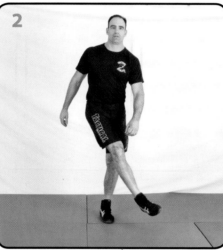

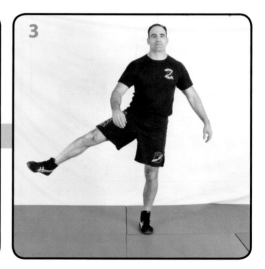

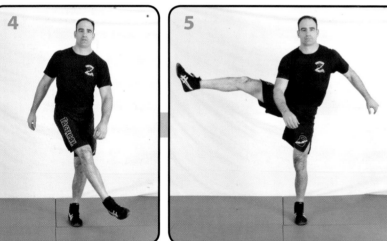

b. Arm Swings—Vertical

— Raise one arm overhead and pinch your shoulder blades together, opening up your chest.
— Alternate arm positions, keeping chest open, and gradually increase ROM.
— Repeat sequence in a smooth, rhythmic fashion.

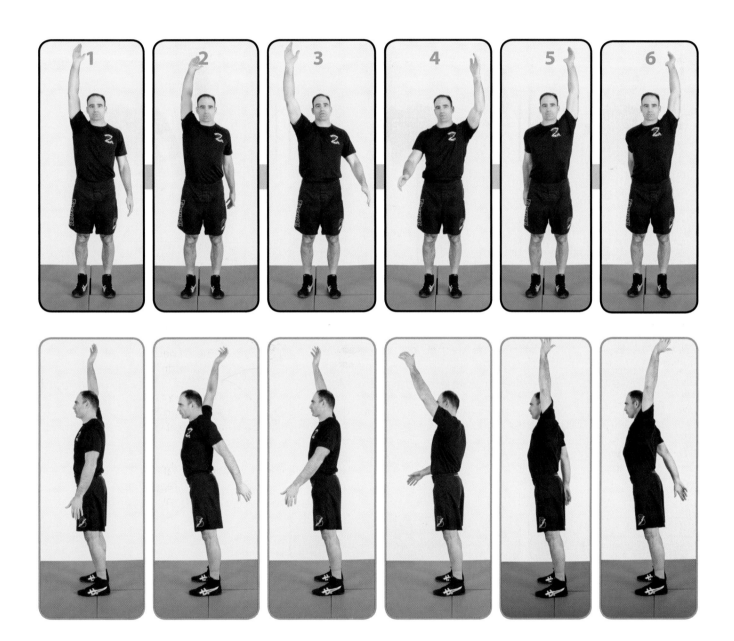

c. Arm Swings—Horizontal

— Cross your arms in front of your chest.
— Drive your elbows back, opening your chest.
— Recoil, then open your arms horizontally while contracting your upper back muscles, allowing your chest to open further.
Note: This is not a ballistic stretch. Do not force yourself into a new ROM!

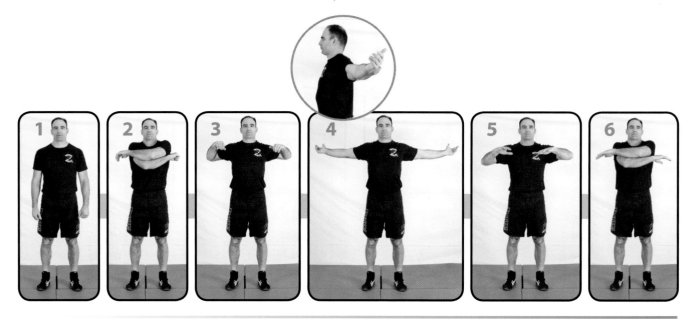

d. Arm Swings—Diagonal

— Cross your arms in front of your chest.
— Drive your elbows back, opening your chest.
— Recoil then open your arms diagonally while contracting your upper back muscles, allowing your chest to open further.
Note: This is not a ballistic stretch. Don't force yourself into a new ROM.

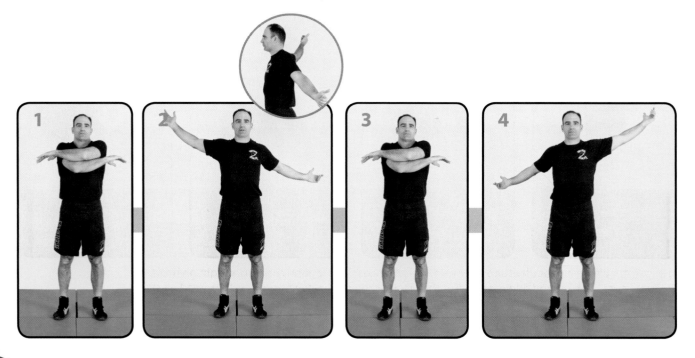

III. POST TRAINING STRETCHING

The following stretching exercises should be saved for the end of the training session. The purpose is to increase flexibility and build strength at extreme ranges of motion. PNF (proprioceptive neuromuscular facilitation) stretching is a combination of passive stretching and isometric contractions. The key is to hold a steady isometric contraction for up to 30 seconds; don't hold your breath; breathe shallowly and then let out a sigh of relief. When your intra-abdominal pressure drops, the exhausted muscles should instantly relax, making quick gains in range of motion.

a. Good Morning Hamstring Stretch

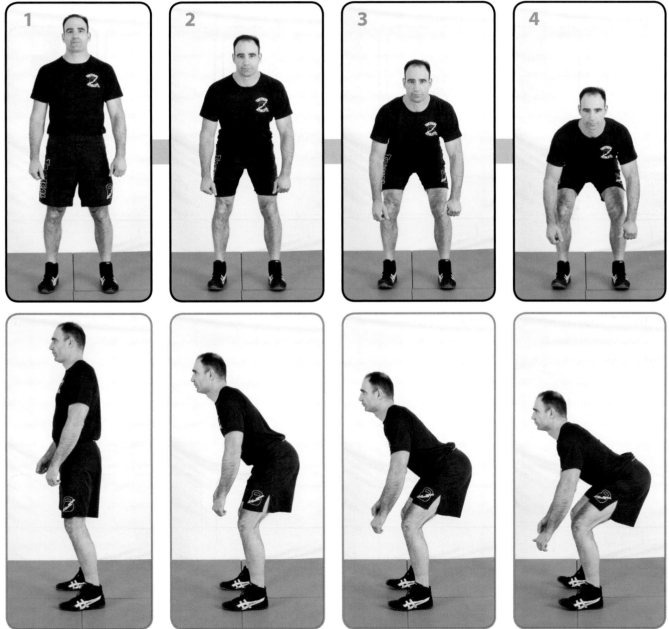

1) Begin standing with your feet shoulder width apart, knees slightly bent, chest up, weight on heels.
2) Move your butt back and down, folding at the hip, keeping back arched, your chest up, head neutral.
3) Inhale, contract your hamstrings, glutes, and lower back as hard as you can and count to 5 (seconds).
4) Exhale and relax your muscles, allowing upper body to drop closer to the floor.
   — Repeat steps 3–4 two more times.

b. Relax-into-Stretch Toe Touch

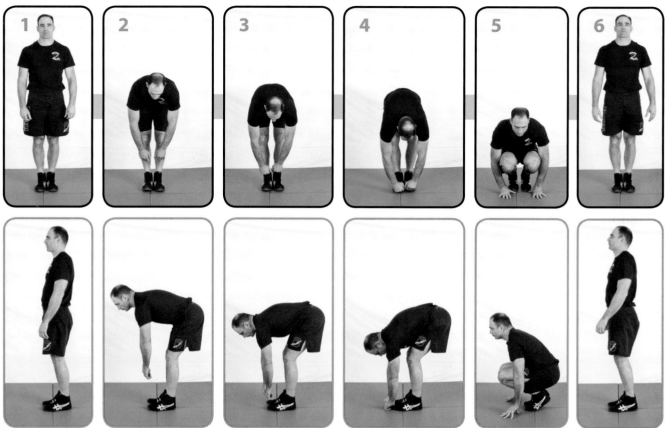

1) Begin standing with your feet together, knees straight (a slight bend is OK).
2) Bend over by folding at the hips and attempt to touch your toes. Don't reach any farther than you can do so comfortably.
3) Inhale, contract your hamstrings and glutes, clench fists, and grip floor with your toes as hard as you can and count to 5 (seconds).
4) Exhale and relax your muscles, allowing upper body to drop closer to the floor.
5–6) Repeat steps 3–4 two more times. When finished, bend your knees and stand up.

Note: Staying in a toe touch is not recommended unless you make an effort to lift your hips and elongate your lower spine instead of forcing it to round. The reason: possible overstretching of the lower back ligaments.

---

c. Kneeling Hip Flexor Stretch

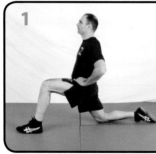 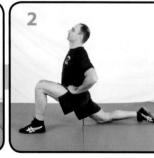 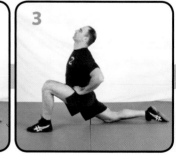 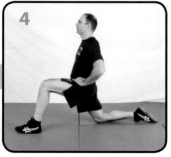

1) Kneel on right knee, toes pointed. Plant your left foot firmly in front of you: keeping your calf perpendicular to the floor.
2) Inhale, keep your hips square, your chest open, and contract your right hip flexor by attempting to bring your heel and knee closer to each other. **Note:** the foot and knee do not actually move. Hold for 5 seconds.
3) Exhale and relax, dropping your hip down closer to the ground. Keep your back arched, chest out, and chin up.
4) Repeat steps 2–3 two more times.
— Switch leg position and repeat steps 1–4.

Spinal Decompression Hangs

The following exercises are a great way to decompress your entire spine during or after a training session. Try them in between heavy sets of swings or deadlifts, or during the cool down.

a. Heels Down:

1. Grip a pull-up bar, hands approximately shoulder width apart, palms facing away. Be sure to keep your shoulders down and in their sockets by actively contracting your lats and scapulae.

2. Flex your foot upward and stretch your heels down. Hold this stretch for 5–10 seconds. This is a good way to stretch the entire spine.

3. Relax, then repeat 2 more times.

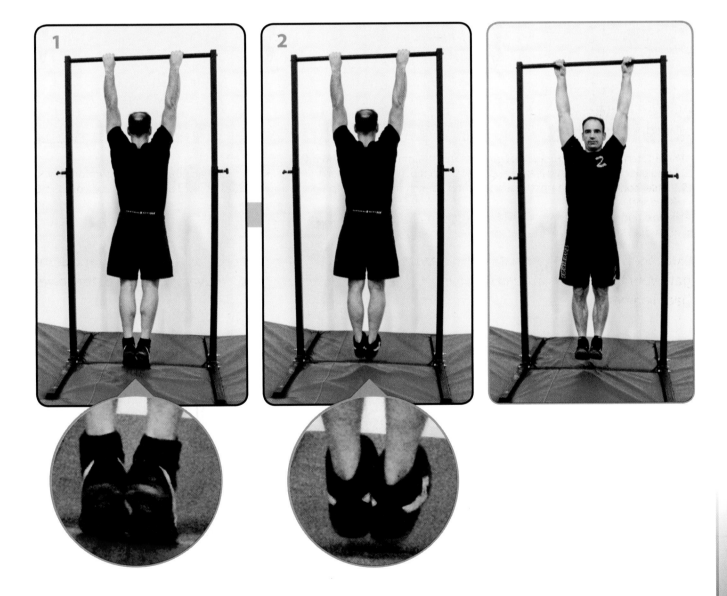

b. PNF Style Decompression:

1. Grip a pull-up bar, hands approximately shoulder width apart, palms facing away. (Note: this exercise works best when your legs are straight, feet dangling a few inches off the ground.)

   -While hanging, keep your shoulders down and in their sockets by actively contracting your lats and scapulae.

   -Inhale, and then forcefully contract all the muscles in your glutes, abs, legs, back, and arms for 3–5 seconds.

2. Passively exhale and instantly relax, allowing the entire length of your spine to elongate.

   -Repeat sequence 2 times.

3. Slowly rotate your hips left.

4. Slowly rotate your hips right.

   -Step down; do not jump down from pull-up bar!

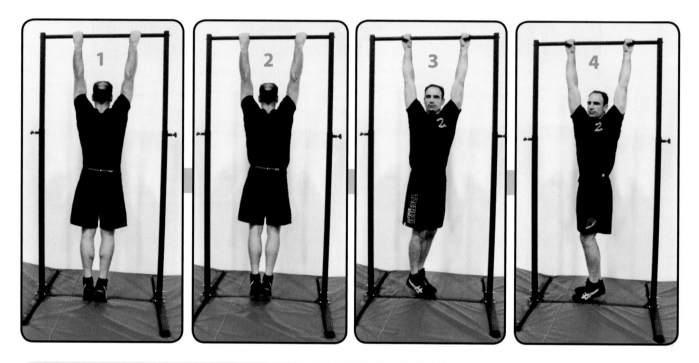

Spine Decompression Is Vital to Spine Health and Mobility

(Excerpt from *Super Joints* by Pavel Tsatsouline)

The authoritative Soviet Physical Culture and Sports Encyclopedic Dictionary states that spine mobility is very dependent on the thickness of the intervertebral discs: the thicker the discs, the greater the mobility. The discs act as shock absorbers. Their spongy core does the job. When a disc absorbs liquid it can get almost twice as thick—which explains height fluctuations of a few centimeters throughout the day.

After fifty years of age, discs dry up and a person shrinks and loses his flexibility. The value of traction or elongation exercises cannot be overestimated. "Just a little time will pass [since you started hanging on a pull-up bar], and you will feel as if the bar has gotten lower, as if you have ground up or rather stretched out a centimeter or two," promises Russian coach Mark Tartakovsky.

In a free hang, Tartakovsky advises various leg and torso movements to amplify the effect: moving the legs back and forth or side to side, together and separate, non-ballistic turns of the torso and with the feet held together.

Section 2
Swing Series

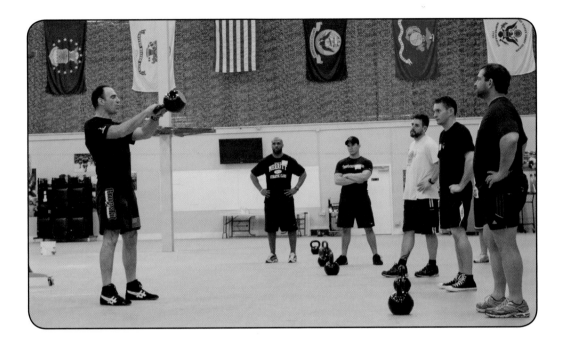

It doesn't mean a thing if you can't do a swing! That's really the bottom line. Any technical flaws left uncorrected while learning the swing will only become magnified as you progress to the more dynamic cleans and snatches. As noted previously in the "Rules of Engagement," it is essential to practice the following exercises in the order they are presented. Everybody needs to begin with the Russian swing.

In this section, you will learn how to perform the:

Russian swing—The foundational movement.

Power swing—Pressure tests your foundation.

American swing—CrossFit swing of choice.

Two-and swing release—Dynamic, hand-to-eye coordination.

Wall-ball substitute—Very dynamic and challenging exercise.

One-hand swing—Assistance exercise for the snatch.

Half-rotation switch—Simple way to switch KB from one hand to the other.

H2H switch—reinforces arm movement for snatch.

"The most important aspect of training, when coaching beginners, is technique."

—Sergey Rudnev,
Honored Coach of Russia, 5x World Champion

In gymnastics, there's something called virtuosity. Virtuosity, as defined by Coach Glassman, founder of CrossFit, is "doing the common, uncommonly well." It is the pinnacle for which gymnasts strive. In the GPP world of kettlebell lifting, there is nothing more "common" than the Russian swing. Strive to perform it "uncommonly well."

Conditioning Benefits of the Swing

Most people who have never lifted kettlebells have a hard time comprehending the enormous cardiovascular and metabolic conditioning benefits associated with practicing the kettlebell swing. After a kettlebell workout or demonstration, it is not uncommon for a spectator to ask, "What muscle group does that exercise work?" This is usually followed by "That looks like a good way to injure your lower back!" As I catch my breath, gather my thoughts, and wipe the sweat that's dripping off my face, one more question gets fired my way: "What do you do for cardio?" Before answering, I try to discern if the questioner is really serious or just playing a game of "stump-the-chump."

What muscles does the swing work?

Kettlebell swings are multijoint compound movements that build strength and endurance in the muscles along your entire posterior chain (i.e., glutes, hamstrings, abs, back extensors, etc.). These are the muscles that develop athleticism (e.g., the ability to run faster, jump higher, and hit harder). They are the "go" muscles, not your "show" muscles. As an athlete, honestly, I couldn't care less if I have a tight butt or shapely legs. My goal is to have the ability to generate, apply, and sustain maximum power output. Nonetheless, if you value possessing a tight butt, shapely legs, and a nicely developed back, then a prescription of kettlebell swings will help you achieve that goal.

Are kettlebell swings bad for your back? No! Correctly executed kettlebell swings are probably one of the best lower-back rehabilitation or pre-habilitation exercises you can do. Swings build serious strength and endurance in the muscles of your lower back and core, which is one of the major factors in maintaining back health. Your focus needs to be on proper lifting mechanics and the nuances of generating maximum speed and power from your hips. It's all about technique. If you swing your kettlebells like Quasimodo (aka The Hunchback of Notre Dame), not using your hips and moving at the speed of a three-toed tree sloth, then you might have a few issues.

What about cardio?

Keep it simple. High-intensity interval training with kettlebells will burn the butter off your body in less time than you thought possible. Personally, I avoid long, slow, distance running like the plague. If you can't run, don't like to run, don't want to run, are too heavy to run, or just don't have the time to run, then I have the program for you! Each exercise in this section will end with an exercise prescription that follows the Tabata Protocol established by Izumi Tabata.

Tabata intervals consist of 20 seconds of maximum intensity exercise, followed by 10 seconds of rest. This cycle is repeated 8 times (for a total of 4 minutes). This is an extremely time-efficient method of training. During the initial study, after 6 weeks of testing, Dr. Tabata noted a 28 percent increase in anaerobic capacity along with a 14 percent increase in maximal oxygen consumption (VO_2 max). This also proved to be a very effective method for post-workout fat loss. Intense interval work raises the body's metabolic rate long after the exercise session is completed. Recent studies have confirmed that interval training is more effective for fat loss than low-intensity, continuous exercise. To achieve these results, you must apply a maximal effort.

I. RUSSIAN SWING

The Russian swing (i.e., two-arm swing to chest or eye level) is the foundational exercise upon which all the other swings in this series are built. There is a time and place for the overhead swing (aka American swing), but not until the Russian swing is mastered. Take your time and carefully follow all the teaching progressions, by the numbers, step-by-step. This will take mental focus and discipline, but the results will be worth it. Most common errors are preventable and correctable through good practice. Create the habit of constantly analyzing every movement you practice and why it's important.

It takes me anywhere from 1 to 1.5 hours to cover all the teaching progressions of the Russian swing at the Kettlebell Trainer Courses. This is with people who are highly motivated, in great shape, and already have a solid foundation in functional movements. For the average Joe or Jane walking off the street, it may take several training sessions to get through the teaching progressions for the Russian swing alone. That's OK!

Consider it time well invested.

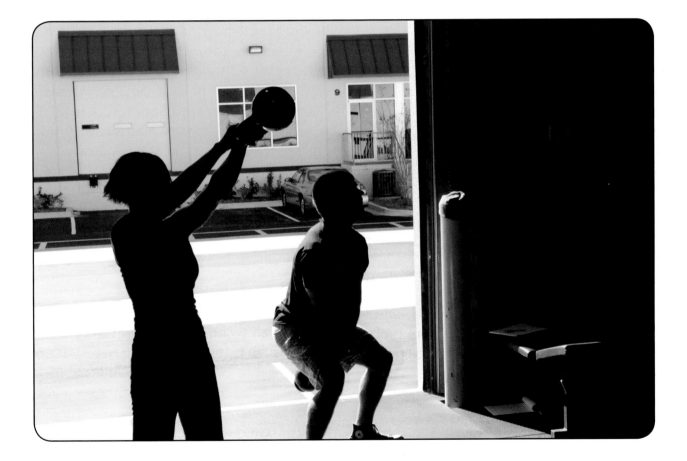

I. Russian Swing (standard)

Familiarize yourself with the picture sequence below and read the captions to get an idea how the movement is performed. Right now it is for demonstration purposes only, to show the end result or standard of performance. You will have an opportunity to refer back to and practice the Russian swing later, as you move through each skill-building exercise as outlined under "Drills and Skills."

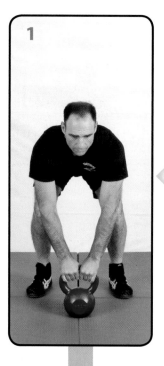

Start position:

- Feet between hip and shoulder width apart, toes pointing in the direction you're facing.

- Kettlebell is centered, 3–6 inches in front of your toes.

- Keep your chest open, shoulders back and down.

- Fold at the hips (i.e., sit back and down), shift your weight to your heels, and keep your neck in a neutral position.

- Establish a two-handed grip on the kettlebell.

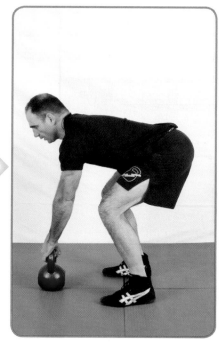

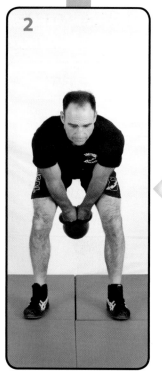

Perform the back swing:

- Inhale through your nose; tighten your abs and glutes.

- Keeping your weight on your heels, slightly extend your legs and back angle, contract your lats, and hike the kettlebell back between your legs.

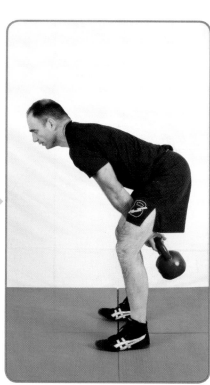

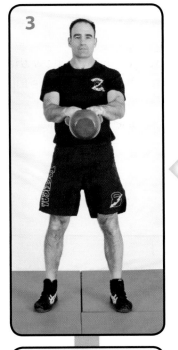

3

As the kettlebell reaches the end of the back swing, press through your heels and extend your legs, hips, and back until you are in the upright position. This action should launch the kettlebell to hip or chest height. Note: Arms must be relaxed; shoulders stay back and down. The shoulders provide the pivot point. This is not a front deltoid exercise!

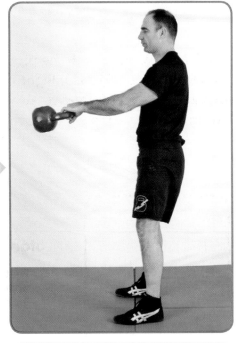

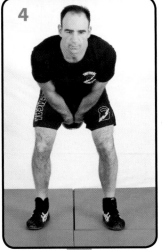

4

Allow gravity to take the kettlebell back down. Just before your forearms crash into your pelvic area, fold at the hips (i.e., sit back and down) and shift your weight to your heels.

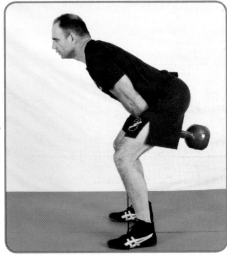

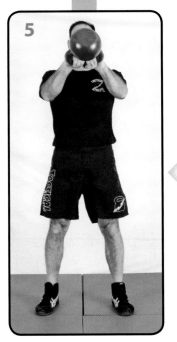

5

As the kettlebell reaches the end of the back swing, drive through your heels and extend your legs, hips, and back until you are in the upright position. This action should launch the kettlebell to chest or eye level.

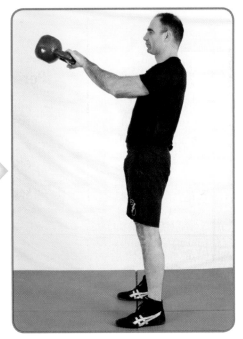

Swing Series

Drills and Skills

The Drills and skills section follows the crawl-walk-run training approach. You will master the drills in each phase, apply them, and then move on to the next. In the crawl phase, the Russian swing will be reduced to its most basic elements, concentrating on correct posture and movement. In the walk phase, correct posture and movement will be applied to the deadlift. During the run phase, mechanics of the deadlift are applied to the Russian swing moving at full speed. The difference is in the details—apply the drills and enhance your skills. It's that simple.

Movement Prep
Drill #1: Front, Back, Middle of Foot

Many people aren't really kinesthetically aware of where their heels are or how to balance through them. This ability is extremely important in kettlebell lifting, weightlifting, and other sport activities because it increases posterior chain muscle recruitment, transferring into greater power.

Here's an amazingly simple yet effective kinesthetic awareness drill I learned when training with Olympic weightlifting coach Don McCauley, author of *Power Trip: A Guide to Weightlifting for Athletes, Parents and Coaches.*

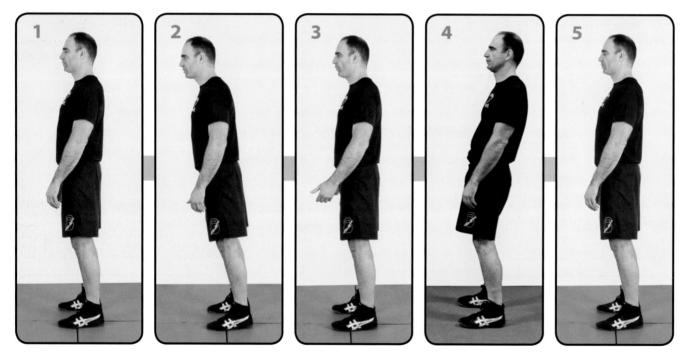

1) Stand straight, heels just wider than your hips and toes pointed forward. Arms should be hanging down normally. Knees should stay comfortably straight during this lesson.

2) Shift your weight to the balls of your feet without causing your heels to rise from the floor ("front"). Hold that position for about 5 to 10 seconds.

3) Move back to the mid-foot and hold position for the same duration of time ("middle").

4) Shift to your heels without causing the front of your feet to rise from the floor. Again hold this position for 5 to 10 seconds ("back").

5) Stand straight and sway to the same three positions, holding each particular one for the same duration of time as above and watching yourself in the mirror as you do it. Repeat these three positions until you're as comfortable on your heels as you are on the balls of your feet.

Movement Prep
Drill #2: Good Morning (Mobility)

This exercise is straight from the Joint Mobility Section. It serves as a quick warm-up, increasing the ROM throughout the hips and back, emphasizes sound mechanics (i.e., open chest, straight back, weight on the heels, etc.) and reinforces correct movement patterns that are directly applicable to the swing.

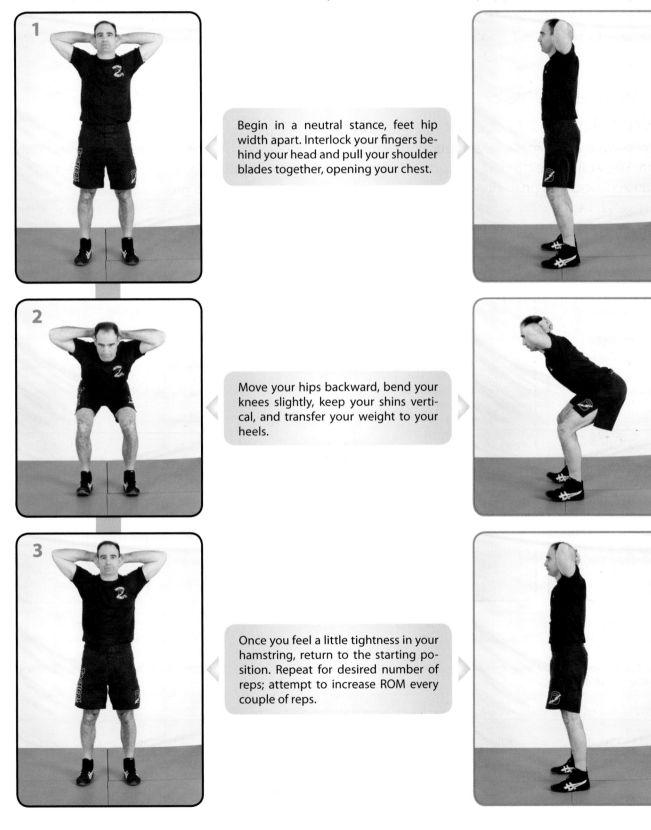

1

Begin in a neutral stance, feet hip width apart. Interlock your fingers behind your head and pull your shoulder blades together, opening your chest.

2

Move your hips backward, bend your knees slightly, keep your shins vertical, and transfer your weight to your heels.

3

Once you feel a little tightness in your hamstring, return to the starting position. Repeat for desired number of reps; attempt to increase ROM every couple of reps.

Movement Prep
Drill #3: Straight Back—Round Back Drill

Don't Slouch! This is a great kinesthetic awareness drill to help you distinguish the difference between what a straight back and a rounded back feels like. It is also a good mobility drill for your spine and will aid your ability to keep good posture (i.e., a straight back) while lifting.

The importance of a straight back (i.e., extended or arched) cannot be over emphasized. It is critical to success in all types of lifting. There are seventeen vertebrae in your spinal column; twelve make up your thoracic and five for your lumbar area. A strong back arch "fuses" them together so they become one solid piece, creating tremendous leverage critical to safe and effective lifting. Generally speaking, females develop this arch quicker than males and younger athletes adapt this position quicker than older ones. The following three-part drill was adapted from Tommy Kono's excellent book *Weightlifting, Olympic Style*.

PART 1

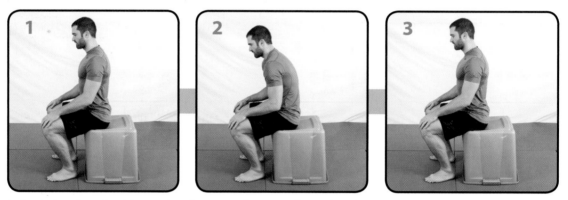

1) Sit at the front end of a chair or bench with your hands on your knees and your feet flat on the ground. Your feet should be spread between hip and shoulder width apart.
2) On purpose, exaggerate the slouch position.
3) Now, sit tall—tall as you can. Repeat steps 2–3 a few more times to get the feel of it and note how flexible your back is. Also note that your pelvic girdle tilts when you perform this movement. Now, perform steps 2–3 again but this time in front of a mirror so you can see and feel the difference.

PART 2

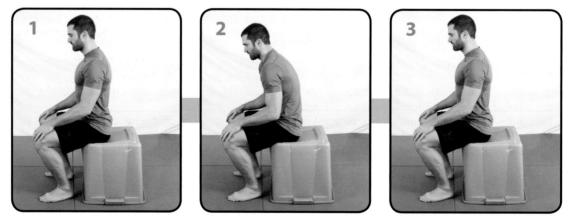

1) Sit tall as you can with your hands on your knees and feet flat on the ground, between hip and shoulder width apart. This time, while sitting as tall as you can, breathe in as deep as possible so your ribcage lifts up. To prevent your shoulders from rising as you inhale and to activate your lats, cup your fingers tightly against the front of your knees and pull your shoulders back and down. Repeat the deep breathing again and try to cram in more air than before. Attempt to raise the top of your chest to touch your chin.
2) Exhale and relax, allowing your back to round. Pause between the deep breaths so that you do not hyperventilate.
3) Sit tall, breathe in deep and raise your upper chest as high as possible. Performed correctly, you should feel a very strong tightening of your mid- and lower-back muscles. There will be also a very strong tightening of the two cords that gather at the base of your lower back. Repeat for 3–5 reps.

PART 3

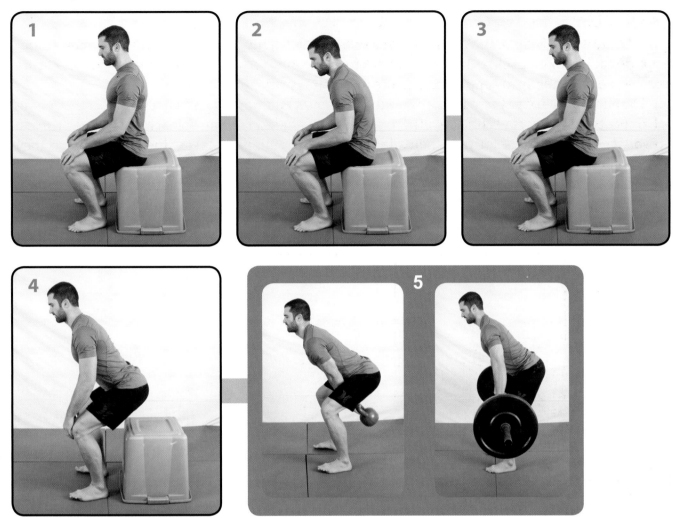

1) Sit tall as you can with your hands on your knees and feet flat on the ground, between hip and shoulder width apart. Once again, while sitting as tall as you can, breathe in as deep as possible so your ribcage lifts up. To prevent your shoulders from rising as you inhale and to activate your lats, cup your fingers tightly against the front of your knees and pull you shoulders back and down. Repeat the deep breathing again and try to cram in more air than before. Attempt to raise the top of your chest to touch your chin.
2) Exhale and relax, allowing your back to round. Pause between the deep breaths so that you do not hyperventilate.
3) Sit tall, breathe in deep and raise your upper chest as high as possible. Performed correctly, you should feel a very strong tightening of your mid- and lower-back muscles. There will be also a very strong tightening of the two cords that gather at the base of your lower back. Repeat for 3–5 reps.
4) Then drive off your heels and slightly extend your knees and hips, rising off the bench. Note: the shin is perpendicular to the floor, the back is arched, and shoulders are projecting beyond the knees. Repeat this drill 2–3 of times.
5) This is the ideal bottom position for the kettlebell swings and it is the launch or power position for the triple extension in Olympic lifting.

In this day and age it seems that more and more people are developing poor postural habits due to prolonged time sitting in front of the computer, in their cars, or on their butts in front the "boob tube" (i.e., TV). You will reap dividends by applying the above three-part drill throughout the day, at your workstation, at the dinner table, in the classroom, and so on. Actively fight and kill the slothful slouch monster! If you need inspiration, find a toddler. Observe how straight a toddler sits on the floor when playing with blocks. That's how we're designed. Don't let gravity or the weight of the world weigh you down. Sit and stand tall!

Movement Prep
Drill #4: Wall Squat

The wall squat can be used as part of a warm-up to reinforce good mechanics, or it can be used as a remedial drill to thwart bad habits such as allowing your knees to track in front the toes. Perform 1–3 sets of 5–10 repetitions as a warm-up or in between sets of deadlifts or swings.

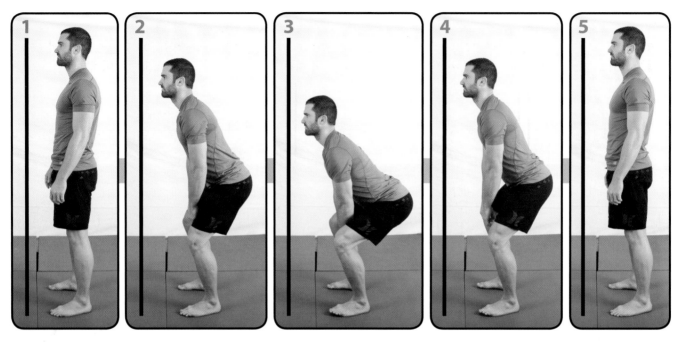

1) Stand facing a wall, toes about 3 to 6 inches away from the wall. Keep your feet parallel and between hip and shoulder width apart. Keep your chest open, pull your scapula together and down.

2) Jack-knife at the hips and slowly move them back and down, keeping your weight on your heels. Maintain an "open" chest throughout the movement by pinching your shoulder blades together. Proper technique will keep your kisser from hitting the wall. Fight the urge to look up. Maintain a neutral neck position.

3) Continue to sit back and down until you reach the "bottom position." The bottom position, for our purpose, is the same as that of a deadlift or swing. It is not parallel or below parallel. This is the same stance you would take prior to performing a swing, deadlift, or standing vertical jump, etc. Hold the bottom position for 1–5 seconds, feel the glutes activate. Note: Do not allow your shoulders to round forward (i.e., chest sink in) or lower back to round (i.e., "tail tuck under").

4) Slowly return to the standing position.

5) It is critical that you "lock out" at the top. In other words, your knees and hips should be straight, quads and glutes maximally contracted. Some find it helpful to imagine pinching a coin between their cheeks (glutes). Repeat for 1–3 sets of 5–10 reps before proceeding to the deadlift. As you become stronger and more flexible, you'll be able to perform this drill with your toes touching the wall.

Wall Squat Common Errors

Here are a few common errors to watch for when practicing wall squats. The first one is obvious and the second is subtler.

✕ Common Error #1: Too Wide, Too Deep

The depth of the wall squat, for teaching the mechanics of the swing, should be the depth of your swing. The middle of your forearms should contact the middle of the inside of your thighs.

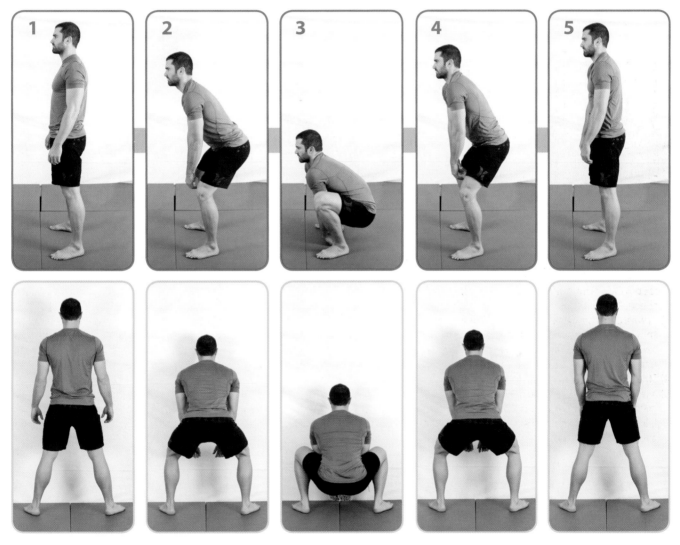

1) Feet wider than shoulder width apart.
2) Upper shoulders slightly rounding.
3) Squat too deep and back is totally rounded.
4) Shoulders still rounded.
5) Shoulders still rounded.

✓ Wall Squat Corrective Action:

Verbally correct their foot position and depth of squat.

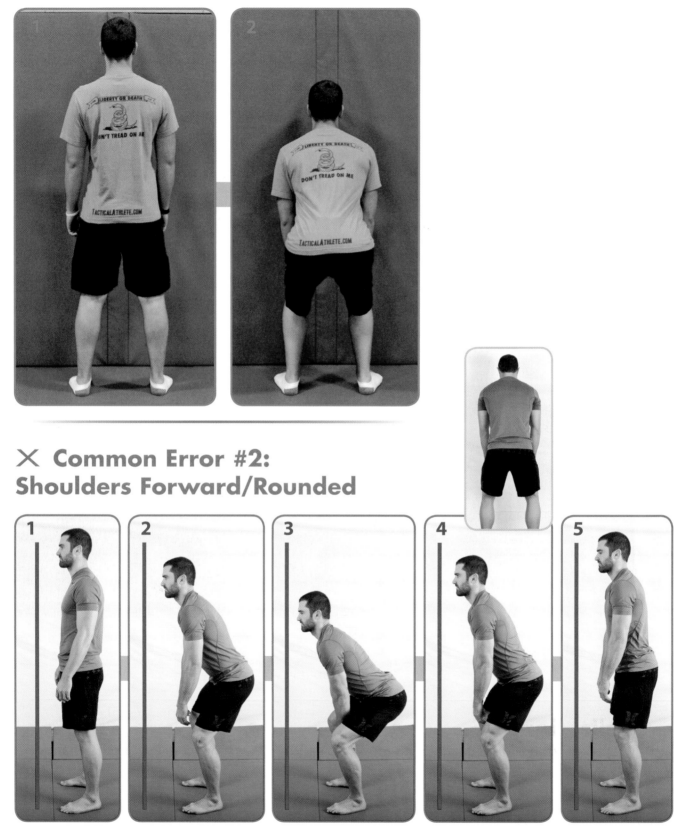

✗ Common Error #2:
Shoulders Forward/Rounded

1) So far so good. 2–5) As Glen descends, his shoulders round forward, hollowing out his chest. He maintains that position throughout the movement.

√ Wall Squat Corrective Action:

1) Place your hand on the trainee's back with thumb and forefingers touching the protruding shoulder blades, and
2) pinch them together.
3) Keep it there for the entire movement down and up.

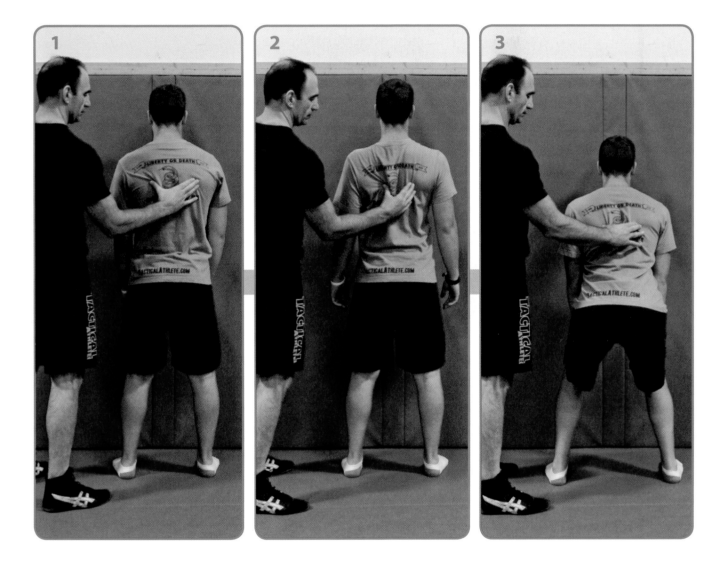

Application:
Now that you've established consistent movement patterns, it's time to apply it to the deadlift.

Movement Prep
Drill #5: Deadlift

If you slow down and analyze the mechanics of the Russian swing, you will find that the movement is almost identical to that of the deadlift (DL). If form deficiencies are not identified and fixed when practicing the DL, then those same deficiencies will magnify and transfer to the more dynamic Russian swing. Our goal of teaching the DL is to establish correct, consistent movement patterns, and then apply those movement patterns to the Russian swing. The more time you invest now, the more headaches and reprogramming you will avoid later.

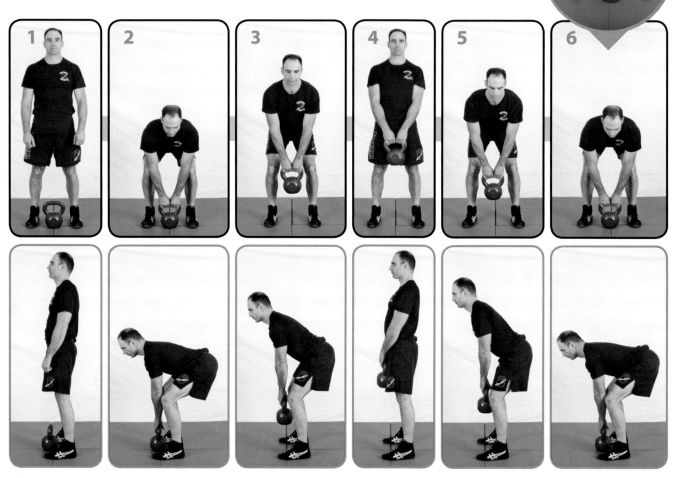

1) Start position:
   • Stand with your feet between hip and shoulder width apart, toes pointing in the direction you're facing.
   • Kettlebell is centered between your feet. Handle is in line with the base of your toes.
2) Keep your chest open, shoulders back and down. Fold at the hips (i.e., hips move back and down), shift your weight onto your heels, keep your neck in a neutral position, and look out, not up. Secure a two-handed grip on the kettlebell, keeping your arms straight.
3) Inhale through your nose; tighten your abs and glutes. Drive off your heels and extend your legs and hips.
4) Continue to drive through your heels, fully extending your legs and hips until you are in the upright position. Chest remains open, keep shoulders pulled back and down. Note: Arms are relaxed and do not lean backward!
5) Fold at the hips, (i.e., hips move back and down), slightly flex your knees, and shift your weight back to your heels. Note: Kettlebell path is vertical (straight up/down).
6) Continue moving your hips backward, maintain a straight back, and return the kettlebell to its original starting position. Repeat for 3–5 reps.

✗ DL Common Error #1: Looking Up

For some reason, most people want to look at the ceiling when performing a deadlift (squat or swing). Regardless of their reasoning, it's wrong and we need to correct it for their safety ASAP. Actions speak louder than words. Instead of arguing your point, do a simple kinesthetic awareness drill that will make your point for you. I learned this amazingly effective drill when training with Mark Rippetoe, author of *Starting Strength*, a number of years ago.

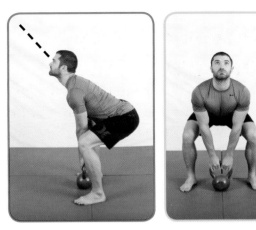

√ DL Corrective Action: Ripp's Head Position Drill

PART 1

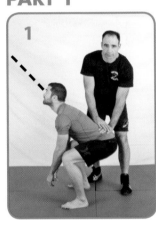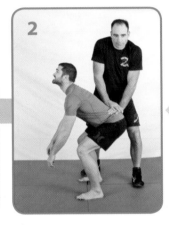

1) Have a client or training partner assume the bottom position of the deadlift and look up. Place your hands on the small of his back.

2) Instruct him to drive off his heels and stand up, as if performing a deadlift. Keep your arms locked and resist his upward movement. The partner performing the drill will feel off balance and weak as he attempts to stand up.

PART 2

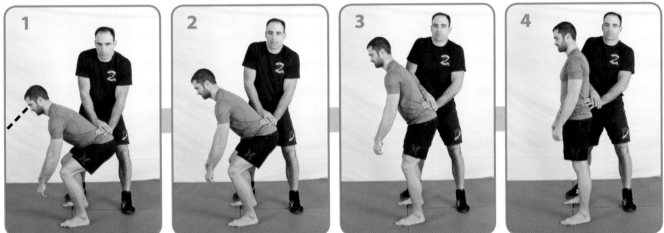

1) Have a client or training partner assume the bottom position of the deadlift. This time have him keep a neutral head position, looking a few feet in front of him. Place your hands on the small of his back.

2) Instruct him to drive off his heels and stand up, as if performing a deadlift. Keep your arms locked and resist his upward movement.

3–4) The partner performing the drill should feel much better balance, muscle recruitment, and power from the hips as he drives to the standing position. Actions speak louder than words. Once you experience the difference, you'll never look back . . . or in this case, up.

Proper head/eye position is essential for balance, stability, and neck safety. This is one of many common threads found in all the athletic lifts, regardless of implement (i.e., kettlebell or barbell).

Swing Series

Application: Deadlift

Apply the above principles to the deadlift. Deadlift the kettlebell for 5 reps. Do not worry about the weight (or lack thereof). Just keep your neck neutral, pick a spot on the floor 5–6 feet in front of you, and look at it.

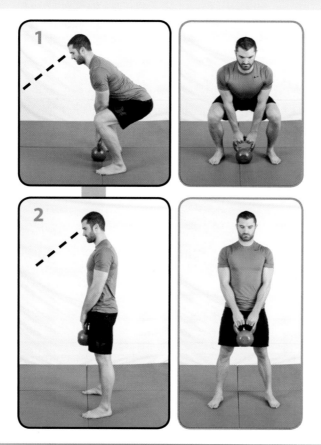

✕ DL Common Error #2: Knees Forward

Instead of moving the hips back and then down, which effectively loads the big muscles of the hams and glutes, folks tend to move their hips straight down. This will cause the knees to move forward past their toes, which then transfers their body weight to the balls of their feet.

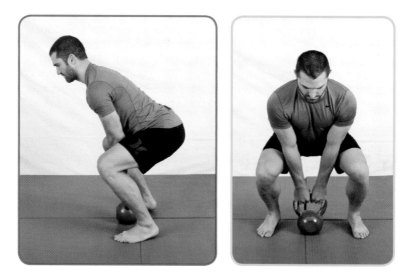

√ DL Corrective Action: Hip Flexor Recruitment Drill

This drill will teach you how to effectively activate your hip flexors during the "loading," or descending phase of the deadlift. It will also teach proper back alignment and optimum hip flexor activation.

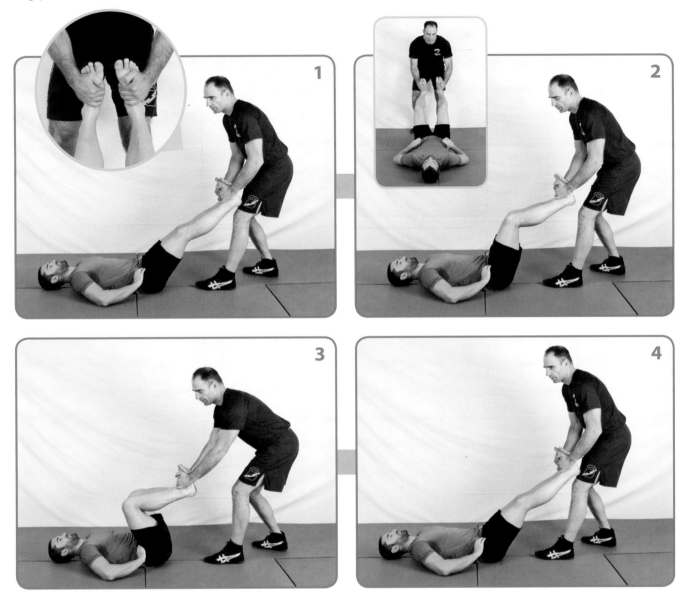

1) Begin by lying on your back. Place the fingers of each hand on the creases of your hips. Raise your feet off the ground and flex your feet back toward you. Have a partner hold your feet by grabbing the top of your foot with a thumbless grip, palms down. Note: You won't get the right stimulus if he holds your feet by the heels with palms up. If a partner isn't available, use a resistance band to assist. 2) With your legs straight and feet flexed, slowly pull your knees to your chest. Your partner is to provide a little resistance. 3) Continue pulling your knees all the way to your chest. As you reach this point, the hip flexors should almost feel like they are cramping. Hold this isometric contraction for about 3 to 5 seconds and make a mental note of that sensation. 4) Slowly extend your legs until you are back in the starting position. Repeat for 3 reps. Take a short break and then proceed to the wall squat.

Application 1: Wall Squat

Go back to the wall and perform one set of 5 reps of the wall squat. This time purposefully engage the hip flexors every time you descend. In other words, pull yourself down into the bottom position. Don't just yield to gravity. If you can't feel your hip flexors firing, repeat the hip flexor recruitment drill until you can. Shake out any tension, and then proceed to the deadlift.

Swing Series

Application 2: Box Squat

The box squat reinforces the idea of moving your hips back and down, rather than straight down with knees sliding forward. The box acts as a physical target to aim for.

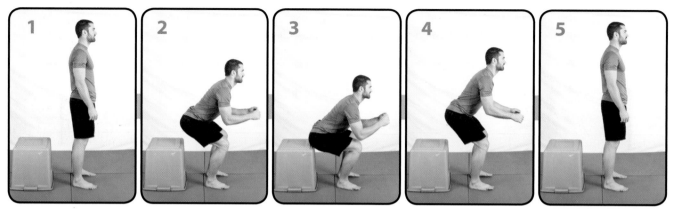

1) Stand with feet between hip and shoulder width apart, heels approximately 6 inches from the front of a plyo box or bench. This is a target for your butt.
2) Actively engage your hip flexors, moving your hips back, weight shifting to your heels.
3) Continue until your butt makes light contact with the box.
4-5) Drive off your heels and return to the starting position.

✕ DL Common Error #3: Round Shoulders

Rounding the shoulders is a common error in the bottom position, the top position, or both.

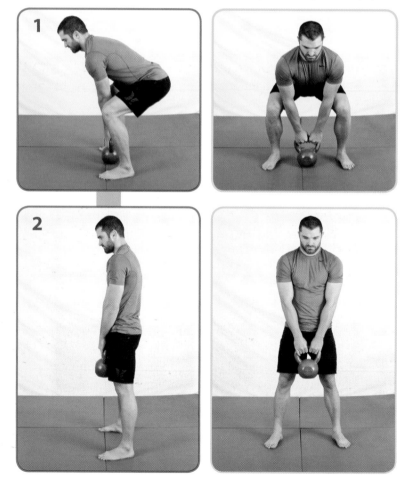

√ DL Corrective Action:

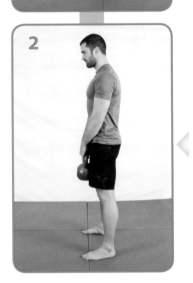

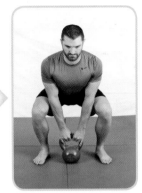

Make a conscious effort, when placing your hands on the kettlebell, to straighten your arms by flexing the triceps, then pull your shoulders back and down, lifting your chest.

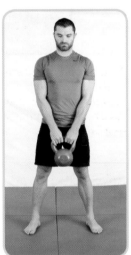

Continue to keep your chest open as you move to the top position.

NOTE: If verbal instructions fail, place your hand on the trainee's back with thumb and forefingers touching the protruding shoulder blades, and pinch them together. Hold them together throughout the entire movement

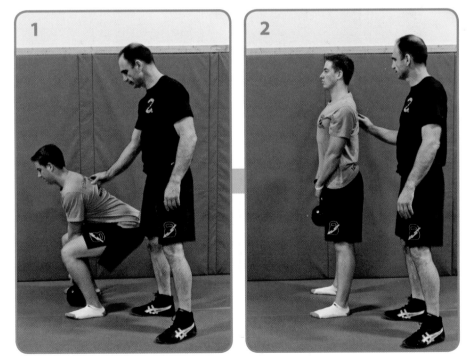

Swing Series

✕ DL Common Error #4: Round Back (i.e., lumbar flexion)

All the previous exercises from the beginning until now should have automatically fixed this problem before it started. Regardless, if the start of the deadlift looks like the picture here, immediately stop and take the following remedial action.

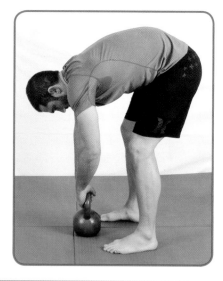

1. Review the hip flexor recruitment drill (see pg 71).
2. Review the Good Morning Mobility Drill (see pg 75), active hip flexors upon descending.
3. Review the seated Straight Back—Round Back Drill (see pg 62).
4. Practice 5 more reps of the DL.

Note: If there is still some roundness in the lower back at the bottom position, tight hamstrings could be a contributing factor.

√ DL Corrective Action: DL from Blocks

Place the kettlebell on blocks to a height where the trainee can maintain proper back extension in the bottom position. As strength and flexibility increase, you can eventually decrease the height of the blocks until you can pull from the floor in good form.

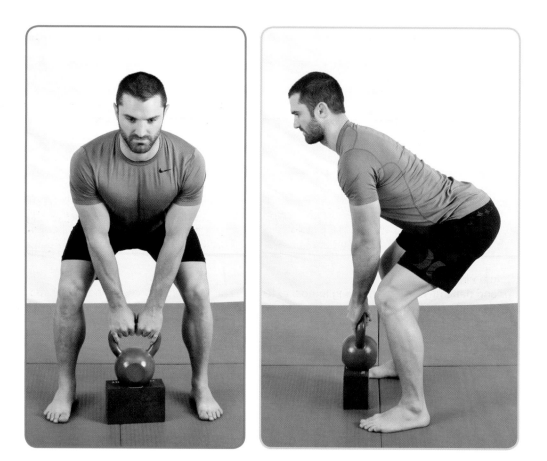

√ DL Corrective Action: Good Morning Stretch

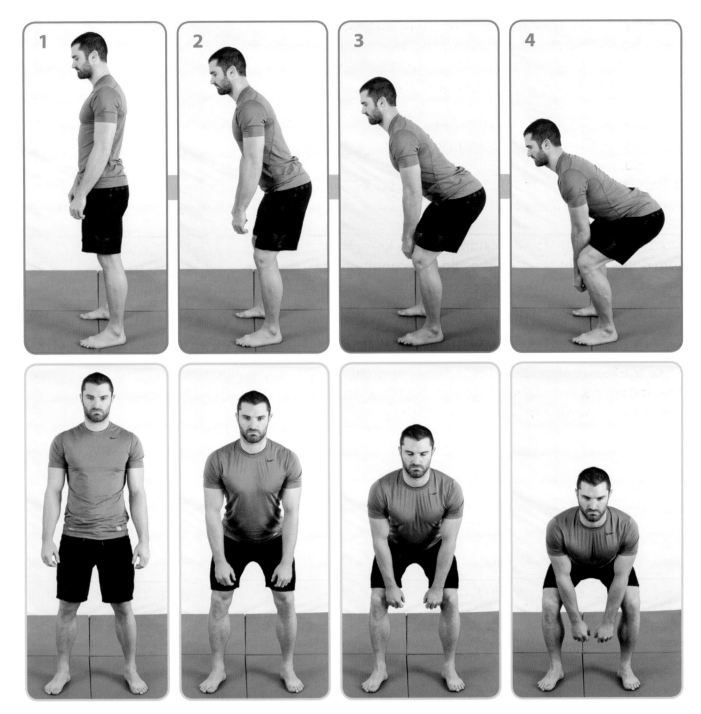

1) Stand with feet hip width apart.

2) Hinge at the hips and bend forward, maintaining lumbar extension and keeping your chest open and head up.

3) Once you feel a little tightness in your hamstrings, hold that position and isometrically contract all the muscles of your lower body (i.e., grip floor with toes, contract hamstrings, quads, glutes). Hold for 5 to 10 seconds, then exhale and relax.

4) Lower your body and repeat the isometric contraction. Repeat the drill 2 more times. Practice DL for 5 reps.

Note: If the good morning stretch doesn't correct the problem, then you must deadlift the kettlebell from blocks.

Application:

Now that you've established consistent movement patterns in the deadlift, it's time to apply a little speed and turn it into the Russian swing (RS).

Russian Swing

Perform a set of 10 Russian swings. Start with very low swings and gradually build up the height with every rep. Keep your chest open, arms straight, shoulders relaxed, and allow the kettlebell to swing freely.

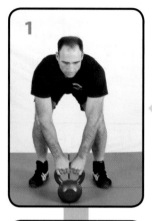

1) Start position:
- Feet between hip and shoulder width apart, toes pointing in the direction you're facing.
- Kettlebell is centered 3–6 inches in front of your toes.
- Keep your chest open, shoulders back and down.
- Fold at the hips (i.e., sit back and down), shift your weight to your heels, and keep your neck in a neutral position.
- Establish a two-handed grip on the kettlebell.

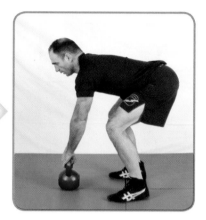

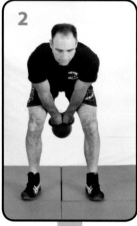

2) Perform the back swing:
- Inhale through your nose, tighten your abs and glutes.
- Keeping your weight on your heels, slightly extend your legs and back angle, contract your lats, and hike the kettlebell back between your legs.

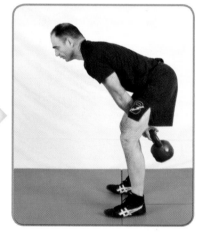

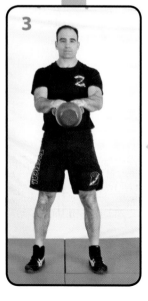

3) As the kettlebell reaches the end of the back swing, drive through your heels, rapidly extending your legs, hips, and back until you are in the upright position. This action should launch the kettlebell to hip or chest height. Note: Arms must be relaxed; shoulders stay back and down. The shoulders provide the pivot point. This is not a front deltoid exercise!

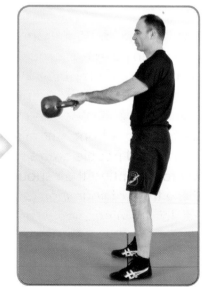

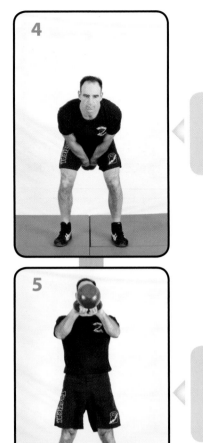

4

4) Allow gravity to take the kettlebell back down. The moment before your forearms crash into your pelvic area, fold at the hips (i.e., sit back and down) and shift your weight to your heels.

5

5) As the kettlebell reaches the end of the back swing, drive through your heels and extend your legs, hips, and back until you are in the upright position. This action should launch the kettlebell to chest or eye level.

✕ RS Common Error #1: Droopy Bell Syndrome

The "Droopy Bell Syndrome" is a common error that occurs when people use their front delts to raise the kettlebell instead of their hips. Most people do not know how to properly use their hips to maximize power. To compensate, the kettlebell is lifted to chest or eye level by performing a front delt raise. This is very common. I've even heard people brag about how great the KB swings are for sculpting their shoulders. All I have to say is that if the front of your shoulders are getting smoked doing kettlebell swings, you're doing them wrong!

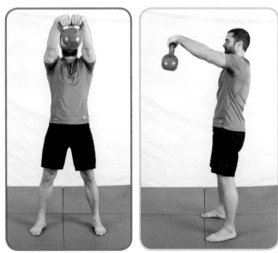

√ RS Corrective Action:

Part 1: Partner Hip Flexor Stretch

The combination of a hip flexor stretch followed by a couple standing vertical jumps will dramatically increase your ROM (range of motion) and power output. Both drills must be performed in tandem, one right after the other, then immediately applied to the Russian swing. The total time invested is only 2–3 minutes. So, get ready to release the "parking brake" and unleash the power.

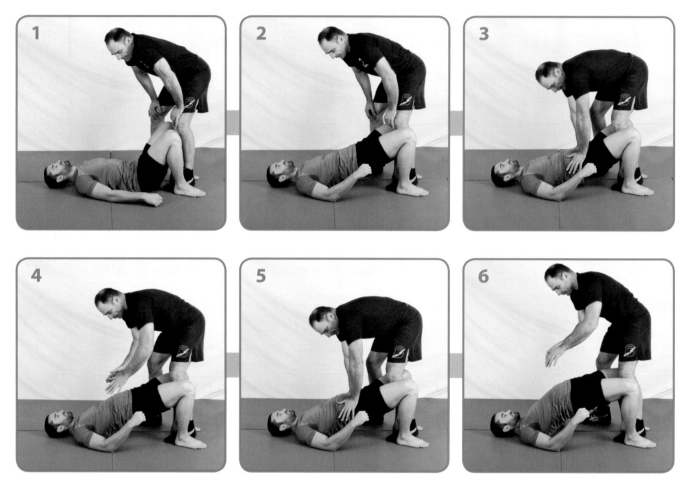

1) Your partner lies on his back, feet flat and heels close to his glutes. Step in between his feet.

2) Partner performs a shoulder bridge by raising his hips toward the ceiling, shoulders and head remains on the floor. Once his hips reach the limit of his ROM, have him pinch your leg with his knees and contract his glutes.

3) Place the palms of your hands on his hipbones and apply downward pressure. The goal is for your partner to maintain an isometric contraction at that range of motion.

4) Hold for 5–10 seconds, and then lift your hands off his hips. Your partner should immediately exhale (out his mouth) while continuing maximal glute contraction. Executed properly, his hips should float up to a new ROM. The harder he holds the isometric contraction, the greater the ROM gain will be when his hips are released.

5–6) Repeat this sequence 3–5 times, and then stand up. He should notice an immediate change in his posture when standing. He will feel taller as his posture returns to its original vertical alignment. Immediately perform 3 standing vertical jumps.

Solo Hip Flexor Stretch

If a partner is not available, you can modify and perform this essential stretch by yourself.

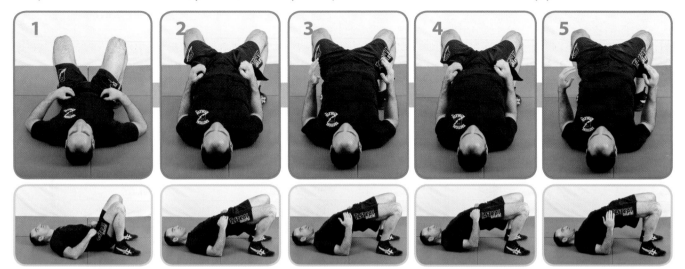

1) Lie on your back, feet flat and heels as close to your butt as possible. Rest your fingers over the top of your hipbones.
2) Perform a shoulder bridge by raising your hips toward the ceiling; your shoulders and head remain on the floor. Once your hips reach the limit of your ROM, apply downward pressure on your hipbones with your fingers cupped together. Maintain an isometric contraction for 5–10 seconds without dropping your hips.
3) Release your fingers and exhale (out your mouth) while continuing maximal glute contraction. Executed properly, your hips should float up to a new ROM. The harder you hold the isometric contraction, the greater the ROM gain will be when your hips are released.
4–5) Repeat this sequence 3–5 times, and then stand up. You should notice an immediate change in your posture when standing. Immediately perform 3 standing vertical jumps.

Part 2: Standing Vertical Jump (SVJ)

Always follow the hip flexor stretch with SVJs. If you don't, you will unwittingly create a common error known as "water skiing" or leaning back at the top position. This happens because your body will mimic the last position it was in. To counter that tendency; immediately perform the SVJ as soon as you stand up. It is also important to understand that the hip drive and extension used in performing the Standing Vertical Jumps are identical to the hip drive, extension and speed of movement when performing the kettlebell swings.

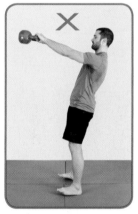

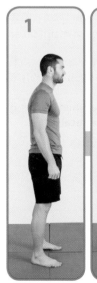
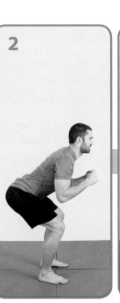
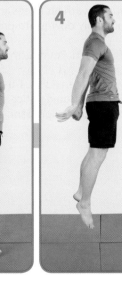

1) Start by standing with your feet between hip and shoulder width apart. 2) Sit back as if you're getting ready to jump as high as you can; shift your weight to your heels and load your glutes and hamstrings. 3) Drive through your heels, rapidly extending your hips and legs. Note the full extension of the legs, hips, and vertical body position. 4) Don't get hung up on the height of your SVJ. Pay attention to your body position in the loading phase, driving off your heels, and what rapid, full extension of your hips and legs feels like. Repeat for 3–5 reps. Immediately perform 10 Russian swings, using the same rapid hip extension.

Box Squat SVJ

The combination of the box squat and standing vertical jump is a great kinesthetic awareness drill that reinforces getting the hips back during the loading phase, then full leg and hip extension during the exploding phase (i.e., rapid extension of knees and hips). This is also a great drill to use right after practicing the hip flexor recruitment drill. Some people need a tangible target to aim and move toward.

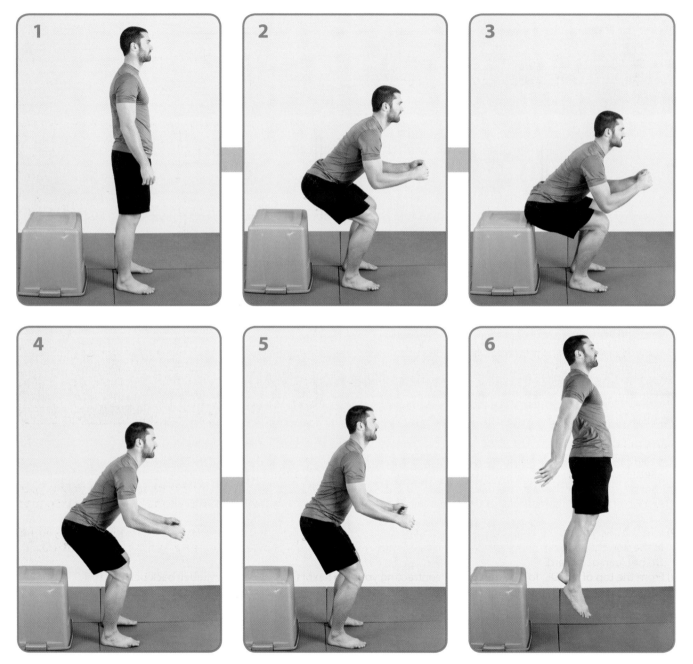

1) Stand with feet between hip and shoulder-width apart, heels approximately 6 inches from the front of a plyo box or bench. This is a target for your butt.
2) Actively engage your hip flexors, moving your hips back, weight shifting to your heels.
3) Continue until your butt makes light contact with the box.
4–5) Drive off your heels, rapidly extending your hips and legs.
6) Note the full extension of the legs, hips, and vertical body position. Don't get hung up on the height of your SVJ. Repeat for 3–5 reps.

Application: Russian Swing

Immediately after performing the box squat SVJ, practice the Russian swing. Concentrate on applying the same mechanics while you swing the kettlebell, except your feet do not leave the floor.

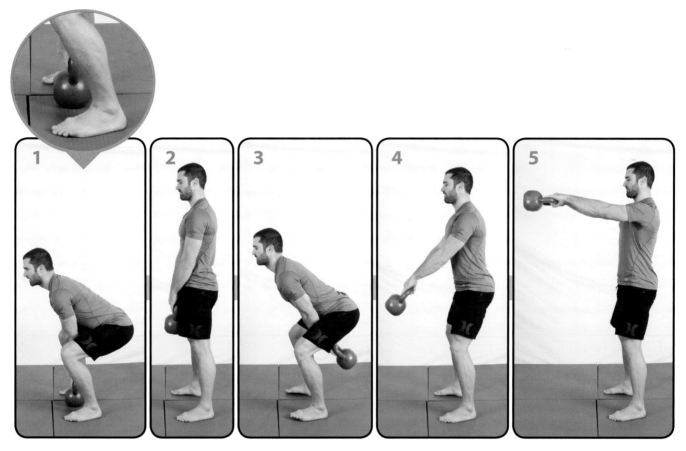

Start position:
- Stand with your feet between hip and shoulder width apart, toes pointing in the direction you're facing.
- Kettlebell is centered between your feet. Handle is in line with the base of your toes.
- Keep your chest open, shoulders back and down. Fold at the hips (i.e., hips move back and down), shift your weight to your heels, keep your neck in a neutral position, and look out, not up. Secure a two-handed grip on the kettlebell, keeping your arms straight.

2) Inhale through your nose; tighten your abs and glutes. Drive off your heels, fully extending your hips and legs until you are in the upright position. Chest remains open, keep shoulders pulled back and down, glutes are tight. Note: Arms are relaxed. Do not lean backward!

3) From the top of the DL, fold at the hips by contracting your hip flexors and hike the kettlebell back between your legs.

4) Rapidly extend your hips and legs by driving off your heels, as you did in the SVJ.

5) Keep driving through your heels until your legs and hips reach full extension. Note: The KB should float up. Keep the arms relaxed and chest up. Think of your shoulders as a pivot point, your arms are like lengths of rope or chain, and your hands are hooks attached to a wrecking ball. The height of the KB is determined by power transferred from your hips not the strength of your arms. Repeat for 10 reps. Start with very low swings and gradually build up the height with every rep. You should feel an immediate sense of freedom of movement and power from your hips.

If you do not feel more power from your hips, then repeat another cycle of hip flexor stretches and standing vertical jumps. This should yield noteworthy results.

I cannot overemphasize the importance of these drills. They will serve you well if applied prior to each training session or workout of the day.

Swing Series

Breathing Tips

Breathing patterns affect force production and performance. Beginners have a tendency to stop breathing during repetitive lifts of low-moderate intensity. It is important to develop the habit of always inhaling and exhaling during exercises. Kettlebell sport coaches constantly remind beginners to "breathe, breathe, always breathe" then mimic proper respiratory cycles.

There are basically two ways to match your breath to the movement while strength training: anatomically and biomechanically. In movements with small efforts such as the mobility exercise for spinal flexion/extension exhalation coincides with trunk flexion (bending) and inhalation coincides with trunk extension. This is called an anatomical match. In contrast, when high forces are generated the expiration should match the forced phase of movement, regardless of its direction or anatomical position. Rowers exhale or use the Valsalva maneuver during the stroke phase when the trunk and legs are extended. This breathing is termed a biomechanical match. For strength exercises, CrossFit kettlebell exercises (Part 1), and H2H Drill (Part 2), the breathing should be matched biomechanically. This is the simplest, safest approach for beginners or athletes who use a wide variety of strength and conditioning implements while performing high-intensity, low-duration circuit training (GPP).

Part 1: Inhale Phase

There are two phases to the breathing cycle, inhale and exhale. It is important to develop the habit of inhaling as 60–85 percent of your lung capacity prior to loading your muscles. Inhale through your nose on the descent prior to the deadlift or while descending during the swing.

High intra-abdominal pressure is useful because it reduces the compressive force acting on the intervertebral disks and may lessen the probability of spinal disk injury; and, ultimately, increase your lifting ability. When inhaling, it is preferable to increase intra-abdominal pressure over intra-thoracic breathing (i.e., chest breathing) or holding your breath.

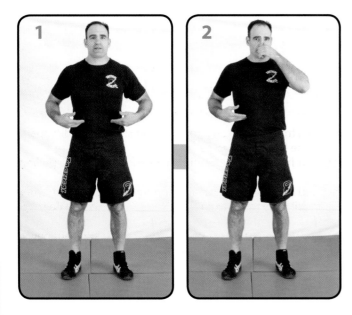

Inhale Drill #1
1) Inhale through your nose:
   • Stand tall and place your fingertips into the sides of your stomach just under your ribcage.
   • Inhale deeply, paying attention to how far your hands move with each breath.

Inhale Drill #2
2) Remove one hand from your stomach and using the thumb from your free hand press in and completely close off one side of your nostrils.
   • Inhale as deep as you can through your one nostril and notice how much more air seems to fill your diaphragm.
   • The good news is as we are swinging a kettlebell, we don't need to take one hand off the kettlebell to close one nostril. Just by inhaling sharply and deeply, your nostrils will automatically collapse, restricting the airflow and causing it to go where your body needs it when you need it the most.

Part 2: Exhale Phase

Rather than exhaling all of your air at once, or holding your breath, forcefully exhale a tiny stream of air through your clenched teeth while pressing your tongue to the roof of your mouth. This will contract the diaphragm and the muscles of the abdominal cavity and increase your intra-abdominal pressure, thus increasing the stability of the trunk and the transfer of force through it. Forced expirations, rather than the Valsalva maneuver (i.e., expiration efforts with a closed glottis), should be used whenever possible.

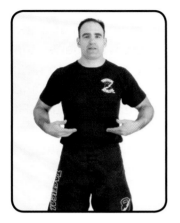

Dynamic Exhale Drill
1) Exhale through your teeth.
   • Stand tall and place your fingertips into the sides of your stomach just under your ribcage.
   • Inhale then exhale a quick short blast of air through your teeth. This should be similar to a fighter exhaling upon making contact.

On the upward portion of the swing, exhale a little bit of air, similar to a fighter exhaling on contact. Employ proper breathing in all exercises.

The difference is in the details, so work toward achieving perfect form. Think of each training session as just that: a "training" session, not a workout. Once you've mastered the kettlebell swing and these basics, you'll be ready for the many variations and challenging routines that will be discussed later in the text.

Application: Pick-Up/Swing/Put-Down Drill

From this point forward this is how we will pick up and put down the kettlebell for all two-handed swings. Concentrate on matching your breath with your movement. This is the safest, most efficient means of getting the kettlebell in action and the safest manner to return it to the starting point. This method will be applied to all the dynamic kettlebell lifts (i.e., one-arm swings, cleans, snatches).

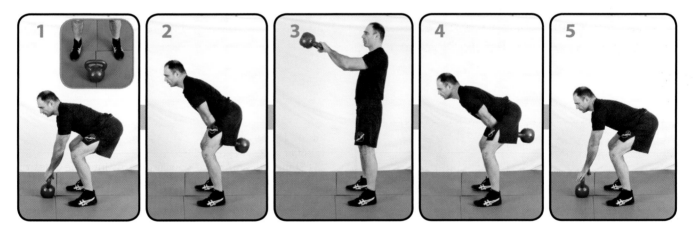

1) Position the kettlebell few inches in front of your feet, centered. Begin from the starting position: feet shoulder width apart, knees bent, back straight, head neutral, with a two-handed grip on the kettlebell handle.
2) Inhale through your nose; tighten your abs and glutes. Drive off your heels, slightly extending your legs and back, pulling (i.e., hiking) the kettlebell backward between the legs.
3) Rapidly extend your hips and legs by driving off your heels, as you did in the SVJ. Keep driving through your heels until your legs and hips reach full extension. Exhale through your teeth upon full hip and leg extension. Note: the KB should float up. Keep the arms relaxed and chest up.
4) As the kettlebell begins its descent, keep your hips straight until the last moment before your forearms crash into your pelvic region. At that point, pull your hips back allowing a full back swing. Repeat for 2–3 more reps.
5) Finish by allowing the final back swing (be sure to inhale), lowering your hips, and then allowing the kettlebell to come to a controlled stop right in front of your feet (i.e., starting position). Repeat this drill for 3–5 sets.
*I cannot over emphasize the importance of this exercise. Repetition establishes habit. Drill this exercise so that you can't do it wrong! Don't be a safety violator!

Major Malfunction
When Putting the Weight Down

The sequence that follows is very common when people are in a rush or careless or choose to sacrifice form for time or reps. This scenario can easily be avoided. I wish I could say it never happened to me but then I'd be just another big fat liar. Here's how it plays out:

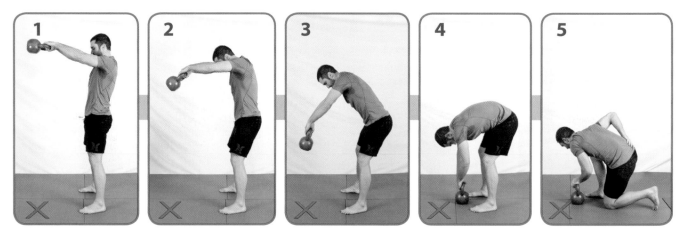

1) You finally reach your final rep or time and you are thinking to yourself, "Whoo-hoo I made it!" 2) Instead of keeping good form and disciplining yourself to keep your back straight, fold at the hips, allow a good back swing, and so forth, you choose to allow the kettlebell to drop straight down. 3) As the kettlebell is going down you decide to allow your back to round. 4) The final "death nail" is as your back is rounding you let out a big sigh of relief "Aaaah," passively exhaling through your mouth. 5) This is usually followed by a rapid series of events that includes but is not limited to a sharp breathtaking pain in your lower back, an instant buckling of the knees, a series of screams, cuss words, threats, and moans, followed by even more drama that can last up to several hours, days, weeks, or even months. "An ounce of prevention is worth a pound of cure."

√ Corrective Action: The Pick-Up/Swing/Put-Down Drill

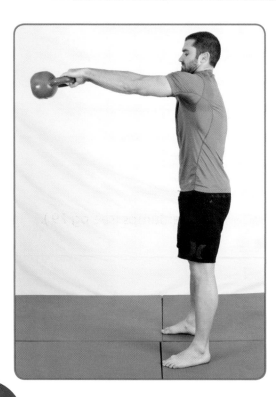

✕ RS Common Error #2: Locked Elbows, Rounded Upper Back

√ Corrective Action: Partner Drill

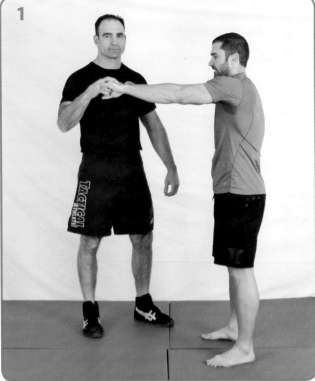

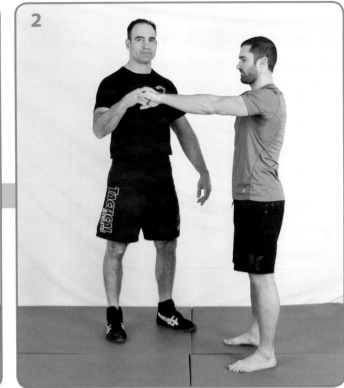

1) Have your partner assume the top position without a kettlebell. Have him grab your hand like a kettlebell.

2) Provide a little resistance and have him pull his shoulders back and down.

Application: Russian Swing

Perform 10 Russian Swings, emphasizing open chest with your shoulders back and down.

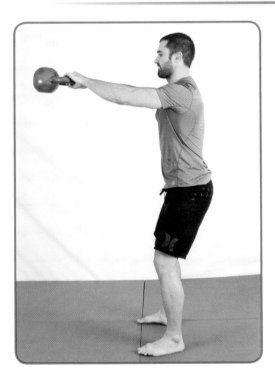

✕ RS Common Error #3: Short Stroke

Hip not fully extended (open).

√ Corrective Action #1:

Hip Flexor Stretch/Standing Vertical Jumps (see pg 79).

√ Corrective Action #2: Butt Kicking Drill

This is a great kinesthetic awareness drill that will help people lock out and get full hip and leg extension. Activating the glutes is the key to this drill.

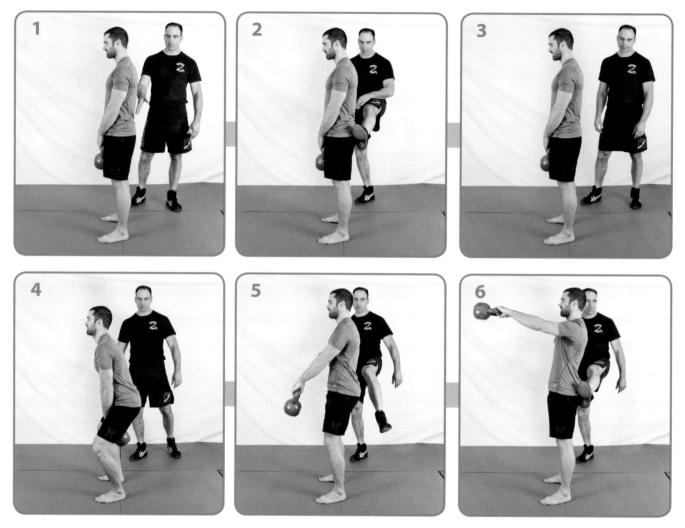

1) Have your partner deadlift the kettlebell to full upright position. Have him maximally contract his glutes and legs.

2) Lightly tap him on the butt with your foot to ensure it's actually tight. This gives him kinesthetic body awareness and helps him realize what tight is.

3–4) Have your partner turn the top of the DL into a swing.

5–6) Lightly tap them on the butt with your foot to emphasize tight glutes and full hip extension.

Word to the wise: If you don't feel comfortable using your foot to check tightness then use a clipboard or the knuckles of your fist. Avoid at all costs slapping the trainee on the butt with the palm of your open hand! Even in jest, this would be unprofessional and inappropriate. No good comes from that!

Application: Russian Swing

Perform 10 Russian Swings, emphasizing full hip extension.

✕ RS Common Error #4: Leaning Back

Aka water skiing.

√ Corrective Action #1: PVC Pipe

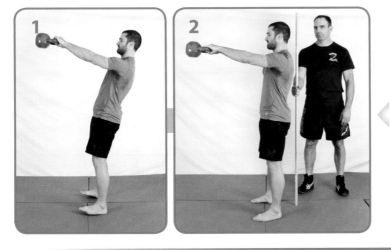

Hold a piece of PVC pipe vertically, behind his heel while swinging. Be sure to lean it or pull it to the side to allow his hips to move backward for the back swing.

Conclusion

At this point, your movement should be more consistent and efficient. As an athlete, you must focus your attention on the photo sequences that show you how to do it right. As a coach, if your athlete's movement doesn't look right, match it to the common error sequence then follow the corrective action. Keep it simple. You now have a vast array of tools to get the job done. Be patient, continually assess the situation, and cycle through the corrective actions and all will be well in your world.

Once the Russian swing is mastered here are a couple of simple exercise prescriptions. Full work-outs will be addressed in Section 6, Program Design, but for now, we'll just focus on a simple routine with the exercise you just learned. This is great for beginners or folks who are extremely limited on training time.

Russian Swing Rx:

10 x 10
10 sets of 10 reps, 30 seconds rest in between sets or
10 sets of 10 reps, 30 seconds of jump rope in between sets or
10 sets of 10 reps, light jog 200 meters or

Tabata Swings 20/10:
• 20 seconds of work, followed by 10 seconds of rest
• 8 rounds = 4 minutes

Tabata Mod 45/15
• 45 seconds of work, followed by 15 seconds of rest
• 8 rounds = 8 minutes

Is that all? Yep. Don't forget to warm up with either joint mobility or movement prep exercises and cool down with the post-stretching exercises.

■ II. Power Swing ■

The power swing increases the tempo and power output of the Russian swing. By shortening the up stroke and pushing down on the down stroke, it allows you to perform more reps in less time. This exercise is very grip, core, and anaerobic intensive. In addition, it will pressure test your form, reinforcing your ability to keep a straight back. This is truly a self-correcting exercise.

The limiting factor of learning from a book is that you cannot see speed, rhythm and timing. Even though the photos look similar to the Russian swing, pay close attention to the captions below.

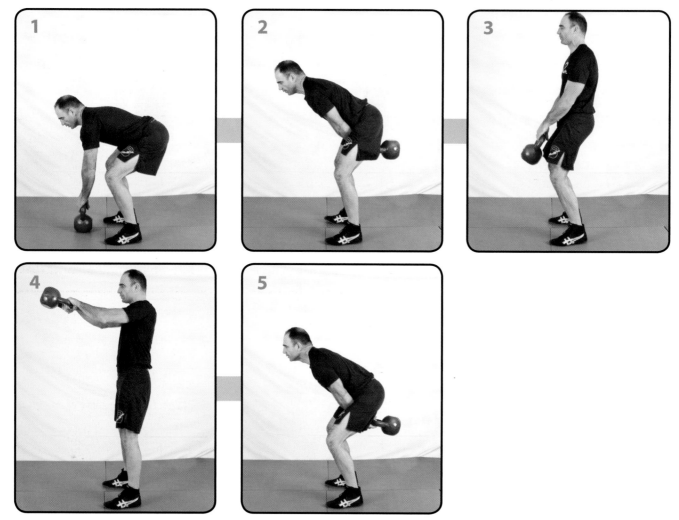

1) Begin from the starting position; kettlebell should be centered a few inches in front of your feet. Your feet are shoulder width apart, knees bent, back straight, head neutral, with a two-handed grip on the kettlebell handle.
2) Inhale through your nose; tighten your abs and glutes. Drive off your heels, slightly extending your legs and back, pulling (i.e., hiking) the kettlebell backward between the legs.
3) Drive off your heels, rapidly extending your legs and hips.
4) Actively exhale through your teeth as your legs and hips reach full extension, and consciously tighten your glutes. At this point there is a sequence of events that happen in quick succession. Timing is everything!
   • Engage your lats, chest, and abs to slow and stop the kettlebell at shoulder level.
   • Simultaneously death grip the kettlebell handle.
   • Push the kettlebell down as you would a ball slam.
   • Note: Do not hinge at the hips either before or when you push the kettlebell down. This is critical! Keep your glutes tight and hips straight when you push the KB downward.
5) Keep a straight back, tight abs, and neutral head alignment. When the kettlebell reaches its lowest point, explode out of the hole. You will notice a lot more kinetic energy built up at the bottom of your swing and more power throughout your extension. Try to move faster with every rep. Repeat for 10 repetitions. Be aware that your grip will be heavily taxed during this exercise. Be sure there is a clear impact zone in front and in back of you.
Caution: before performing the power swing for the first time, practice the following partner dill as outlined below.

Drill #1: Partner Assisted Power Swing

Before jumping straight into the power swing, get with your training partner and practice this drill first. It is important to keep a straight back and pressure test your form with a gradual increase of downward pressure.

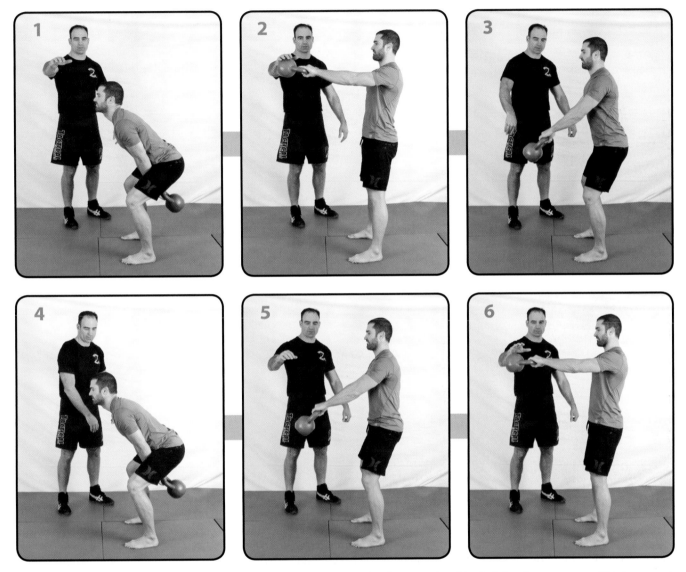

1) Stand to the side of your training partner. Hold your hand out, palm down, at shoulder height of your partner. This is a target for him to aim for. From the starting position, have him perform a back swing.

2) As he extends to the top of the swing, allow the kettlebell to touch the palm of your hand. Watch his mechanics and ensure everything is correct (straight back, breathing, full extension, etc.).

3) Lightly push the kettlebell down.

4) Watch his mechanics (hips back, weight on heels, neutral neck, etc.) as the kettlebell swings to the back position.

5) Reset your hand to his shoulder height.

6) As the kettlebell touches your hand, push it down a little harder than the rep before. Repeat this sequence and gradually increase the downward pressure with each repetition. Be a good coach. Look for form deviations and provide constant feedback.

After one or two sets of the partner-assisted power swing, try a couple of sets of the unassisted power swing.

Power Swing Common Errors

When coaching the Power Swing, you must be "Johnny on-the-spot" with detecting and correcting errors. Errors are magnified because of the increased velocity of the kettlebell. If you practice without the aid of a coach or training partner, be extra sensitive to what your body is telling you. If at any time you feel a "whiplash" effect or see quick flashes of bright light; STOP, place the kettlebell on the ground and make a "note to self": Something is wrong! Reassess the situation, fix what needs fixing, and move on.

✕ Common Error #1: Floppy Top

Floppy top is when the kettlebell flops on the top of the power swing. The cause is a combination of a weak grip and an aggressive push down of the KB.

√ Corrective Action:

Instantly tighten your grip on the KB handle before you aggressively push the KB down. You want the aggressive push down, just not the flop on top. Grip it as if your life depends on it.

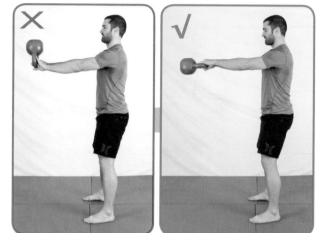

✕ Common Error #2: Floppy Bottom

The floppy bottom is the opposite problem of the floppy top. In this case the kettlebell is whacking you on the bottom. The cause is usually a weak grip. Don't let it smack you anywhere on your body!

√ Corrective Action:

The grip sequence is tight/loose/tight. Where the kettlebell changes directions, you must put the death grip on it. In between each directional change, slightly relax your grip.

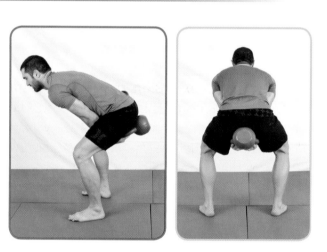

✕ Common Error #3: Short Stroke

Hip not fully extended (open). Experience has shown that whenever people do something different with their hands, they tend to forget about their hips. Should look like this:

√ Corrective Action:

Deadlift to full extension, contract glutes, kick butt. Standing vertical jumps or box squat SVJs.

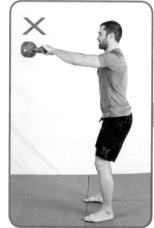
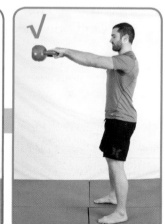

✕ Common Error #4: Improper Hip Sequence

From a coach's perspective, you'll notice a strange "slinky" effect on the spine and a little head snap on the bottom position. Neither is a desired outcome. From a practitioner's perspective, you'll feel a "whiplash" affect . . . that is a big a problem. Stop and reassess. Here's what's happening:

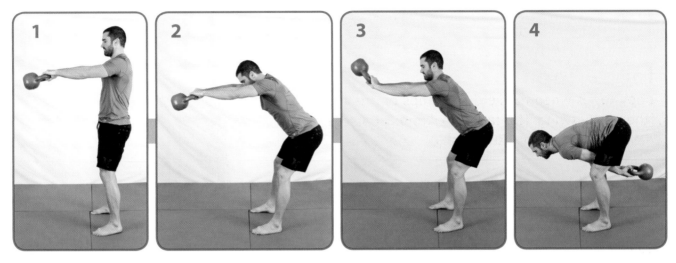

1) You reach the top position; so far so good.
2–3) You unhinge your hips, then push down on the kettlebell, and that's the crux of the problem.
4) The kettlebell will then jump speed and cause a shock wave through your spine . . . not good!

Corrective Actions:

• Deadlift to full extension, maximally contracting your glutes. Explain while the trainee is holding that contraction: "This is what you should feel at the top position. Continue to keep your glutes tight as you push the kettlebell down. Do not pull your hips back until the last fraction of a second (i.e., before your hands and KB crash into your groin). Got that?"

• Perform the partner-assisted power swing. Verbally coach. As the trainee extends, say "hip extension"; when you push the kettlebell bell down, say "push"; wait a split second, "then hips." Be sure the trainee doesn't move his hips back until you say "then hips." Repeat the coaching cues and push down for a few reps.

• Once the trainee gets the sequence down (with proper breathing), have him perform the regular power swing. Do a few reps of Russian swings first, ensure good movement and proper breathing, and then perform the power swing, gradually pushing each rep down a little harder by himself. Continue giving verbal coaching cues "good hip extension . . . push, then hips back."

Power Swing Rx:

Tabata Swings:
• **20 seconds of work, followed by 10 seconds of rest**
• **8 rounds = 4 minutes**

III. American Swing

This is CrossFit's swing of choice because the kettlebell moves through a longer range of motion. The swing culminates at top with the kettlebell directly overhead. From a teaching standpoint, if you have taken the time to learn, practice, and master the Russian swing and power swing first, then it will be much easier make a safe and effective transition to the American swing.

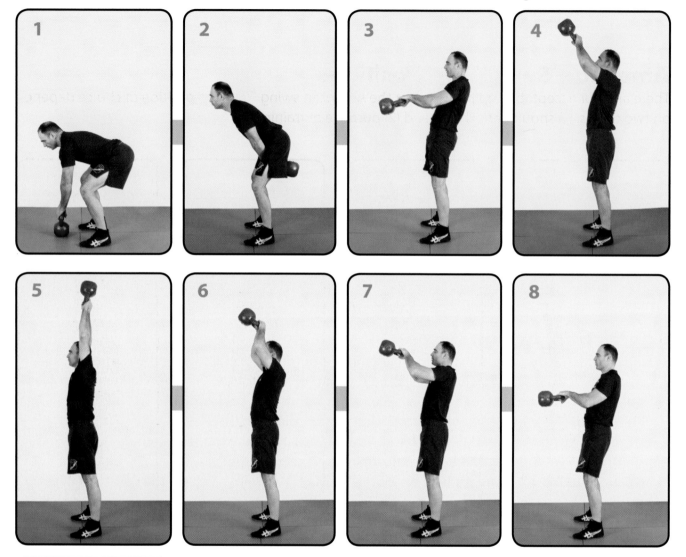

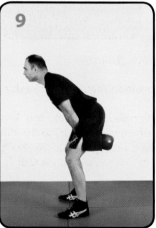

1) Begin from the starting position; kettlebell centered, but a few inches forward of your feet. Your feet are shoulder width apart, knees bent, back straight, head neutral, with a two-handed grip on the kettlebell handle.
2) Inhale through your nose; tighten your abs and glutes. Drive off your heels, slightly extending your legs and back, pulling (i.e., hiking) the kettlebell backward between the legs.
3) Drive off your heels, rapidly extending your legs and hips. Actively exhale through your teeth as your legs and hips reach full extension, and consciously tighten your glutes.
4) As the kettlebell moves overhead, straighten your arms and tighten your grip.
5) Your biceps should be in line with your ear, similar to a handstand. Keeping the arms relaxed, allow the kettlebell to float to the overhead position.
6) Slightly lean back, unlock your elbows, and begin the KB descent.
7) Keep your arms relaxed on the way down. This shortens the arc or kettlebell path and assists in better balance.
8) The slight lean backward will help a smooth transition to the back swing.
9) Allow your arms to fully straighten, and then pull your hips backward at the last moment. Repeat for desired time or reps.

It is important to note that there are two positions where it is essential to keep your arms locked straight. Your arms must be straight whenever you have weight overhead (i.e., top of the military press, jerk, snatch, handstand, etc.) and they must be straight when pulling weight off the ground (i.e., deadlift, BB clean, BB snatch, KB back swing). As in most athletic lifts, the arms should be relaxed in between these two positions. Please understand that if you get into the practice of keeping your arms locked straight throughout the entire ROM of the American swing, it will only make learning the KB cleans and snatch more difficult later on.

American Swing Top Positions

There are four acceptable top positions for the American swing. Your top position of choice depends on two things: (1) shoulder flexibility and (2) purpose of training.

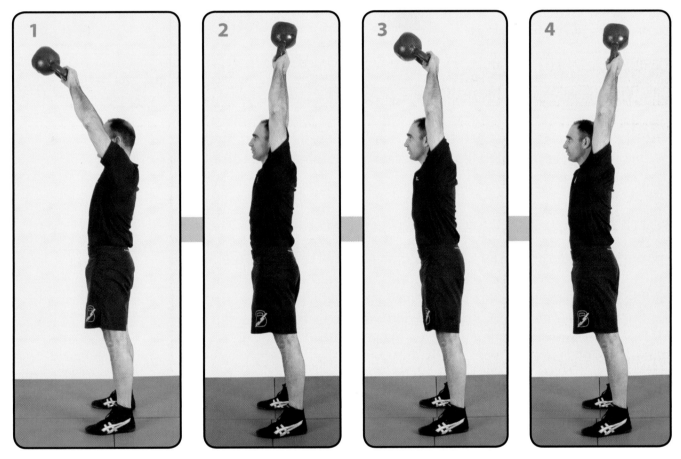

1) If an athlete or client has inflexible, injured, or unstable shoulders, then the top position could look like this:

2) If you are using kettlebells to enhance your fitness level or sports performance, then your top position should look like this.

3) If you want increase the power of the American swing and decrease the cycle time, the top position should look like this: The reason being is that you can quickly reverse directions overhead and accelerate the kettlebell downward, reducing the risk of it flipping overhead. A note of caution when turning the American swing into a power swing; it is very grip intensive. Keep that in mind when coupling this exercise with pull-ups or rope climbs. Just because you can does not mean you should!

4) Lastly, if CrossFit is your sport, then you must follow the rules for competition and show your ear to get credit for your swing.

American Swing Common Errors

Here are some of the most common errors in regards to the American swing.

✕ Common Error #1: Arms Bent Overhead

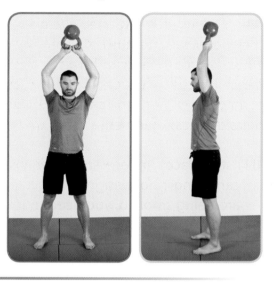

For safety and effectiveness, there are two positions where your arms need to be locked straight; the first is whenever you have weight overhead (i.e., top position) and second, when pulling weight from the floor, back swing (i.e., bottom position).

√ Corrective Action:

Verbally cue the trainee to straighten his arms on the top position. If it's a flexibility issue, then adjust his height to a comfortable ROM.

✕ Common Error #2: Overhead Flip

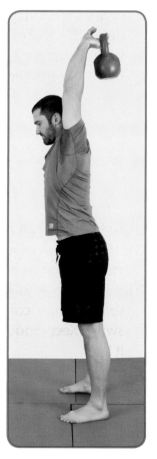

You want to avoid this malfunction at all costs! Due to the momentum of the kettlebell and the fact that you have to balance it upside down, there is a potential for the kettlebell to flip over backward. Nothing good comes from that! Here are a few contributing factors:

• Weak grip.

• Fatigued grip.

• Sweaty hands.

• Wrong KB handle dimensions. This is a biggie. Not all kettlebells are created equal. If the distance between handle and bell is either too long or if the handle is too thick, the ability to stabilize the kettlebell overhead becomes exponentially harder. The combination of these two factors attributed to the numerous "overhead flip" issues that were experienced at the 2009 CrossFit Games.

√ Corrective Action:

Replace poorly designed kettlebells with better ones. I don't care how great of a deal you got when you bought them; scrap them! It's just not worth injuring yourself or others with unsafe equipment.

• Maximally tighten grip on top, but keep your grip relaxed as much as possible the rest of the time.

• Shorten the arc by relaxing your elbows. This will reduce the force pushing against the bell.

• Use chalk. I normally "just say no to chalk" unless it becomes a safety issue, which in this case, it is. Use just enough to get the job done. Chalk is not magic pixie dust. You don't need to rub it over your entire body, nor should you let it become a mental crutch.

✕ Common Error #3:
Too Much Delts, Not Enough Hips, and Arched Back

When taking the kettlebell overhead, most people have a tendency to overcompensate by using their deltoids to get the kettlebell from waist or chest level to overhead. This is common in beginners who are unfamiliar with how to use their hips properly. Experienced kettlebellers can also fall prey to this error, especially toward the end of a tough routine. Overcompensating with the deltoids is less than desirable for three reasons.

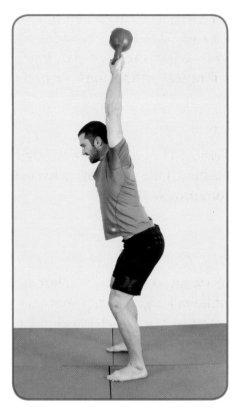

1) First, it places unnecessary strain on the deltoids. The American swing is not designed to "sculpt your delts." If your delts are being smoked, you need to reassess what you're doing because it's wrong.

2) The momentum created by pulling with your delts may be difficult to overcome in the overhead position. This is especially true if you wait until the last second to "put on the brakes." If you have a history of shoulder injuries, it is safer to apply "the brakes" a little sooner and end the top of the swing just in slightly in front of your head.

3) There's a tendency to unhinge your hips as you pull with your delts. This places undue stress on your shoulders and lower back. It causes even more stress if you try to "throw your head through" your arms as the weight moves overhead.

√ Corrective Action:

1) Use more hip drive. Refer to corrective exercises for the Russian swing.
2) If the hips are used correctly, you should be using your lats to slow down and stop the bell as it floats to the overhead position.
3) Once your hips fully extend, keep them there. Make a conscious effort to be sure to powerfully contract your glutes, abs, and armpit muscles at the top of the swing. Keep good alignment. Your shoulders, back, and neck will thank you for it later.

Note the similarities of the top position of the American swing and the handstand.

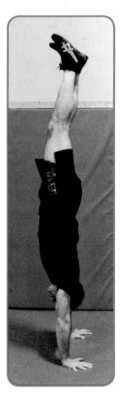

✗ Common Error #4:
Arms Locked Throughout Entire Movement

Keeping your arms locked throughout the entire movement is problematic for a few reasons.

• It's inefficient. The kettlebell travels a longer distance.

• The large arc makes it harder to stop the kettlebell overhead, causing more stress on the shoulders.

• It's harder to maintain the open chest, (i.e., shoulders back and down) throughout the mid-range movements, causing unnecessary stress on your shoulders.

• It will make learning the snatch more difficult.

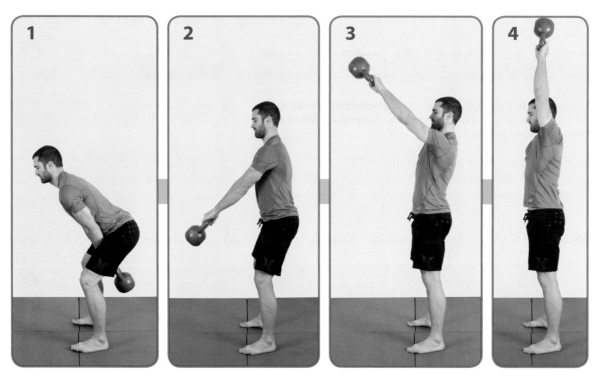

1) This is a good start position.

2–3) Not optimal. Elbows locked, slight round in upper back

4) This is a good finish position.

√ Corrective Action:

1) Practice a few Russian swings and concentrate on keeping your shoulders pulled back and down while keeping your elbows relaxed.

2) Alternate one Russian swing with one American swing until your movement becomes consistent.

✗ Common Error #5: High-Pull and Pressing Overhead

This is an interesting adaptation of the American swing I've seen growing within the CrossFit community since the 2009 CrossFit Games. As I mentioned earlier, the kettlebells with the longer handles, as used in the 2009 Games, made stabilizing the kettlebell overhead (i.e., without flipping) extremely difficult. It was problematic to all the competitors. Let's take a look at the modification of the American swing and analyze the movement.

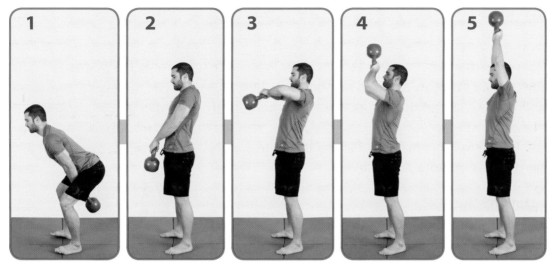

1) Good back swing.
2) Kettlebell path is tighter to the body, similar to a barbell clean or snatch.
3) Keeping the KB handle close to the body, ensuring a vertical kettlebell path.
4) Kettlebell transitions to bottom-up position.
5) Kettlebell is pressed or punched straight up into the overhead position. Then the kettlebell is quickly pulled straight down following the same path right into the hang position/back swing.

√ Corrective Action: Use more hip drive. Don't press.

There's no question of the extreme efficiency of this hybrid movement or the logic behind the adaptation. It facilitates more reps in the same amount of time and eliminates the possibility of kettlebell flip and yet seems to stay within the rules. It makes perfect sense within the competitive "gaming" context. This movement mimics more of a high-pull-press combination from the hang position than a true American swing. Is it wrong? No, it's just different. If you can perform the movement without pressing it to the top, then rock on. If you feel you have to press, then come up with a cool name for that movement because it's really not an American swing.

American Swing Rx

The easiest way to transition into the American swing is to perform one to three Russian swings, and then take it overhead. Once it goes overhead, then continue with the full range of motion American swings for some time or reps.

10 x 10
10 sets of 10 reps, 30 seconds rest in between sets or
10 sets of 10 reps, 30 seconds of jump rope in between sets or
10 sets of 10 reps, light jog 200 meters or

Tabata Swings 20/10:
• 20 seconds of work, followed by 10 seconds of rest
• 8 rounds = 4 minutes

Tabata Mod 45/15
• 45 seconds of work, followed by 15 seconds of rest
• 8 rounds = 8 minutes

IV. Swing Release

The first question people have when they see me demonstrate the two-hand swing release is: "Why, why, why in the world would I ever want to let go of the kettlebell?" There are actually a few good reasons:

1) It reinforces correct hip drive. You can't fake the funk. You must aggressively extend your legs and hips to accelerate the kettlebell to above head level to get the hang time.
2) It reinforces proper arm movement that will be essential to performing a proper snatch.
3) It forces you to break the habit of swinging the KB with locked straight arms, which slows down the learning process for the snatch.
4) It creates more power output, making it very challenging anaerobically.
5) It develops hand-to-eye coordination
6) It's fun!

It is best to practice the swing release in an area where you can freely drop the kettlebell without worrying about causing property damage. It's better to practice multiple sets of low reps. This will keep you fresh, facilitating faster learning.

Two-Hand Swing Release: (Standard)

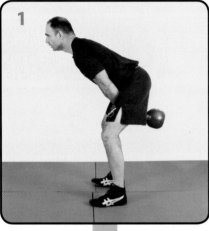

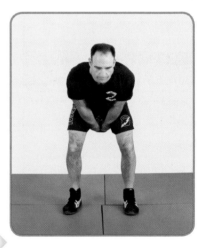

Begin by performing a Russian swing.

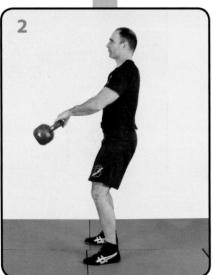

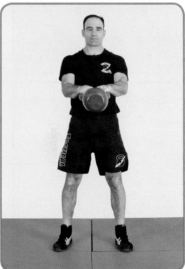

3

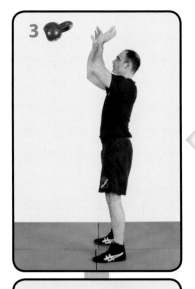

When the kettlebell reaches chest height, purposefully "drag" the fingers of both hands up and off the handle at a 45-degree angle. This will keep the kettlebell handle within hands' reach. Allow the kettlebell to rise to its highest position. The handle should remain horizontal and parallel to the ground while the kettlebell is airborne.

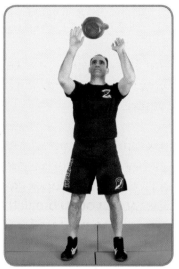

4

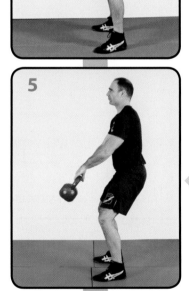

Grab the handle with both hands as it begins to descend. Be sure to secure it before it reaches your shoulder level. Any lower and it will jerk you out of your tennis shoes.

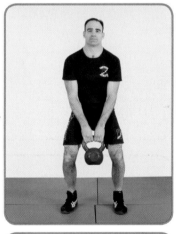

5

Guide the kettlebell on its way down and begin to fold at the hips.

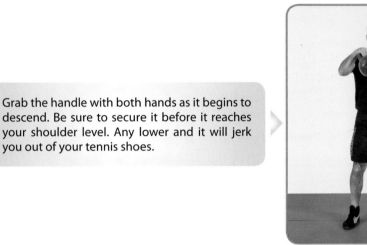

6

Flow right into the back swing, maintain a straight back, an open chest, and keep your weight on your heels. Repeat for desired time or reps.

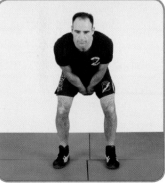

Swing Release Common Errors:

✕ Common Error #1: Kettlebell Flips Over

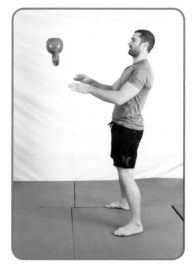

If you swing the kettlebell and then just let go, two things will automatically happen: (1) the bell will move up and away from you and (2) the bell will rotate up, causing the handle to rotate down. Neither is desirable at this point. If this happens, don't try to catch the KB; just let it hit the ground.

√ Corrective Action:

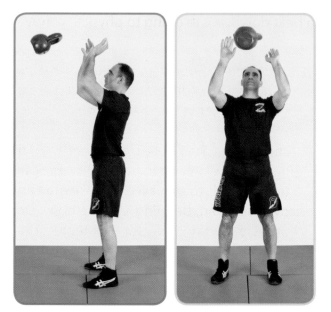

At the top of the swing, pull the kettlebell handle up and toward the ceiling at a 45-degree angle. Actually drag your fingers off the kettlebell handle. This action is very important. It will prevent the kettlebell from flipping and will keep the kettlebell within hands' reach.

✕ Common Error #2: Kettlebell Drifts Away

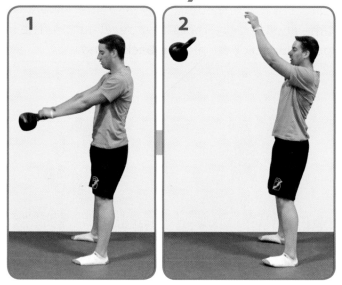

If you release the kettlebell too early, between hip and shoulder level, the kettlebell quickly moves away from your body. Also, if you keep your arms locked straight when you release the handle, it will drift away from you.

Never reach for a kettlebell that is out of arm's reach. It is better to let it fall to the floor than to attempt to grab it and have it pull you forward, out of position, possibly resulting in an injury.

√ Corrective Action:

As the kettlebell reaches shoulder to eye level, consciously bend your arms, dragging your fingers off the handle at a 45-degree angle up and over your head. This will put the kettlebell in perfect position to reestablish your grip.

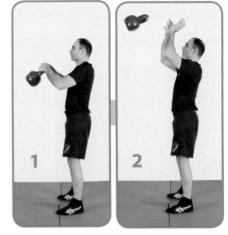

If verbal correction and re-demonstrating the skill doesn't fix the problem, then it's time put the kettlebell down and get physical with your training partner. No, we're not going to give your partner a beat down. We're going to physically move him through the proper movements.

1) Stand next to your training partner, extend your arm to his eye level, then have him grip your pointer and middle finger as they would the kettlebell handle.

2) If necessary, grab his closest forearm with your free hand, physically manipulate his arm in the direction it needs to move (i.e., a 45-degree angle up and over his head, bending at the elbow). Do this a few times, ensuring that your partner just doesn't let go of your fingers but actually drags and pulls them up as he releases.

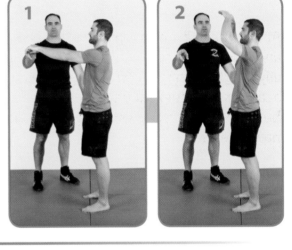

✕ Common Error #3:
Catching the Kettlebell below Shoulder Height

Catching the kettlebell below shoulder height is never a good idea because you don't have enough time and distance for proper deceleration. The kettlebell will either jerk you forward off balance or pull you too deep into the back swing.

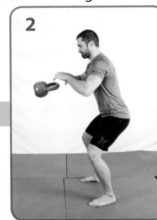
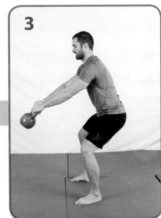
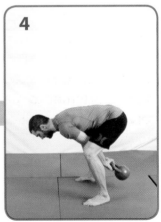

Swing Series

√ Corrective Action:

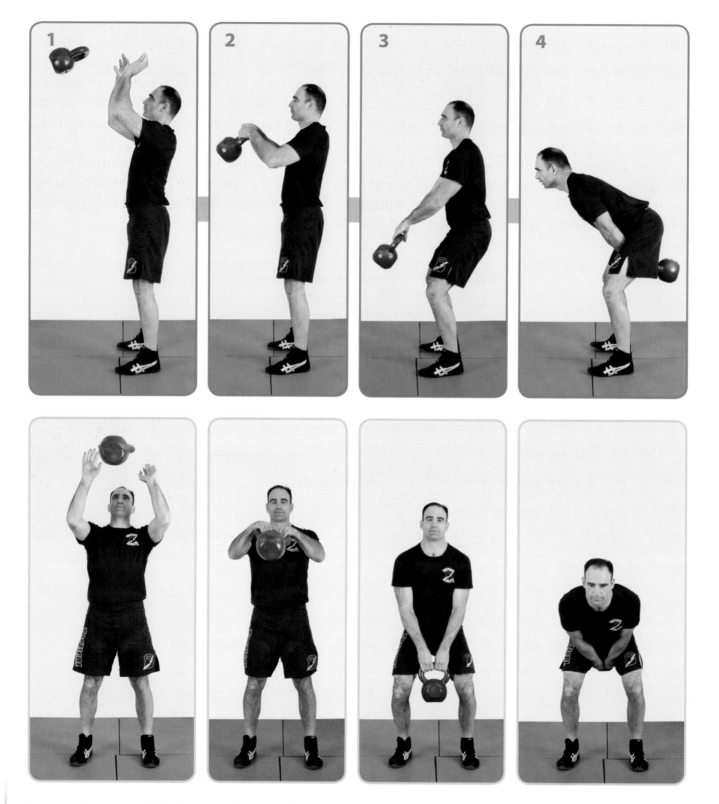

1) Concentrate on your hip drive to get the proper hang time.
2) Secure your grip on the handle before shoulder height.
3) Maintain good posture and balance.
4) Decelerate into the back swing.

Never forget that you always have the option of not trying to catch the kettlebell if something doesn't seem right. Here's a perfect example of a situation that occurred during a photo shoot for the cover of my first DVD. We were trying to take some cool action shots of me doing some H2H Drills (i.e., kettlebell juggling). I was standing on top of an 8-foot-high cinder-block wall, flipping the kettlebell around while my photographer was taking the pictures below me from ground level. At one point toward the end, I was getting tired and I messed up a release that put the kettlebell out of position in front of me. I had a choice to make: attempt to catch the kettlebell and risk being jerked off the wall or just let it go and possibly risk breaking the kettlebell and some concrete below. As I thought through the cost/benefit analysis, I decided to let it go. Instantly after the making that decision, a thought flashed through my mind. "Man, I hope my photographer is clear of the impact zone!" Thankfully, the kettlebell landed a foot or two in front of him, a near miss! The best part was that my kettlebell survived completely unscathed. I dusted it off and inspected it. You could barely notice where the paint chipped!

Swing Release Rx

In the beginning, it's a good idea to alternate 1 Russian swing, then 1 swing release to help reset and maintain good form. Practice multiple sets of lower reps (10–20). Fatigue and sloppy form should be avoided at all costs. Remember: Skill first!

Tabata Swing Releases:
• 20 seconds of work, followed by 10 seconds of rest
• 8 rounds = 4 minutes

■ V. Wall Ball Substitute ■

The wall ball is a staple exercise for CrossFitters. If you are unfamiliar with this exercise, then here's a quick description of the movement. Begin by front squatting a 20-pound Dynamax Medicine Ball, then explosively extend (i.e., jump), push-pressing (i.e., shoving) the ball up and forward to an 8- to 10-foot-high target on the wall in front of you. As the ball rebounds off the wall, immediately catch it, squat, and repeat the process. Now, you might find yourself somewhere in the world where you may not have a 20-pound med ball or even a wall. If you have a kettlebell, then this is the drill for you.

Familiarize yourself with the photo sequence below. It's for demonstration purposes only, to show the flow and end result. For practice, go to the Drills and Skills section. Practice one skill at a time, detect and correct any errors, then move on to the next skill.

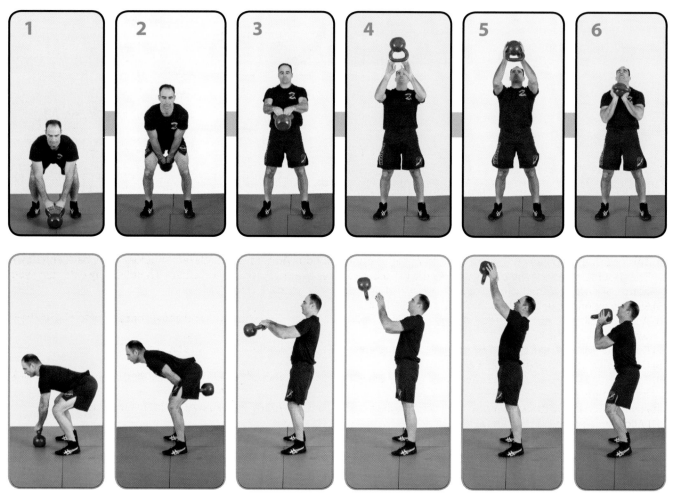

1) Start position:
   • Feet between hip and shoulder width apart, toes pointing in the direction you're facing.
   • Kettlebell is centered, 3–6 inches in front of your toes.
   • Keep your chest open, shoulders back and down.
   • Fold at the hips (i.e., sit back and down), shift your weight to your heels, and keep your neck in a neutral position.
   • Establish a two-handed grip on the kettlebell.
2) Perform the back swing:
   • Inhale through your nose, tighten your abs and glutes.
   • Keeping your weight on your heels, slightly extend your legs and back angle, contract your lats, and hike the kettlebell back between your legs.
3) As the kettlebell reaches the end of the back swing, press through your heels, extending your legs, hips, and back until you are in the upright position.

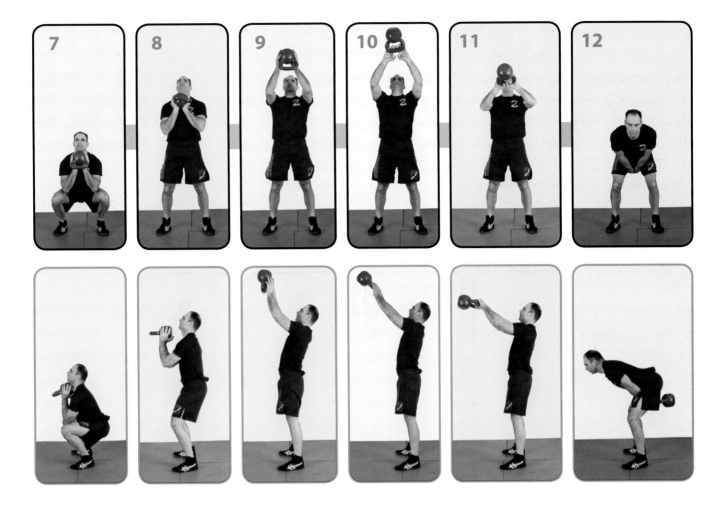

4) This action should launch the kettlebell from hip to eye level. Note: Arms must be relaxed; shoulders stay back and down. The shoulders provide the pivot point. As the kettlebell reaches eye level, release the kettlebell handle, fully extending your hands, allowing the bell to continue its movement upward as the handle rotates downward.

5) Slightly extend your arms and catch the rising bell with both hands.

6) Actively pull and decelerate the kettlebell high into your chest. Keep your elbows in and allow your knees to slightly bend when receiving the KB.

7) Continue to descend into a full front squat, kettlebell resting high on your chest, weight stays on heels.

8) Drive off your heels, extending your legs and hips.

9) The power from your hips, transferred through your core, will launch the weight off your chest. Push the bell up and away as your arms extend.

10) By pushing the kettlebell up and away, the handle will automatically rotate upward directly into your hands.

11) Allow gravity to take the kettlebell back down.

12) Stay upright and well balanced as the kettlebell descends. Just before your forearms crash into your pelvic area, fold at the hips (i.e., sit back and down) and shift your weight to your heels. Repeat for desired time or reps.

Swing Series

Drills and Skills

The wall ball substitute can be broken down into two parts. I strongly recommend that you master each part individually before putting them together into one sequence.

Skill #1: Swing Release, Half-Flip Catch, Push Press

Skill #1 has all the mechanics of the wall ball substitute minus the front squat. The swing release, half-flip catch, and push press are the critical components that must be mastered first. We can increase the intensity later by adding the front squat. All safety rules still apply. When in doubt, push the kettlebell away from your face and allow it to harmlessly land on the floor. Assess the situation, think about what happened and why, make the necessary correction, then move on.

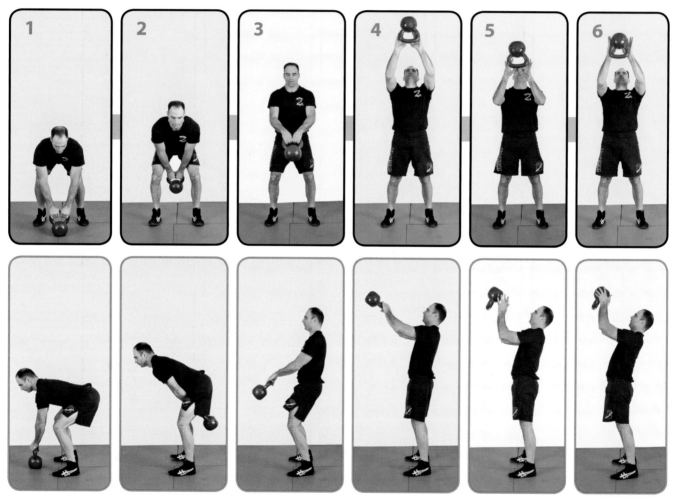

1) Start position:
   • Feet between hip and shoulder width apart, toes pointing in the direction you're facing.
   • Kettlebell is centered, 3–6 inches in front of your toes.
   • Keep your chest open, shoulders back and down.
   • Fold at the hips (i.e., sit back and down), shift your weight to your heels, and keep your neck in a neutral position.
   • Establish a two-handed grip on the kettlebell.
2) Perform the back swing:
   • Inhale through your nose, tighten your abs and glutes.
   • Keeping your weight on your heels, slightly extend your legs and back angle, contract your lats, and hike the kettlebell back between your legs.
3) As the kettlebell reaches the end of the back swing, press through your heels, extending your legs, hips, and back until you are in the upright position.

4) This action should launch the kettlebell from hip to eye level. Note: Arms must be relaxed; shoulders stay back and down. The shoulders provide the pivot point.
5) As the kettlebell reaches eye level, release the kettlebell handle, fully extending your hands, allowing the bell to continue its movement upward and the handle to rotate downward.
6) Slightly extend your arms and catch the rising bell with both hands.
7) Actively pull and decelerate the kettlebell high into your chest. Keep your elbows in and allow your knees to slightly bend when receiving the KB. Note the hand position on the kettlebell. The bases of your thumbs must be close together. Pause for a second or two, think about what you're doing, and then:
8) Drive off your heels, extending your legs and hips. The power comes from your hips, transferred through your core; your arms will launch the weight off your chest.

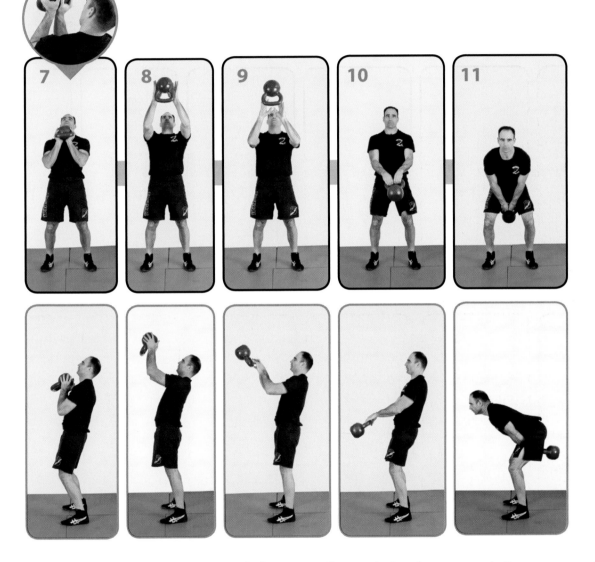

9) Push the bell up and away as your arms extend. This action will cause the handle to automatically rotate upward directly into your hands.
10) Allow gravity to take the kettlebell back down. Stay upright and well balanced as the kettlebell descends.
11) Just before your forearms crash into your pelvic area, fold at the hips (i.e., sit back and down) and shift your weight to your heels. Repeat for desired time or reps.

Swing Series

✕ Common Error #1: Chicken Wing and Thumbs Position

This common error has two parts that go together like "peas and carrots."

The first one is the chicken wing. This is where the elbows are flared out away from the body. Elbows must remain tight against the body for effective power transfer when push-pressing the KB off your chest to arms' reach.

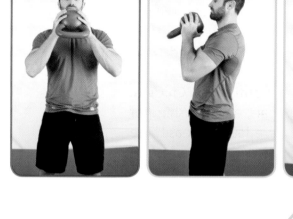

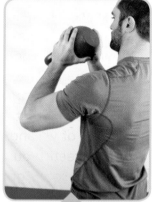

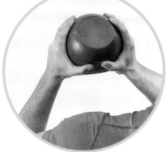

The second issue is the position of the thumbs. Thumbs aren't that strong. It won't take much for the kettlebell to blast through them, impacting you in the face or chest. Neither outcome is positive.

√ Corrective Action:

Catch the kettlebell with the bases of your thumbs touching each other. This creates an impervious barrier and decreases the stress on your thumbs. In addition, it forces you to move your elbows closer together. So, you fix both problems with one correction by keeping your thumbs oriented vertically and close together!

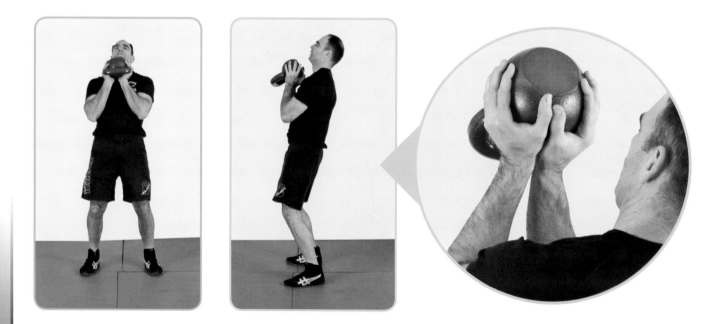

✕ Common Error #2: Over-Rotation

Over-rotation is common when you allow too much space between the kettlebell and your hands or if you release the handle like a maniac. Regardless, no good will come from catching the kettlebell like this. It usually ends with the handle smashing you in the grill, followed by you spitting out a mouthful of Chiclets. This scene of wailing, tears, and gnashing of what few teeth you have left can easily be avoided by some good old-fashioned common sense.

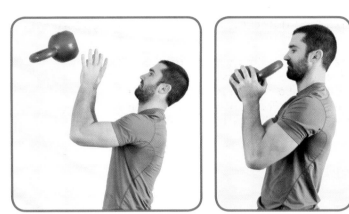

√ Corrective Action:

Keep your hands close to the kettlebell as you release and catch it. Ensure the kettlebell rotates slowly. It doesn't need to be a lightning-fast rotation. It's a big, loopy release with a slow rotation. If at any time the kettlebell rotates too fast or appears to be moving uncomfortably close toward your face, don't attempt to catch it, just push it away with both hands and step back.

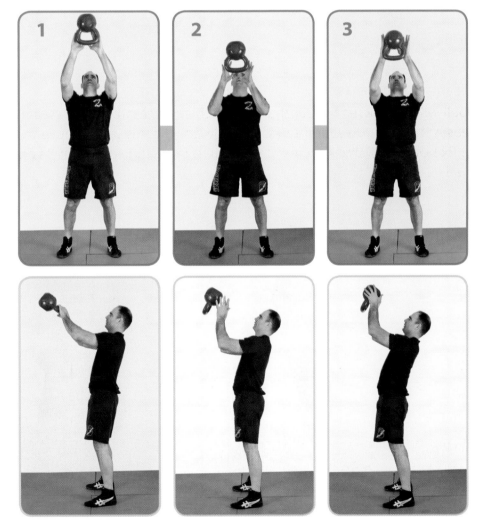

✕ Common Error #3: More Bad Catches

Here are two more bad catches to avoid.

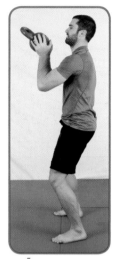

This is another form of over-rotation. There's no fear of getting hit in the teeth with the handle, but it's going to make reestablishing your grip on the handle a lot more difficult.

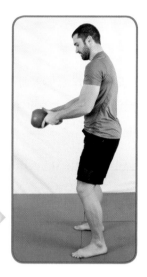

This is the classic underhand catch (i.e., palms up). A lot had to go wrong to get to this point. Always catch with your palms facing away from you. If the kettlebell is so low that you have to flip your palms up to catch it, you're better off just to let it fall to the ground.

√ Corrective Action:

Just say no to catching any poorly released and out-of-position kettlebell! It's that simple. I won't make you do burpees or punishment PT for dropping a kettlebell. If it's out of position, I want you to drop it! On the other hand, if you catch one that you should have dropped, now that's a different story; you just violated an important safety rule! Don't be a safety violator!!

Skill #2: Front Squat

The second part of the wall ball substitute is the front squat. Practice the front squat in the following manner.

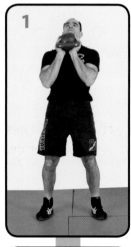

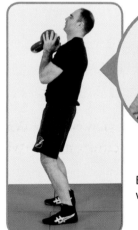

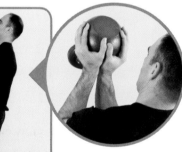

Begin in the standing position, feet shoulder width apart, holding the bell with both hands, handle down, elbows tight against your sides.

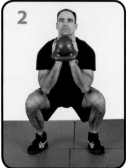

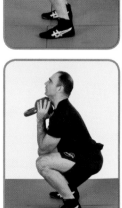

1) Actively contract your hip flexors, pulling your hips back and down. As you are descending, keep your chest up and attempt to spread your knees apart, opening your hips.
2) Inhale on the way down and exhale on the way back up.
3) Isolate and practice the front squat until it feels comfortable. This may take a while, but through consistent practice your range of motion and strength will increase.

Be sure to keep a straight back and an open chest when performing a front squat. As to common errors, if your profile looks similar to a dog pooping in an open field, then you're doing it wrong! Squat only as deep as you can while keeping good back position.

Skill #3: Wall Ball Substitute

If you feel comfortable with skills 1 and 2, then it's time to link them together and practice the full exercise. Perform multiple sets of low reps to get the feel of this exercise.

Wall Ball Substitute Rx

Continuing on with the Tabata theme, we'll look at three workouts.

1. Tabata Skill #1: Flip, Catch, Push-Press, repeat
   - 20 seconds of work, followed by 10 seconds of rest
   - 8 rounds = 4 minutes

2. Tabata Skill #2: KB Front Squats
   - 20 seconds of work, followed by 10 seconds of rest
   - 8 rounds = 4 minutes

3. Tabata Skill #3: Wall Ball Substitute
   - 20 seconds of work, followed by 10 seconds of rest
   - 8 rounds = 4 minutes

Congratulations, you have built a solid foundation of two-arm swings! When you train, always remember that repetition establishes habit. Strive for perfection and you will achieve excellence.

VI. One-Arm Swing

Up until now, we've covered the mechanics and fundamental movements of the various two-arm kettlebell swings. Through proper, regular practice, your swing should now be more efficient, consistent, and powerful. Now it's time to move to the next progression: the one-arm swing.

Performing the kettlebell swing with one arm is more demanding. From the waist down your movement and hip drive is the same as for the two-arm swing. Here are a few benefits of practicing one-arm swings:

- Increased demands on your grip strength
- Increased core activation and stabilization
- Develops tremendous strength endurance in your lower back
- The best assistance exercise for learning the mechanics for the kettlebell snatch.

In addition, any previously undetected technical deficiencies will soon become obvious. For these reasons, I highly recommend that you practice one-arm swings with a lighter kettlebell. If one is not available, then it is better to practice more sets with fewer repetitions in each set. Strive to work as hard as possible, while staying as fresh as possible. Remember, fatigue is counterproductive when learning new skills.

One-Arm Swing

Familiarize yourself with the picture sequence below and read the captions to get an idea how the movement is performed. Right now it is for demonstration purposes only, to show the flow and end result. In a few moments, we will break it down into easily digestible pieces for practice toward mastery.

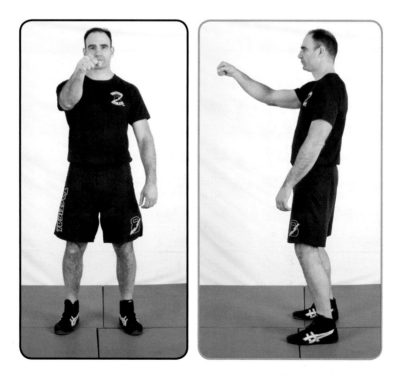

Note: Hand position must be at a 45-degree angle at the top of the swing. This means your hand externally rotates as it swings upward.

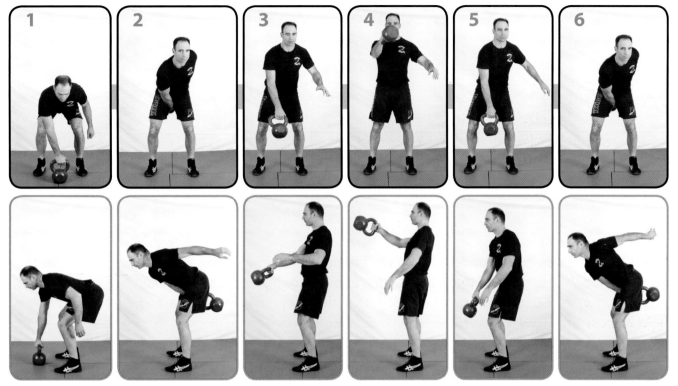

1) Start position:
   • Feet between hip and shoulder width apart, toes pointing in the direction you're facing.
   • Kettlebell is centered, 3–6 inches in front of your toes.
   • Keep your chest open, shoulders back and down.
   • Fold at the hips (i.e., sit back and down), shift your weight to your heels, and keep your neck in a neutral position.
   • Establish a one-handed grip on the kettlebell.
   • Note: Hand position is near the corner closest your thumb and forefinger.
   • Free hand stays off the body.
2) Perform the back swing:
   • Inhale through your nose, tighten your abs and glutes.
   • Keeping your weight on your heels, slightly extend your legs and back angle, contract your lats, and hike the kettlebell back between your legs.
   • Internally rotate the hand gripping the kettlebell at least 45-degrees so that by the end of the back swing it's pointing up toward your butt.
   • Free arm mimics the direction of kettlebell.
3) As the kettlebell reaches the end of the back swing, press through your heels, extending your legs, hips, and back until you are in the upright position. Be sure to square your shoulders (i.e., pull the working shoulder back) as your torso becomes upright.
4) This action will launch the kettlebell from hip to eye level. Note: Arms must be relaxed; shoulders stay back and down. Ensure that the kettlebell travels up and down your centerline.
5) Allow gravity to take the kettlebell back down. Stay upright and well balanced as the kettlebell descends.
6) Just before your forearm crashes into your pelvic area, fold at the hips (i.e., sit back and down) and shift your weight to your heels. Repeat for desired time or reps.

Drills and Skills

Drill #1: Alternating One- and Two-Arm Deadlift

It is important to master the mechanics of the one-arm deadlift before attempting the one-arm swing, since the common errors are similar for both movements. If technical deficiencies are not identified and fixed when practicing the one-arm DL, then those same errors will only magnify and transfer to the more dynamic one-arm swing. Let's continue with the crawl-walk-run approach and concentrate our efforts on consistency of movements before intensity.

By alternating one- and two-arm deadlifts, you will:

- Reinforce good mechanics.
- Realize that the movement from the hips down is the same regardless of whether you are performing a one-arm or two-arm deadlift.
- Establish the habit of proper hand position in the corner of the KB handle. This hand position is the same for all one-handed exercises (i.e., cleans and snatch).
- Get used to rotating the shoulders in the bottom position while keeping your back straight.
- Get used to actively squaring up the working shoulder in the top position.
- Keeping your nonworking hand off any part of your body.

The way this drill works is that you perform a one-arm deadlift (right), then a two-arm deadlift, then a one-arm deadlift (left), then two, then right, then two, left, and so on.

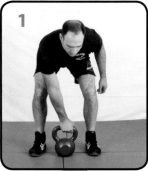

Start position:
- Feet between hip and shoulder width apart, toes pointing in the direction you're facing.
- Kettlebell is centered, 3–6 inches in front of your toes.
- Keep your chest open, shoulders back and down.
- Fold at your hips (i.e., sit back and down), shifting your weight to your heels; keep your neck in a neutral position.
- Establish a one-handed grip with your right hand in the corner nearest your thumb and forefinger. Keep your arm straight.
- Free hand stays off the body.

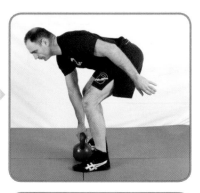

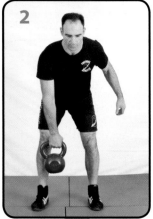

Inhale through your nose; tighten your abs and glutes. Drive off your heels and extend your legs and hips.

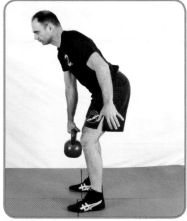

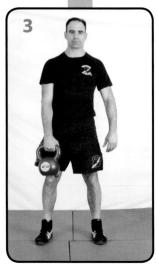

Continue to drive through the heels, fully extending your legs and hips until you are in the upright position. Chest remains open, right shoulder is pulled back and down. Note: Arm is relaxed and kettlebell hangs directly below the shoulder.

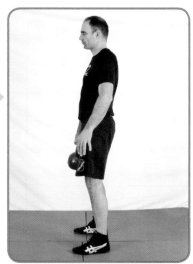

4

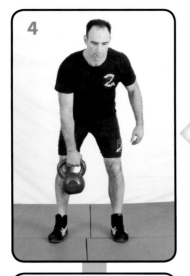

Fold at the hips, (i.e., hips move back and down), knees slightly flex, weight shifts back to heels.

Note: Kettlebell path is vertical (straight up/down).

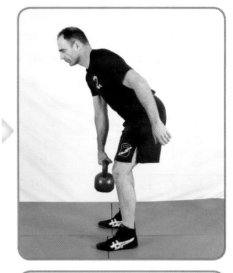

5

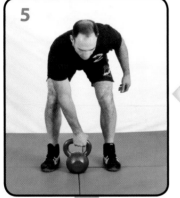

Continue moving your hips backward, maintain a straight back, and return the kettlebell to its original starting position.

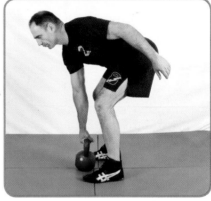

6

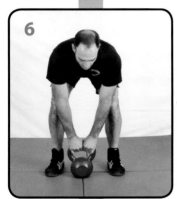

Secure a two-handed grip on the kettlebell, keeping your arms straight.

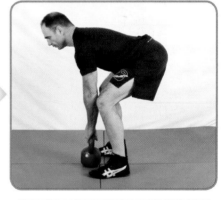

7

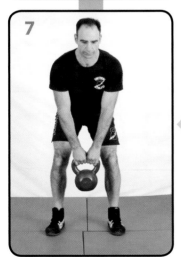

Inhale through your nose; tighten your abs and glutes. Drive off your heels and extend your legs and hips.

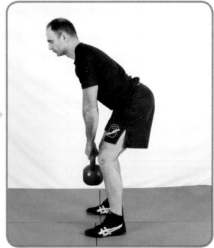

Swing Series

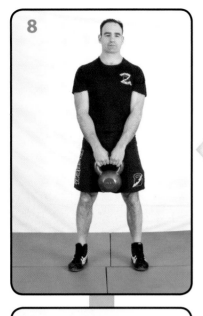

8

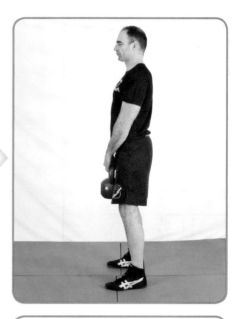

Continue to drive through the heels, fully extending your legs and hips until you are in the upright position. Chest remains open, keep shoulders pulled back and down. Note: Arms are relaxed; do not lean backward!

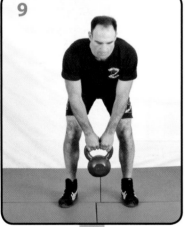

9

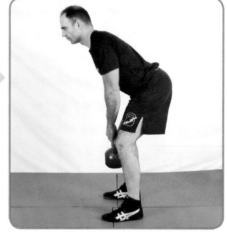

Fold at the hips, (i.e., hips move back and down), knees slightly flex, weight shifts back to heels. Note: Kettlebell path is vertical (straight up/down).

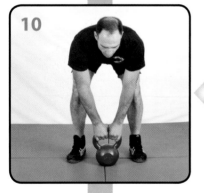

10

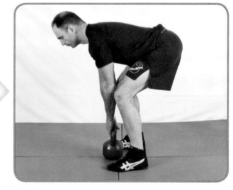

Continue moving your hips backward, maintain a straight back, and return the kettlebell to its original starting position.

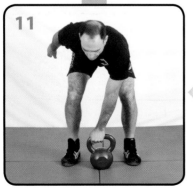

11

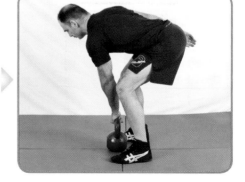

Establish a one-handed grip with your left hand in the corner nearest your thumb and forefinger. Keep your arm straight. Free hand stays off the body.

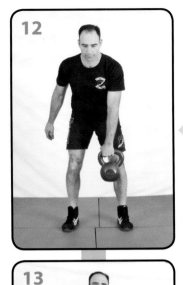

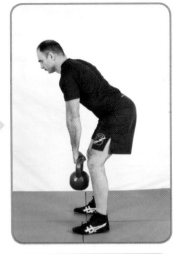

Inhale through your nose; tighten your abs and glutes. Drive off your heels and extend your legs and hips.

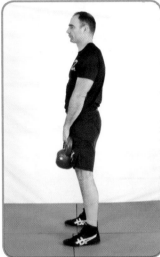

Continue to drive through the heels, fully extending your legs and hips until you are in the upright position. Chest remains open, left shoulder is pulled back and down. Note: Arm is relaxed and kettlebell hangs directly below the shoulder.

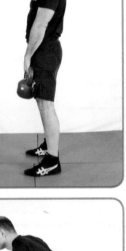

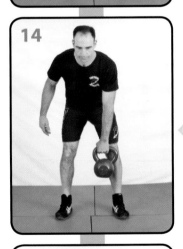

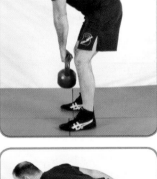

Fold at the hips, (i.e., hips move back and down), knees slightly flex, weight shifts back to heels.

Note: Kettlebell path is vertical (straight up/down).

Continue moving your hips backward, maintain a straight back, and return the kettlebell to its original starting position. Repeat this deadlift pattern until you have performed 5 reps per arm.

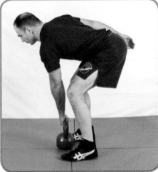

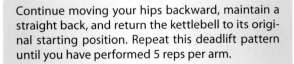

Swing Series

Troubleshooting the One-Arm Deadlift

✕ Common Error #1: Hand in Center of Handle

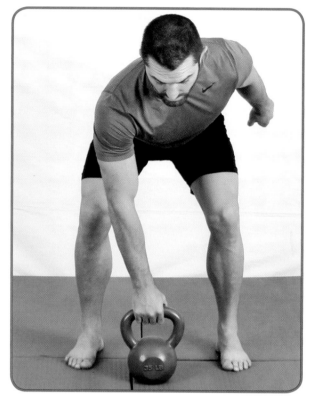

√ Corrective Action:

If you get confused as to which corner your hand should be in; open your hand and let your thumb point the way. The corner your thumb is pointing to is the corner you need to get your hand in.

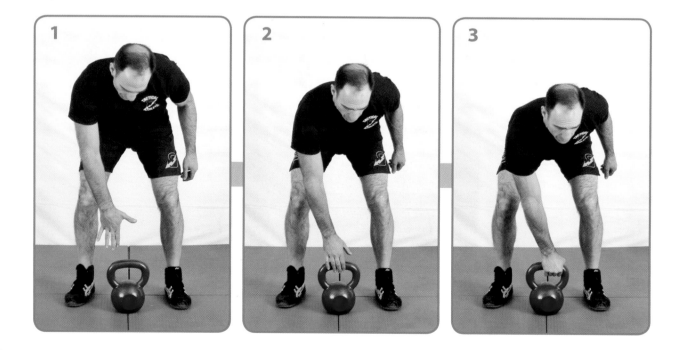

✕ Common Error #2:
Flat Back and Shoulders Totally Squared

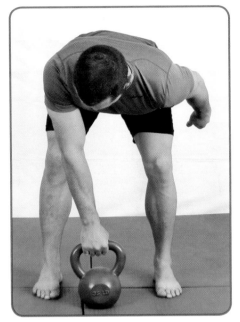

√ Corrective Action:
The hips need to drop slightly to get a better back angle, then the right hand needs to slide into the left corner of the KB handle, allowing the right shoulder to dip slightly.

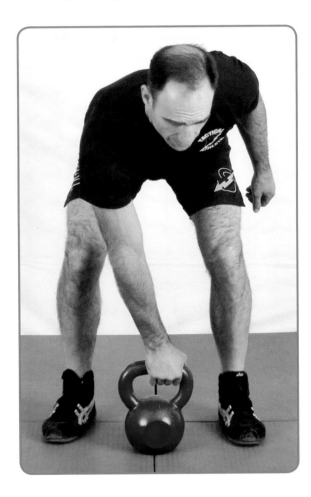

Swing Series

Application: One-Arm Swing

Perform 5 one-arm swings (right), then 5 one-arm swings (left).
Repeat for three rounds (i.e., sets).

✕ Common Error #1: Shoulders Not Square On Top

The kettlebell is pulling you out of position.

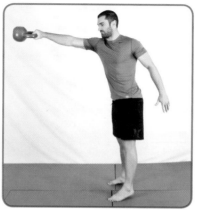

√ Corrective Action:

Actively pull your shoulder back as your torso straightens and your forearm clears your hips. This will help propel the kettlebell upward to eye level. Think to yourself—"hip extension, square my shoulders" while performing each rep.

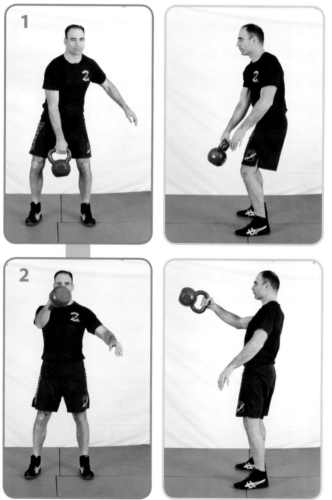

✕ Common Error #2:
Elbow Locked and Hand Angle Wrong

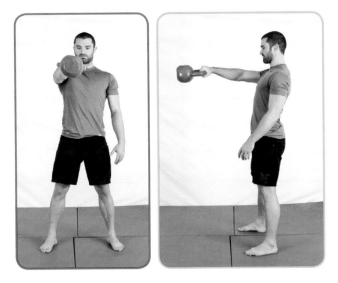

√ Corrective Action:

Keep your arm relaxed and externally rotate your hand to a 45-degree angle. These are two essential elements that will facilitate your learning of the snatch.

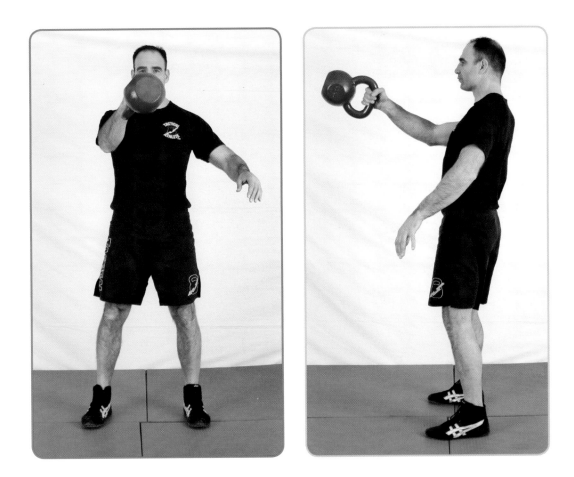

✕ Common Error #3: Flat Back and Hand on Thigh

Going too deep puts unnecessary stress on your lower back and you're a "big fat cheater" if you keep your hand on your thigh.

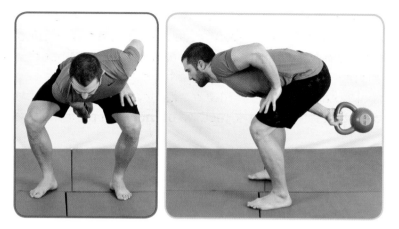

√ Corrective Action:

Maintain correct back angle. The center of your forearm (not the elbow) should be touching the center of the inside of your thigh. Let your off hand track the kettlebell as it swings. Keep it off your thigh!

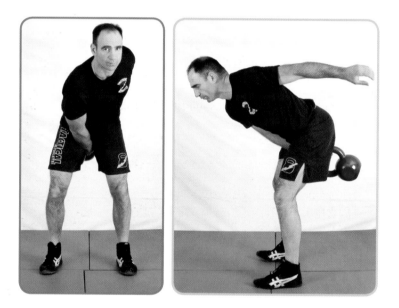

One-Arm Swings Rx

At this stage of the game, it's better to keep things simple. Practice the one-arm swings for multiple sets of 5–10 reps or for time in the Tabata format.

Tabata One-Arm Swings
· 20 seconds of one-arm swings (L), followed by 10 seconds of rest
· 20 seconds of one-arm swings (R), followed by 10 seconds of rest
· 8 rounds alternating arms each round = 4 minutes
· 16 rounds alternating arms each round = 8 minutes

VII. Half-Rotation Switch

The half-rotation switch is the easiest way to transfer the kettlebell from one hand to the other without stopping to put it down. This technique allows for continuous motion, which translates to increased work capacity. It also maximizes safety because you are transferring the KB from hand-to-hand when your spine is in a neutral position. And it reduces the likelihood of grip failure because it makes it nearly effortless to switch from one hand to the other when one becomes fatigued.

Timing is key in the half-rotation switch. Switch the kettlebell from hand to hand when it is at the top end of the swing. The half-rotation switch is the method of choice for performing one-arm swings indoors.

To perform a half-rotation switch:

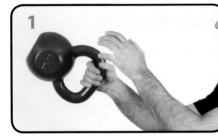
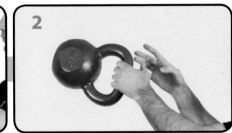
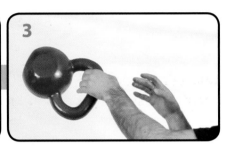

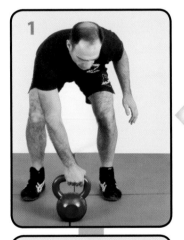

Start position:
- Feet between hip and shoulder width apart, toes pointing in the direction you're facing.
- Kettlebell is centered, 3–6 inches in front of your toes.
- Keep your chest open, shoulders back and down.
- Fold at the hips (i.e., sit back and down), shift your weight to your heels, and keep your neck in a neutral position.
- Establish a one-handed grip on the kettlebell.
- Note: Hand position is near the corner closest your thumb and forefinger.
- Free hand stays off the body.

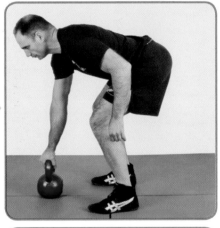

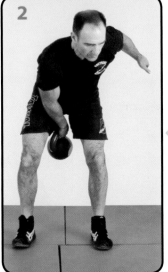

Perform the back swing:
- Inhale through your nose, tighten your abs and glutes.
- Keeping your weight on your heels, slightly extend your legs and back angle, contract your lats, and hike the kettlebell back between your legs.
- Internally rotate the hand gripping the kettlebell at least 45 degrees so that by the end of the back swing your thumb is pointing up toward your butt.
- Free arm mimics the direction of kettlebell.

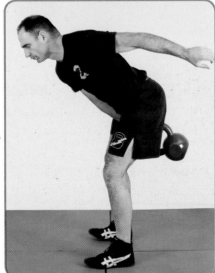

3

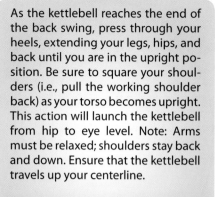

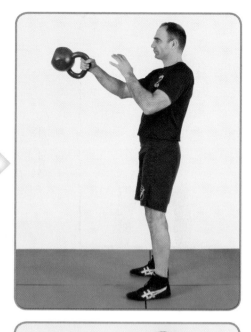

As the kettlebell reaches the end of the back swing, press through your heels, extending your legs, hips, and back until you are in the upright position. Be sure to square your shoulders (i.e., pull the working shoulder back) as your torso becomes upright. This action will launch the kettlebell from hip to eye level. Note: Arms must be relaxed; shoulders stay back and down. Ensure that the kettlebell travels up your centerline.

Note: Hand position must be at a 45-degree angle at the top of the swing. This means your hand externally rotates as it swings upward.

4

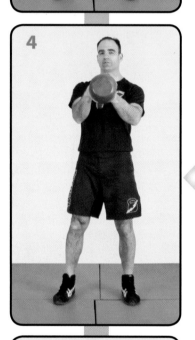

As the kettlebell reaches the top position, simultaneously release your right hand and establish your grip with your left hand. Note: The hands stay in the exact same corner.

5

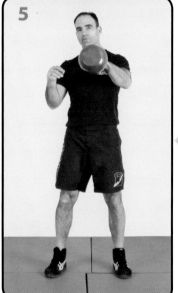

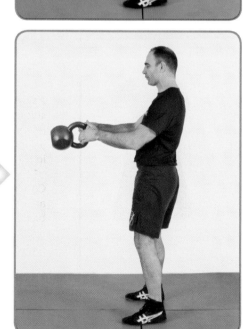

Continue rotating the kettlebell and allow gravity to take the kettlebell back down. Stay upright and well balanced as the kettlebell descends.

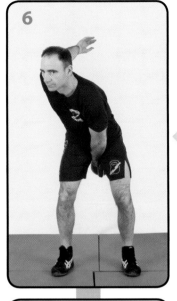

6

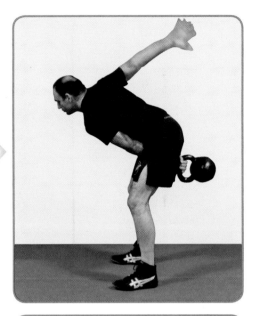

Just before your forearm crashes into your pelvic area, fold at the hips (i.e., sit back and down) and shift your weight to your heels.

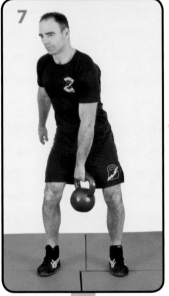

7

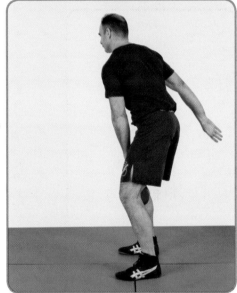

As the kettlebell reaches the end of the back swing, press through your heels, extending your legs, hips, and back until you are in the upright position.

8

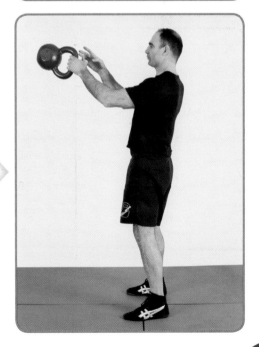

As the kettlebell reaches the top position, simultaneously release your left hand and establish your grip with your right hand. Note: The hands stay in the exact same corner.

Continue rotating the kettlebell and allow gravity to take the kettlebell back down. Stay upright and well balanced as the kettlebell descends. Repeat for desired time or reps.

Swing Series

✕ Common Error: Hand Placement

The biggest common error when first learning the half-rotation switch is placing your hand in the wrong corner of the kettlebell. People have a tendency to see an open spot on the handle then instinctively go for it. In addition, whenever folks do something different with their hands, they have a tendency to forget about their hips and end up "short stroking."

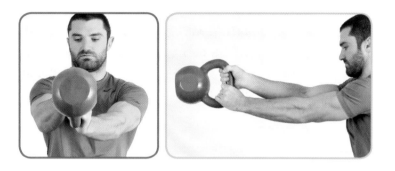
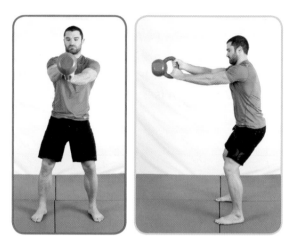

√ Corrective Action:

1. Alternate one-arm swings with half-rotation switches. This will help you reset your hip drive and hand position and give you time to think about what's being done and why. In other words, perform one swing right, then a half-rotation switch, one swing left, then a half-rotation switch.

2. If you are having problems with the hand position, just put your hands together as if clapping. Think "palm to palm." The kettlebell should continue rotating in the same direction.

Half-Rotation Switch Rx

1. Tabata: Swing then a switch
- 20 seconds of performing as prescribed:
- One-arm swing, then a half-rotation switch.
- Repeat with the other hand, one-arm swing then a switch.
- Followed by 10 seconds of rest.
- 8 rounds alternating arms each round = 4 minutes
- 16 rounds alternating arms each round = 8 minutes

2. Tabata: Switch every rep
- 20 seconds of switching hands upon every rep, followed by 10 seconds of rest.
- 8 rounds alternating arms each round = 4 minutes
- 16 rounds alternating arms each round = 8 minutes

The H2H switch is a more versatile and demanding way to alternate the kettlebell from one hand to the other. The main difference with this variation is that the handle does not rotate; it remains horizontal during the hand switch. In the beginning, it is important to practice the H2H switches at a relatively low level, between waist and chest, just to get the feel of the exercise. As you become more comfortable and proficient, add more hip drive and shoulder pull. This will accelerate the kettlebell to eye level and above. This is where you derive the most benefit. The coordinated effort between your hips and shoulder will give you the hang time you need to make the switch. If you think about it, the H2H switch is just a one-handed version of the two-arm swing release.

H2H Switch at Chest Level

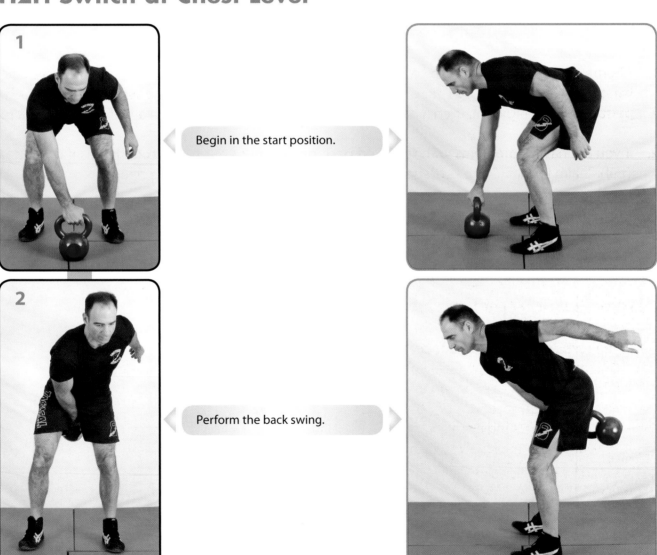

1 — Begin in the start position.

2 — Perform the back swing.

3

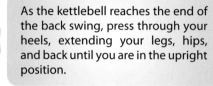

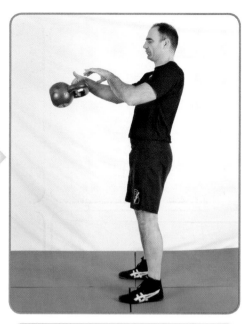

As the kettlebell reaches the end of the back swing, press through your heels, extending your legs, hips, and back until you are in the upright position.

4

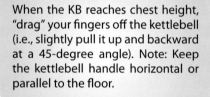

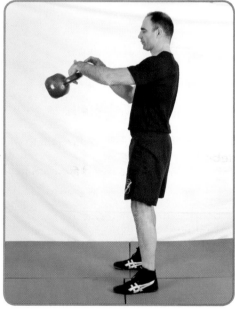

When the KB reaches chest height, "drag" your fingers off the kettlebell (i.e., slightly pull it up and backward at a 45-degree angle). Note: Keep the kettlebell handle horizontal or parallel to the floor.

5

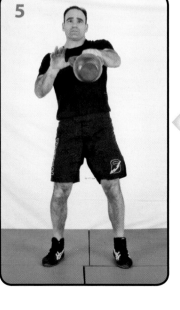

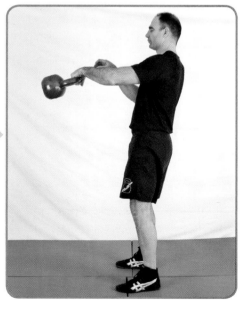

Left hand, palm facing down, goes over the top of your right to establish your grip.

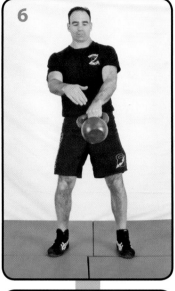

6

Allow gravity to take the kettlebell back down. Stay upright and well balanced as the kettlebell descends.

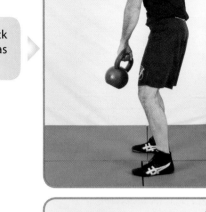

7

Just before your forearm crashes into your pelvic area, fold at the hips (i.e., sit back and down) and shift your weight to your heels.

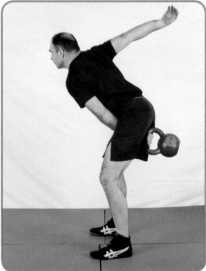

H2H Switch at Eye Level

1

As the kettlebell reaches the end of the back swing, press through your heels, extending your legs, hips, and back until you are in the upright position.

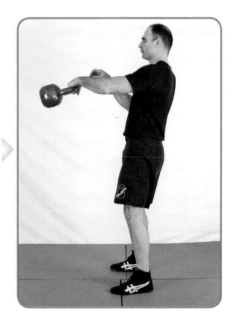

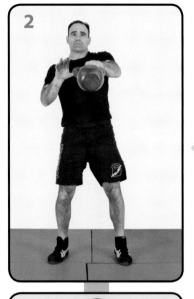

2

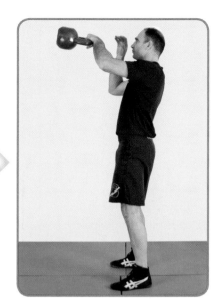

As the kettlebell reaches the top position, pull the kettlebell handle up and back at a 45-degree angle.

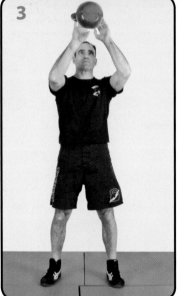

3

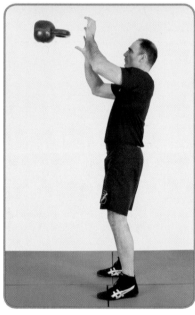

Keep your eye on the handle as you drag the fingers of your left hand off the kettlebell.

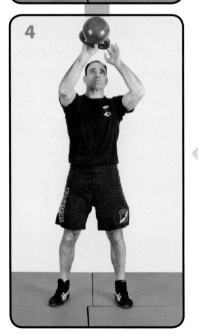

4

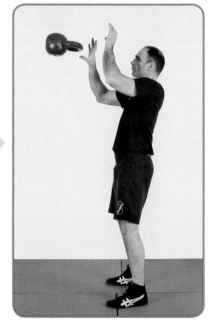

Reach out with your right hand to grab the handle.

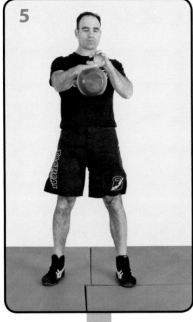

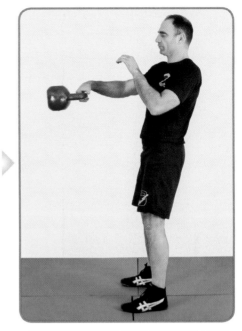

Establish your grip with your right hand.

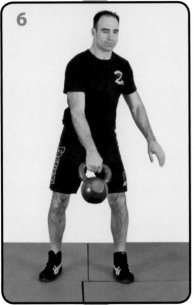

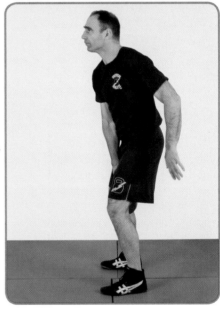

Allow gravity to take the kettle-bell back down. Stay upright and well balanced as the kettlebell descends.

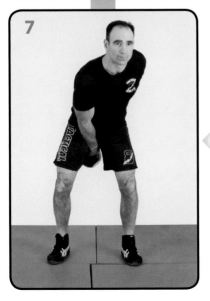

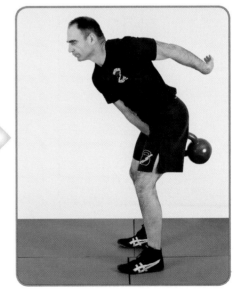

Follow the kettlebell into a good back swing position. Repeat for desired time or reps.

Swing Series

This exercise will really challenge your core and grip strength in a unique way. It will also improve your hand-to-eye coordination and hand speed. More importantly, it sets up the proper arm movement that will be used later when we learn the KB snatch.

Always remember, if something doesn't feel right when you let go of the kettlebell, just let it drop safely to the ground. We all drop it from time to time. It's really not a big deal. If the kettlebell gets too close to your face or body, simply push it away and step back. If the kettlebell moves too far away or rotates, just watch it hit the floor. Remember, quick feet are happy feet.

H2H Switch Rx

By now you are probably getting a little bit tired of the Tabata protocol. Here are a few options to mix things up.

Perform 4 rounds of 25 H2H switches (alternating hands each rep)
One-minute rest in between sets

Perform 1 round of 25 H2H switches
Perform 1 round of 25 half-rotation switches
Repeat above sequence 3 times
One-minute rest in between sequences

Perform 1 round of 25 H2H switches
Perform 1 round of 25 half-rotation switches
Perform 1 round of 25 two-arm swing releases
Repeat above sequence 3 times
One-minute rest in between sequences

Section 3
Turkish Get-Up Series

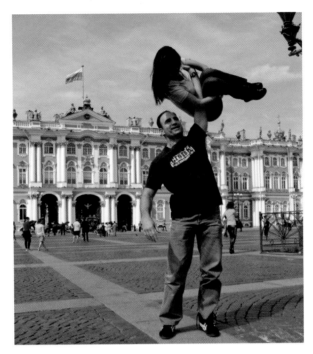

In the Turkish get-up series we will introduce to you some of the most effective methods for building strength, stability, and flexibility throughout the entire body. Over the last ten years, these exercises have especially proven themselves as excellent pre-habilitation and rehabilitation exercises for the shoulders. Through careful and diligent practice, all over-head exercises become safer and easier.

In this section, you will learn how to perform:

The correct methods of picking up/putting down one and two kettlebells while lying in the supine position, which is essential for shoulder safety.

One-arm floor press—assistance exercise for the arm bar stretch and TGU.

Double floor press—bench press substitute.

Arm bar stretch—builds exceptional shoulder strength, flexibility, and stability.

Turkish get-up—A true "no BS" total-body strength exercise.

"One of the brilliant things about the TGU movement is that it teaches external rotation stability of the shoulder joint through an enormous range of motion."

—Kelly Starrett

History

I first learned the movements for the arm bar stretch and TGU in December of 2000. It was part of the curriculum Pavel Tsatsouline taught us during a five-day custom course hosted at the New Mexico Law Enforcement Academy. We used light dumbbells because this was back in the pre-kettlebell days. It is significant to note that, at this point in time, I was seriously considering undergoing a third surgery on my right shoulder. For fifteen-years I experienced chronic shoulder subluxations/dislocations. I diligently practiced every rubber band exercise and rotator cuff program in the realm of physical therapy, but to no avail. My right shoulder was at the point where it would chronically dislocate in my sleep. Talk about a rude awakening!

Anyway, during one of the training sessions, Pavel told a story about the TGU being a staple exercise for old-time strongmen and wrestlers. He said it was one of the first exercises taught to aspiring weightlifters. Supposedly, no other exercises were taught or practiced until the pupil could perform the TGU with a 100-pound weight in either hand. I figured it was just weightlifting folklore, but the story caught my attention and motivated me to make the 100-pound TGU a personal goal. I ended up fabricating two homemade 105-pound kettlebells and a year or so later successfully performed singles with either hand. Now ten years later and by God's grace, I'm even stronger and still surgery free!

For the average healthy male, it may not seem like a big deal, but let me put it in perspective. The 1980s were a bad decade for my shoulders. During my senior year of high school, I dislocated my right shoulder playing football about once every game and twice during the championships. I was a starting offensive and defensive tackle, never missed a play and made All-State that year. My first shoulder surgery was performed in the winter of 1985. Two years and at least a dozen dislocations later, I earned a second surgery on the same shoulder, performed by the same doctor. It was fall of 1987. To my surprise, my surgeon decided at the last minute to perform the exact same procedure, called a Putti-Plat procedure. I wasn't surprised or thrilled when it produced the exact same unstable results! In the spring of 1989, I had a surgery on my left "good" shoulder after experiencing three dislocations. This time I chose a different doctor, who performed a different procedure called a Bankhart procedure. Other than limiting some ranges of motion, I never had another problem with that shoulder.

About a year and a half ago, an orthopedic surgeon participated in one of my kettlebell instructor courses. His specialty is fixing shoulders. Orthopedic surgeons come from all over the world to train under him to learn his technique. It was an awesome opportunity to clarify some nagging questions I had concerning my shoulders. My first question was about the difference between the Putti-Plat procedure performed on my right shoulder in '85/'87 versus the Bankhart procedure performed on my left in '89. His exact words were "They (i.e., orthopedic surgeons) stopped performing the Putti-Plat procedure in the late '80s." Why? "Because it did not work." He explained in detail while drawing pictures on the white board of how the Bankhart procedure anatomically anchors the shoulder into the socket and the Putti-Plat does not. The bottom line: there is nothing anatomically anchoring my right shoulder in the joint. The only thing holding my shoulder in the socket is the muscle that surrounds the joint. He confirmed that the exercises outlined in this chapter are the major contributing factors that enabled me to successfully rehabilitate and strengthen the integrity of my shoulders. He was impressed with the strength, stability, and flexibility I had developed in my shoulders. It's always nice to get confirmation from a reliable source! Knowing what I know today, I'm thoroughly convinced that I could have avoided all three surgeries.

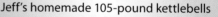
Jeff's homemade 105-pound kettlebells

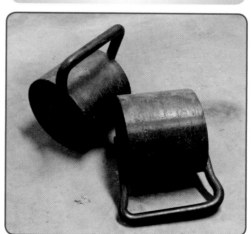

Safety

Safety is paramount when training. Closely follow, practice, and master all exercises as prescribed. Please keep in mind, our goal is to train, not maim our athletes or us. Carelessness and apathy are leading causes of training injuries. There's an old saying; "It's easy to be hard, but it's hard to be smart." Be proactive and pay attention to the details.

Hand Position

Brazilian jiu-jitsu instructors teach and preach "position before submission." In other words, you must establish a solid, advantageous position before securing the submission. Otherwise, your submission attempt will be blocked and quickly reversed. The same holds true with establishing the proper grip on the kettlebell. Every time you grip the kettlebell, make a conscious effort to establish the correct hand position. There's a common theme. The hand position you will learn for the one-arm floor press is identical to the hand position for the double floor press, arm bar stretch, TGU, rack position, military press, push press, and snatch. Learn it right the first time and you'll do it right the rest of your life.

1. Insert your hand, palms up into the kettlebell handle. If you get confused about which corner your hand needs to be in remember: the thumb points the way. Press the web of your hand (i.e., between thumb and forefinger) into the far corner of the handle.

2. Note: The handle should run diagonally across the low part of your hand and wrist, similar to establishing a false grip used on gymnastic rings for the muscle up.

3. Wrap your fingers and thumb around the handle, ensuring your wrist is straight.

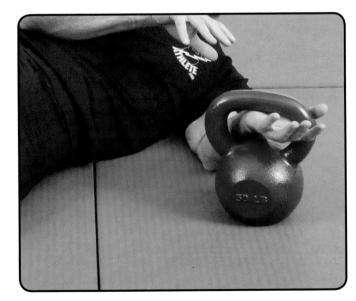 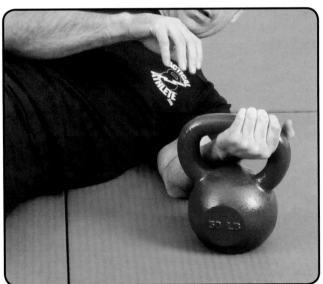

How to Pick Up One Kettlebell

As elementary as this may seem, picking up and placing the kettlebell down is where there is the greatest potential for shoulder injury. The following steps will dramatically reduce the potential for injury. Pay attention to the angle of the kettlebell in relation to the hip and shoulder.

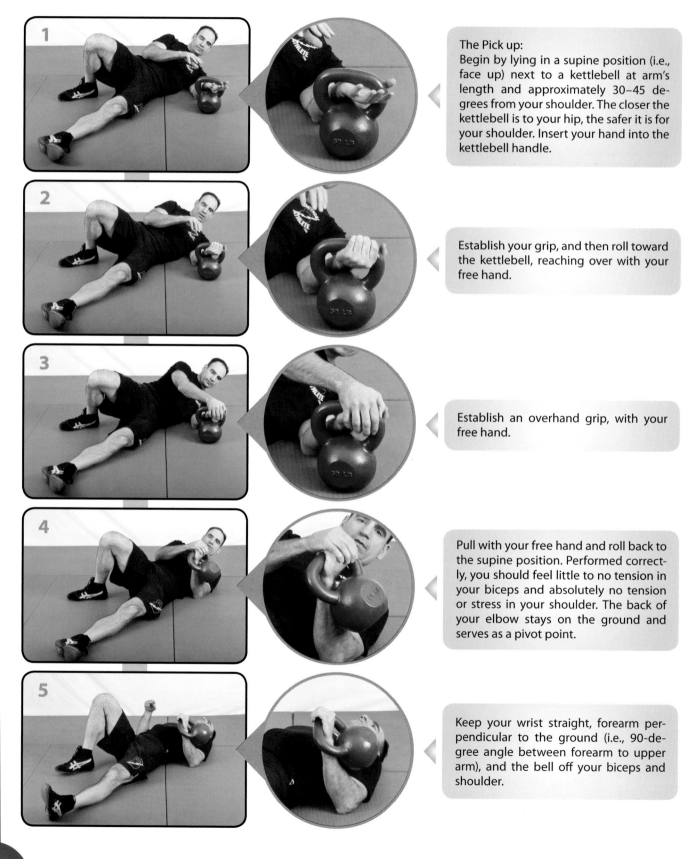

The Pick up:
Begin by lying in a supine position (i.e., face up) next to a kettlebell at arm's length and approximately 30–45 degrees from your shoulder. The closer the kettlebell is to your hip, the safer it is for your shoulder. Insert your hand into the kettlebell handle.

Establish your grip, and then roll toward the kettlebell, reaching over with your free hand.

Establish an overhand grip, with your free hand.

Pull with your free hand and roll back to the supine position. Performed correctly, you should feel little to no tension in your biceps and absolutely no tension or stress in your shoulder. The back of your elbow stays on the ground and serves as a pivot point.

Keep your wrist straight, forearm perpendicular to the ground (i.e., 90-degree angle between forearm to upper arm), and the bell off your biceps and shoulder.

How to Put Down One Kettlebell

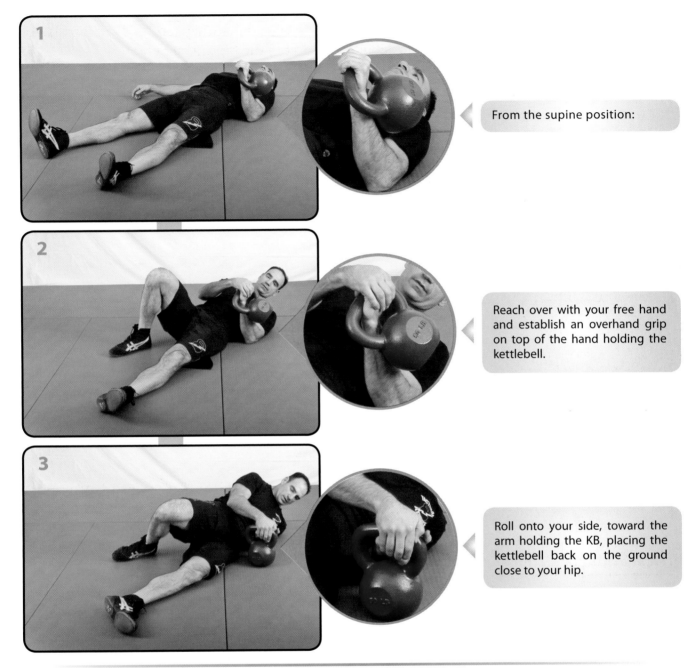

1

From the supine position:

2

Reach over with your free hand and establish an overhand grip on top of the hand holding the kettlebell.

3

Roll onto your side, toward the arm holding the KB, placing the kettlebell back on the ground close to your hip.

Get into the habit of **always** using two hands to pick up or put down the kettlebell when you are on the ground. This will protect your rotator cuff from potential injury. Never ever pick up the kettlebell like this! Safety violation!

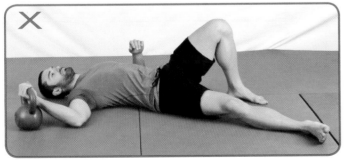

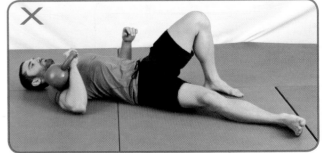

What's wrong with this picture?

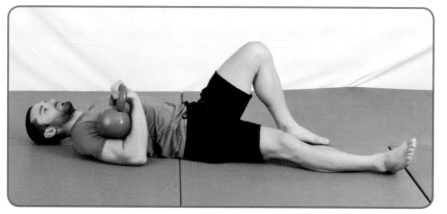
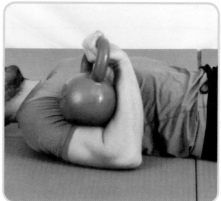

Answer: Wrong grip, bent wrist, and resting KB on his biceps/shoulder.

What's wrong with this picture?

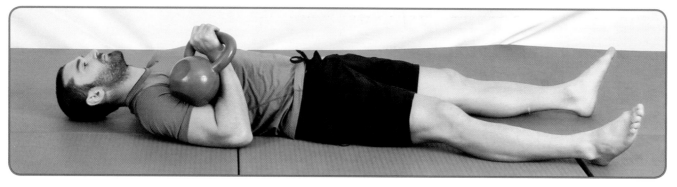

Answer: KB resting on biceps/shoulder.

Floor Press

Floor presses can be performed with one or two arms. The one-arm floor press puts the kettlebell in the correct starting position for the arm-bar stretch and TGU. The double floor press is a safe and effective way to teach the mechanics of the bench press.

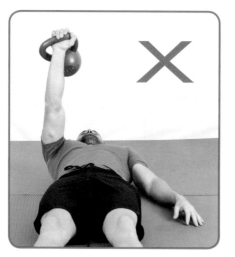
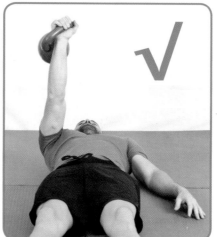

One-Arm Floor Press

The one-arm floor press establishes correct mechanics for pressing weight in the supine position and places the kettlebell in the correct starting position for the arm-bar stretch and TGU.

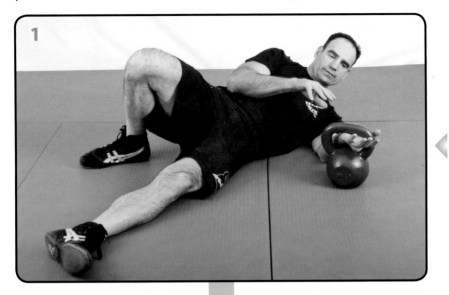

The pick up: Begin by lying in a supine position (i.e., face up) next to a kettlebell at arm's length and approximately 30–45 degrees from your shoulder. Insert your hand into the kettlebell handle.

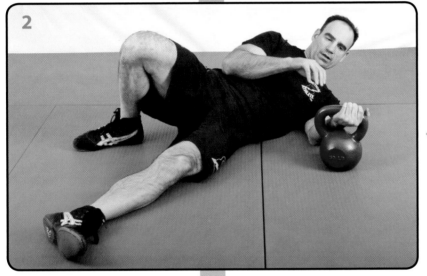

Establish your grip, and then roll toward the kettlebell, reaching over with your free hand.

Establish an overhand grip with your free hand.

Turkish Get-Up Series

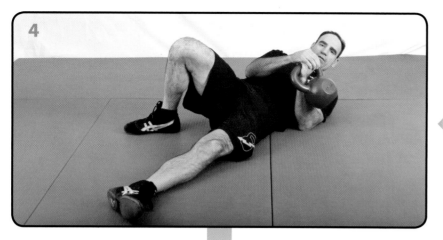

4

Pull with your free hand and roll back to the supine position.

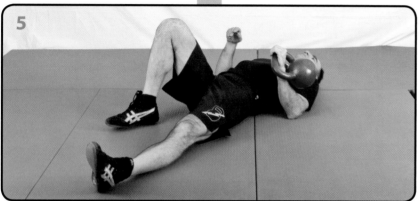

5

Keep your wrist straight, forearm perpendicular to the ground (i.e., a 90-degree angle between forearm and upper arm), and the bell off your biceps and shoulder.

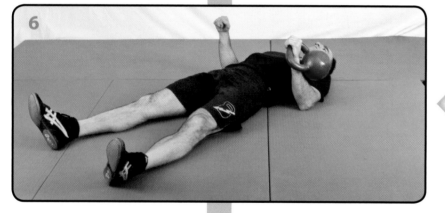

6

Before attempting to press—straighten your legs, pinch your shoulders back and down, lift your chest, and tighten your lat muscles

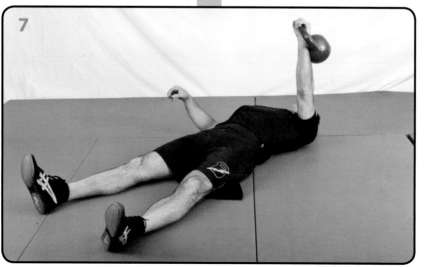

7

Press the kettlebell to arm's length. Note: The center of the kettlebell is directly over the center of my shoulder, wrist is straight, and hand is in neutral alignment (i.e., about a 45-degree angle). Do not allow the kettlebell to turn as you press up or down. Always maintain correct arm angle.

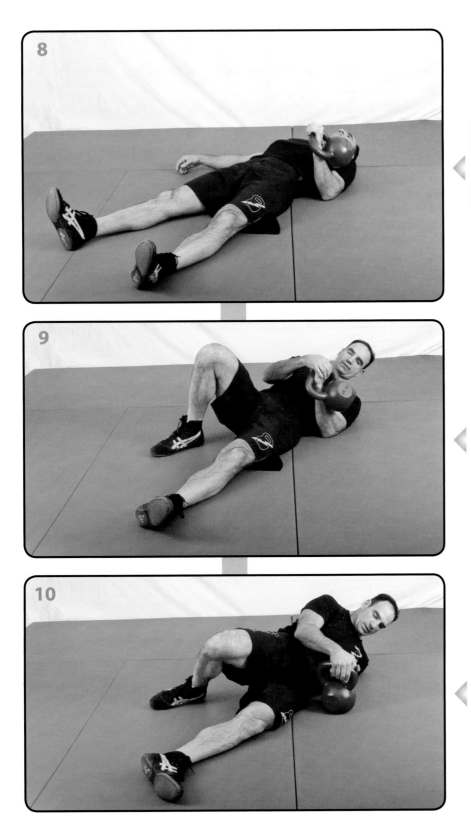

8

Actively pull your elbow to the ground by engaging your lats until you are back at the starting point. Be sure to keep your upper arm close to your torso. Repeat for desired number of reps.

9

After your last rep: Reach over with your free hand and establish an overhand grip on top of the hand holding the kettlebell.

10

Roll on your side, toward the arm holding the KB, placing the kettlebell back on the ground close to your hip.

Double Floor Press

Once you have mastered the one-KB floor press, then it's time to try the two-KB floor press. The exercise is performed exactly the same as you would with one KB. However, close attention must be paid to how you get the kettlebells into position. Practice a few reps of properly picking up and putting down the kettlebells until you feel comfortable with the following procedure.

Picking Up Two Kettlebells, Putting Down Two kettlebells

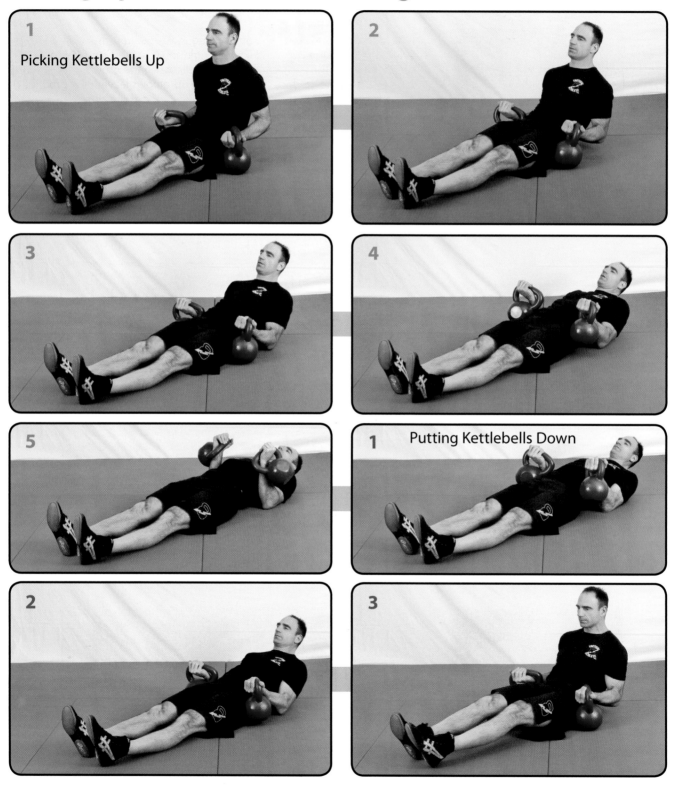

1 Picking Kettlebells Up

2

3

4

5

1 Putting Kettlebells Down

2

3

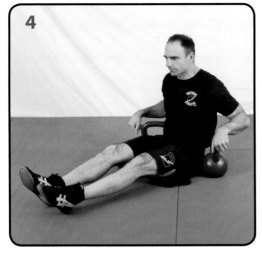

PICKING KETTLEBELLS UP

1–2) Sit between two KBs. Establish your grip on each KB, palms facing up, elbows tight against your sides. Visualize squeezing imaginary tennis balls in each armpit. 3) Sit back slowly until your elbows touch the floor. 4) Keep a 90-degree bend in your elbows and continue to lie backward until your upper back touches the floor. This action will lever the kettlebells up and off the ground. 5) As your shoulders touch the ground and your forearms become perpendicular to the floor, rotate the kettlebells so that your hands are at a 45-degree angle, palms facing away. Note: Wrists are straight, forearms vertical; bells are not touching your shoulders. This is the starting position for the double floor press.

PUTTING KETTLEBELLS DOWN

1) Rotate your hands until you are looking at your palms, maintain a 90-degree bend in your elbow, and slowly begin to sit up. 2) Continue to sit up. Keep elbows on the floor until the kettlebells touch the ground. 3) Once the kettlebell is on the ground, continue sitting up, elbows leaving the ground. 4) Release your grip as you come to the complete upright position.

The Double Floor Press

Follow the procedure above to establish the start position for the double floor press. Once in the start position:

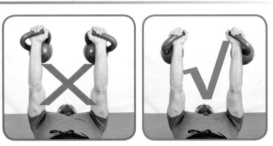

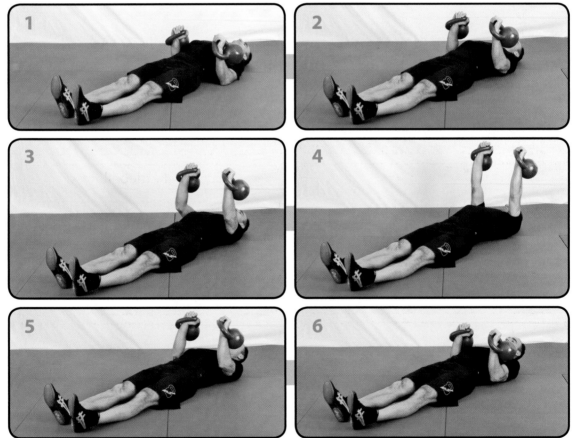

1) Open/lift your chest by pulling your shoulders back and down, activating the muscles of your upper back and lats. 2) Simultaneously, press the kettlebells to arm's length; keeping your shoulders back and down. 3) Maintain 45-degree hand angle as you press. 4) Continue to full extension. Kettlebells are directly over the shoulders, wrists are straight, and hand angle mimics the 10 and 2'oclock hand position on a steering wheel when driving a vehicle. 5) Pull your elbows down, engaging the lats and reversing arm movement. 6) Return to starting point. Note: Elbows stay tight against your sides. Repeat for desired number of reps. Properly and safely return the kettlebells to floor by following the "put down" procedures above.

Double Floor Press Variations:

- Press both KBs with feet spread apart
- Press both KBs with feet together
- Lock out one arm and press the other for reps, then lock out the other arm and press for reps. (SEE SEQUENCE 1)
- Seesaw press: Simultaneously pull one KB down and the other up. (SEE SEQUENCE 2)

SEQUENCE 1

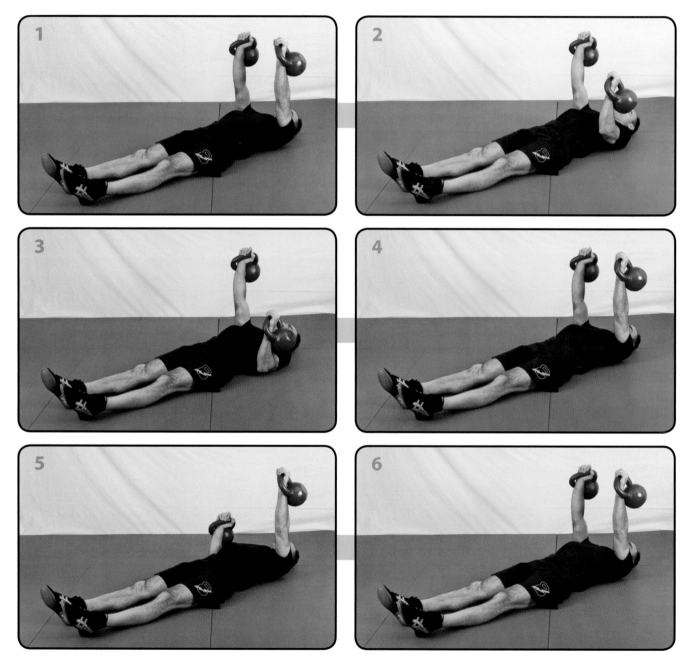

SEQUENCE 2

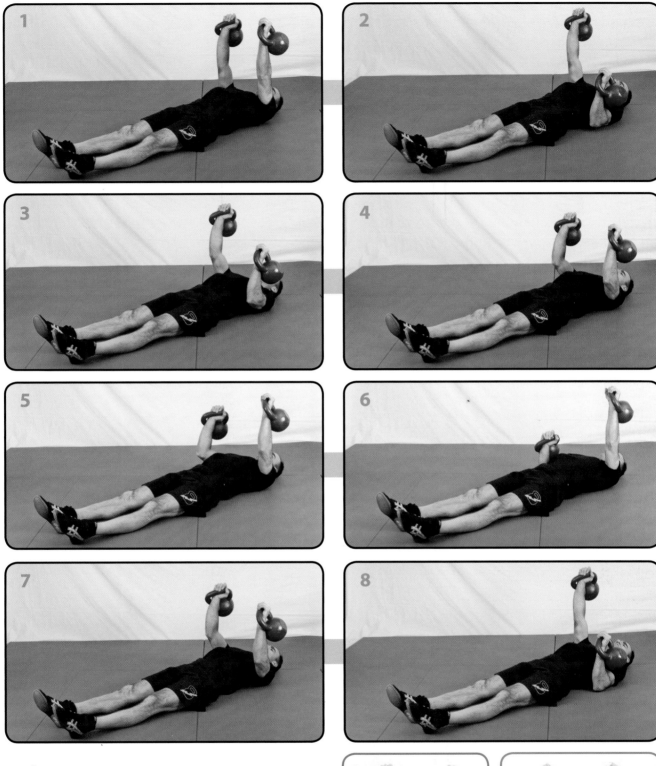

What's wrong with this picture?

Answer: Palms facing away, not angled.

Correct hand position

The Arm Bar Stretch

The arm bar stretch is one of the most effective shoulder rehabilitation and pre-habilitation exercises you can do. It's performed as a static hold. The arm bar stretch is actually more of a static hold strength exercise that effectively strengthens all the stabilizer muscles in the entire shoulder girdle. It does increase flexibility by actively stretching the pectoral muscles, which enhance the ability to maintain good posture. It can be practiced as a standalone exercise or in conjunction with the TGU. Every doctor and physical therapist I have trained immediately fell in love with this exercise and adopted it into their practice.

Begin with a light kettlebell (8 kg–16 kg). I prefer the kettlebell to the dumbbell for this exercise because of the benefit of the offset center of gravity of the bell resting on the back of the forearm. If you lack shoulder flexibility, the offset center of balance will aid your ability to keep your arm in the proper position. Please note that the kettlebell is always directly over the shoulder. Use a spotter and master the movement until you have complete control. Stick with the same size kettlebell until you are confident in your strength and ability to support increased loads.

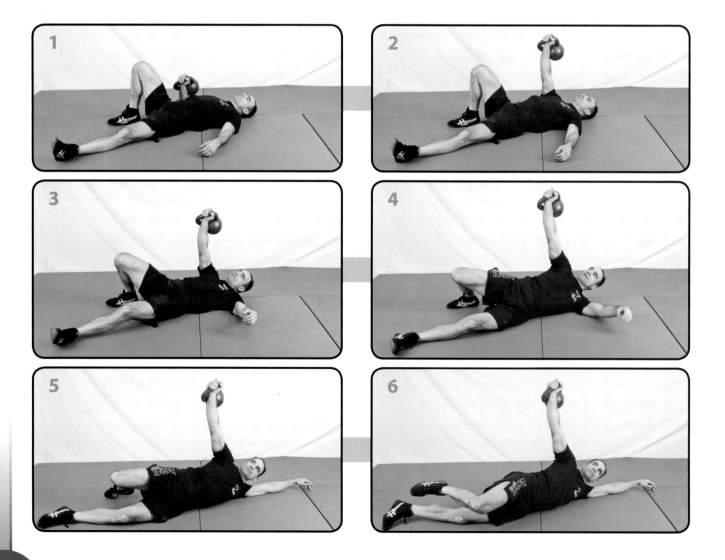

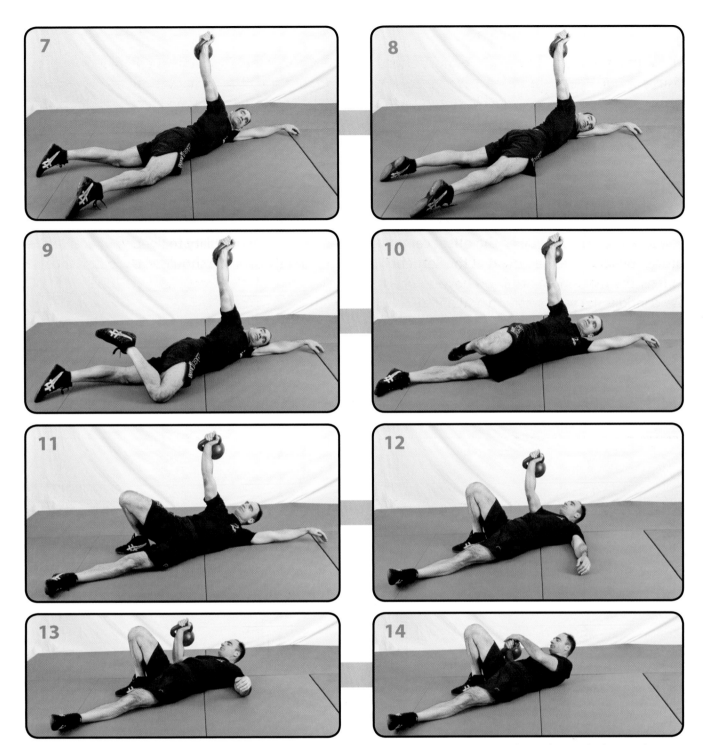

1) Safely pick up the kettlebell, bringing it to the start position, and then post your heel close to your buttocks (i.e., the foot on the same side as your working arm). 2) Press the kettlebell up in front of your chest to arm's length. If necessary, use your other arm to assist the lift or spot the weight. The goal is to get the kettlebell to the locked-out position. Once the elbow is straight, adjust the kettlebell to where it sits deep across the heel of your palm to take strain off your wrist. 3) Drive off your posted foot while keeping your eyes on the kettlebell. 4) Continue driving off your posted foot, slowly rolling over toward your opposite side. Note: your hip and shoulder should move as a unit, maintaining a neutral spine throughout the entire movement. 5) Retract the scapulae of the working arm directly toward your spine. Do not shrug your shoulder! Establish your balance and reposition your nonworking arm so that it's directly beneath your head. 6) Bring your working-side knee across your bottom leg, slowly rolling over. 7) Keep your working arm vertical, your eyes on the kettlebell, and straighten your legs. 8) Continue to flatten your hips and bring your chest toward the ground until you are nearly prone. If the side of your neck gets tired, rest the side of your head on the biceps of your bottom arm. Hold this position for 3–5 seconds. 9) To return to the supine position; bend your working-side knee and lift that foot up. 10) Pull your foot toward its starting position, rolling back onto your side. 11) Continue rolling onto your back, keeping your elbow straight. Repeat steps 1–11 for 3–5 reps, then 12) Pull your elbow down to the floor; keep it tight to your side. 13) Reach across with your free hand, then 14) Lower the kettlebell back to the ground, close to your hip. 15) Switch arms and repeat.

Tips

Active Shoulder Drill

The active shoulder drill is a kinesthetic awareness drill that will help the practitioner to understand how to engage the scapulae to stabilize the shoulder while performing the arm bar stretch. This is a two-part drill. If your training partner has a history of shoulder subluxations or dislocations, then proceed straight to step two, skipping step one.

Step One

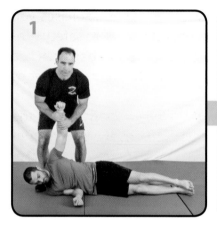

1) Have your training partner lie on his side. Grip his forearm below his wrist with both of your hands. Assume a good deadlift position, keeping a straight back, open chest, etc.

2) Straighten your legs by driving through your heels, lifting your partner up and off the ground. Hold for a second, and then slowly put him back on the ground.

Step Two

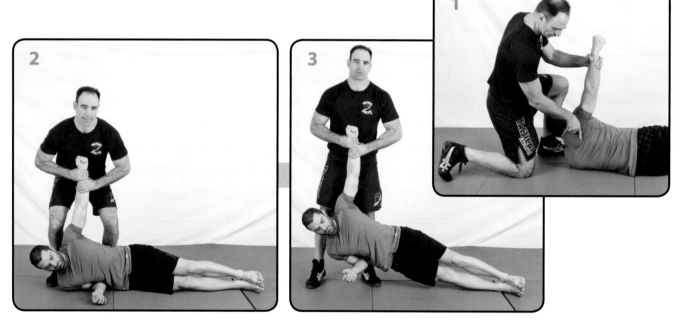
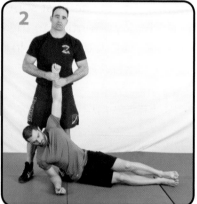

1) Have your training partner actively pull his scapulae straight in toward his spine. Do not shrug the shoulder! Pull it straight and hold.
2) Establish a strong grip on his forearm, below his wrist, and a strong deadlift position.
3) Straighten your legs by driving through your heels, lifting your partner up and off the ground. Hold for a second, and then slowly put him back on the ground. Note: Your training partner will feel noticeably heavier during this lift as compared to step one. That is not the point of the exercise, just a "heads-up." It's the activation of the muscles of the upper back that is important. Repeat step one and step two for the other arm.

Application:

Immediately practice a couple reps of the arm bar stretch with a kettlebell. Be sure to "activate" the muscles of the upper back as you roll to your side and establish your balance, before you bring your top leg over. You should notice that the kettlebell is more stable and that you'll gain more range of motion.

Spotting: You Can't Spot with Your Eyes!

The arm bar stretch, properly implemented, is one of the best shoulder rehabilitation exercises you can do. However, it can cause injury if you don't pay attention to the details and adhere to safety procedures. A good training partner will make or break you, literally. In the case of the arm bar stretch, a spotter is required. The spotter facilitates learning and maximizes safety while the trainee develops spatial awareness, strength, and coordination.

Be a good spotter. Understand that you are in a position of trust and are fully responsible for the safety of your training partner. Constantly assess the situation and anticipate potential problems. Ensure you are always in the right place at the right time in case something goes wrong. Coach Tucker says it best: "You can't spot with your eyes!" You must physically be in position to go hands-on and save the lift and assist your training partner. He's counting on you! Understand, whenever you are out of position physically or mentally, you've changed your role from that of a spotter to a witness.

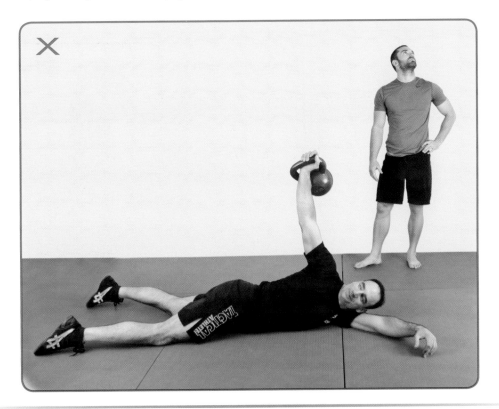

How to Spot/Coach the Arm Bar Stretch

Ensure that your training partner keeps his elbow locked straight throughout the entire movement. If the elbow is straight, any loss of control or balance will be in the lateral plane (i.e., left/right).

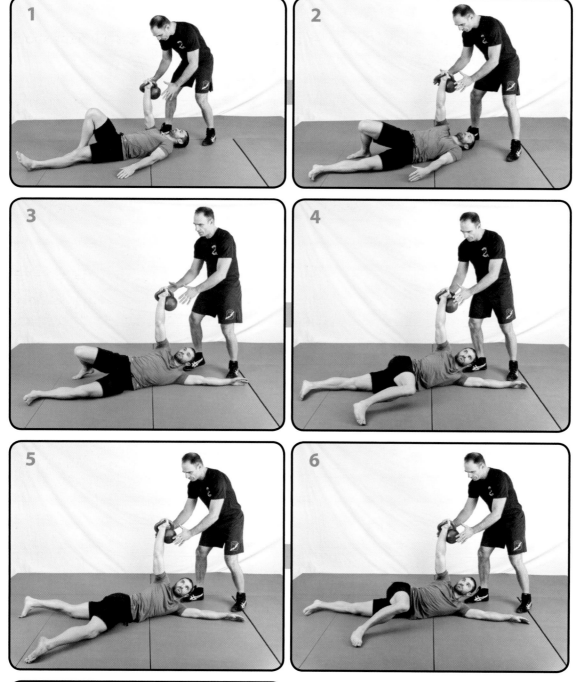

1) Position yourself directly in line with the arm holding the kettlebell. Check for proper grip, straight wrist, straight elbow, and weight being directly over his shoulder. Your hands should be on either side of the KB but not touching the bell.

2–5) Take a small side step as he rolls to his side. Ensure he is driving off the heel, maintains a neutral spine, and his arm stays perpendicular.

6–7) Continue following the KB back to the start position.

- Keep your reps low (i.e., 3–5). Train as heavy as possible but stay as fresh as possible.
- If for some reason you get distracted and begin to lose control or balance of the kettlebell, avoid the temptation to try to save it. Keeping your arm straight, rotate your torso quickly in the direction the kettlebell wants to go and guide it into a controlled crash on the floor. Don't try to fight it. The kettlebell will always win.

What's wrong with this sequence?

Answer: Not driving off posted leg. By throwing the leg across, the hip moves first, leaving the shoulder behind, causing torque on the spine.

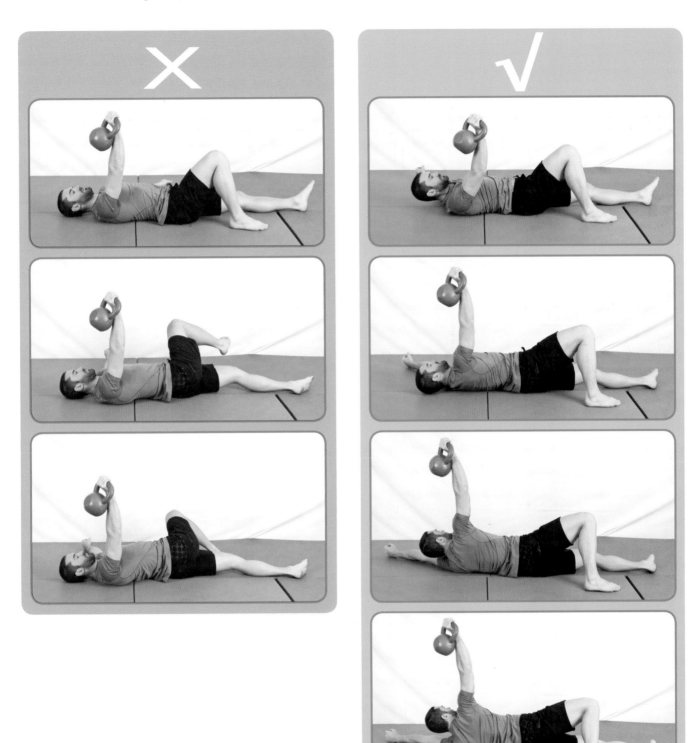

What's wrong with this finish position?

Answer: **Knee bent, hips not flat.**

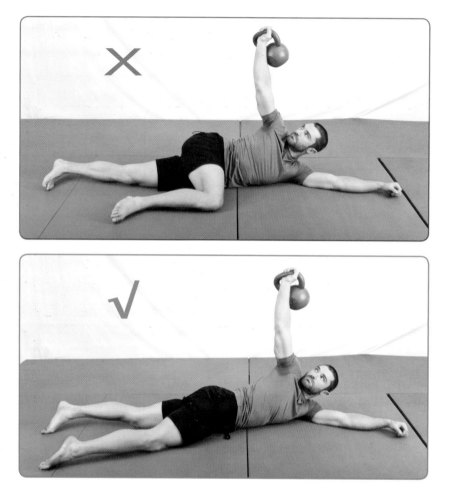

Rx:

Arm bar stretches can be performed for time or reps, but never ever get close to muscle failure. Here are a variety of ways to incorporate this exercise into your current training regime.

Warm up:

· Add one set of arm bar stretches, 3–5 reps per arm, holding the stretch for 3–5 seconds, as part of your warm-up routine (light-medium weight).

Cool down:

· Add one set of arm bar stretches, 3–5 reps per arm, holding the stretch for 3–5 seconds, as part of your cool-down routine (light-medium weight).

Strength:

· Perform 3–5 sets of 1–2 reps per arm (heavy weight).

Static hold:

· Perform 1–3 sets of 1 rep, static hold for 15–60 seconds.

The Turkish Get-Up

There are many ways to perform the TGU. The variation I will share with you is the one that's simple, easy to learn, and has tremendous carryover to any sport or profession. I sometimes refer to it as the tactical TGU because it mimics the tactical way of getting back to your feet if you were knocked down during a fight. This skill is even more important when you find yourself in full kit and level-IV body armor.

To keep it simple, I will teach the tactical TGU in three distinct parts: the sit-up, the transition, and the stand-up. Actively spot and coach each other through each phase. Note: Not all three parts need to be taught or practiced in one training session. Master one part at a time before moving on to the next.

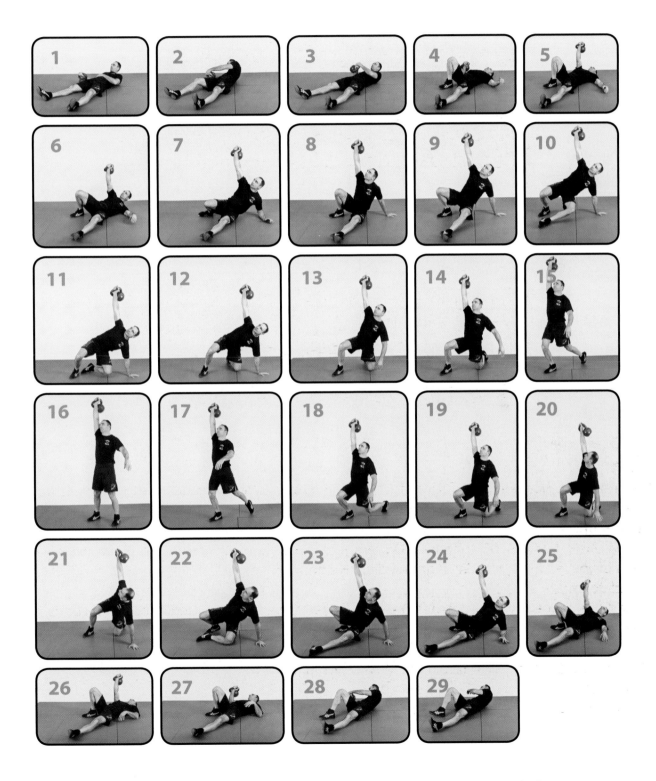

TGU Part 1: The Sit-Up

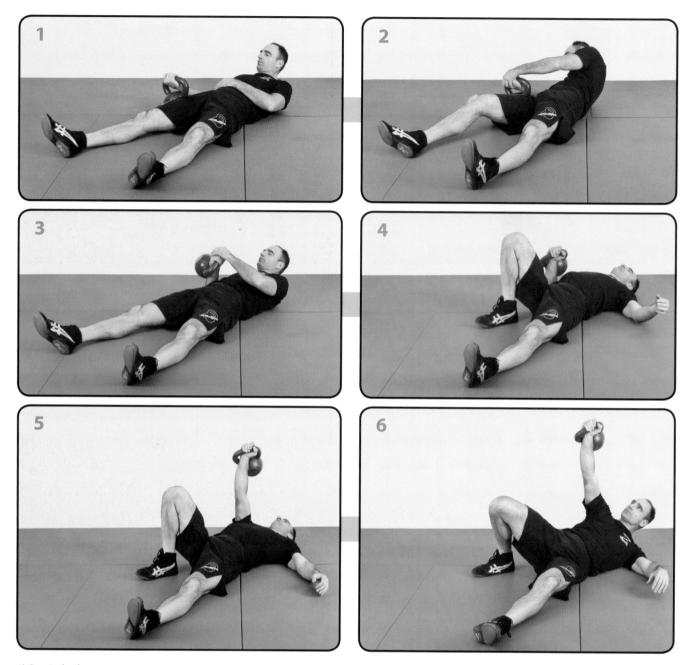

1) Begin by lying in a supine position (i.e., face up) with a kettlebell next to your right hip. Insert your right hand into the kettlebell handle, palm up. Press the web of your hand into the far corner of the handle. Note: The handle should run diagonally across the low part of your hand and wrist, similar to establishing a false grip used on gymnastic rings for the muscle-up. Wrap your fingers and thumb around the handle, ensuring your wrist is straight.

2) Roll toward the kettlebell, reaching over with your free (left) hand placing your palm over the knuckles of the working hand.

3) Pull with your left hand and roll back to the supine position. Keep your wrist straight and forearm perpendicular (i.e., 90-degree angle between forearm and upper arm). Do not allow the KB to rest on your biceps or shoulder.

4) Release your left hand and then post your right foot. The heel must be close to your glutes, but for maximum leverage, the heel must be placed slightly to the outside.

5) Open your chest by pulling your shoulders back and down, then Press the kettlebell to arm's length. Note: The center of the kettlebell is directly over the center of my shoulder, wrist is straight, and hand is in neutral alignment (i.e., about 45-degree angle). Do not allow the kettlebell to turn as you press up or down. Position your free arm at about a 45-degree angle from your hip.

6) Use the knuckle of the thumb gripping the kettlebell as a sight. Pick a spot on the ceiling and keep your gaze fixed there, then sit up by driving off your posted right foot, shifting your weight toward your left (free side) elbow.

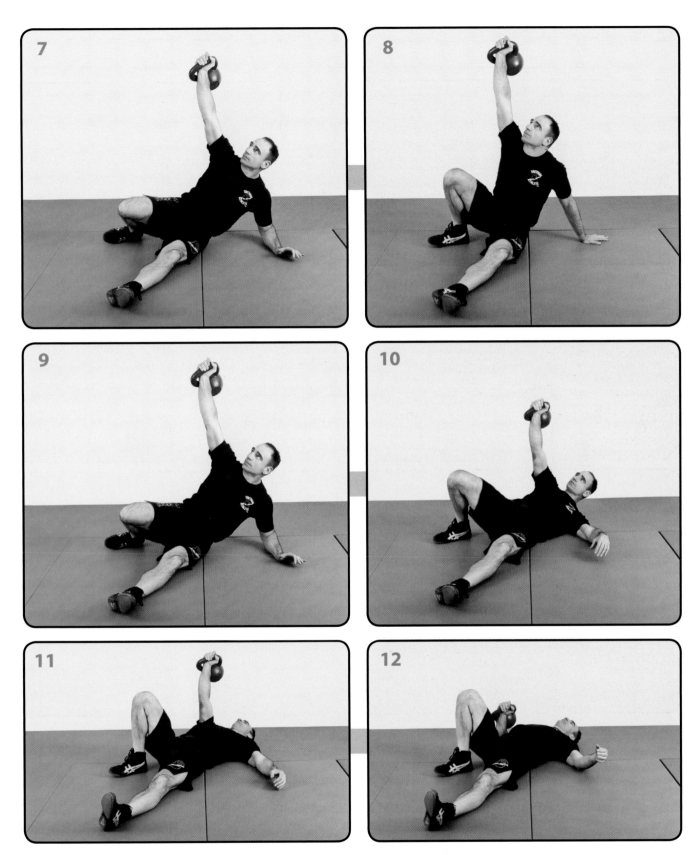

7) Continue pressing through your heel, sitting up, while transferring your weight from your elbow to your forearm.

8) Sit all the way up until your torso is near vertical. The right knee is fully flexed and vertical. Your eyes are on the KB and your left hand is about 45 degrees behind you hip.

9–12) Reverse and retrace the movements in a slow and controlled manner back to the supine position. Note: Be sure to keep working arm locked straight as you descend back to the starting position. Repeat for 3–5 reps for both sides.

✕ Common Error:

Foot Comes Off Ground

It is common for the foot of the extended leg to come off the ground as you try to sit up. Most people hit a sticking point where the leg comes up and then they use it as a pendulum to propel their upper body to the sitting position. Although this is a way to sit up, it's not the preferred way.

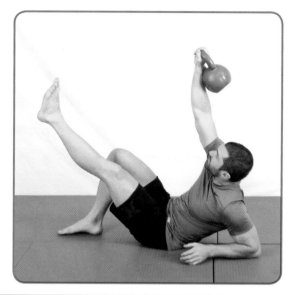

√ Corrective Action:

The reason the foot comes off the ground is because there is a lack of core activation. This is easily fixed by "actively exhaling" as you sit up. Try the following breathing exercise:

Standing Crunch Drill

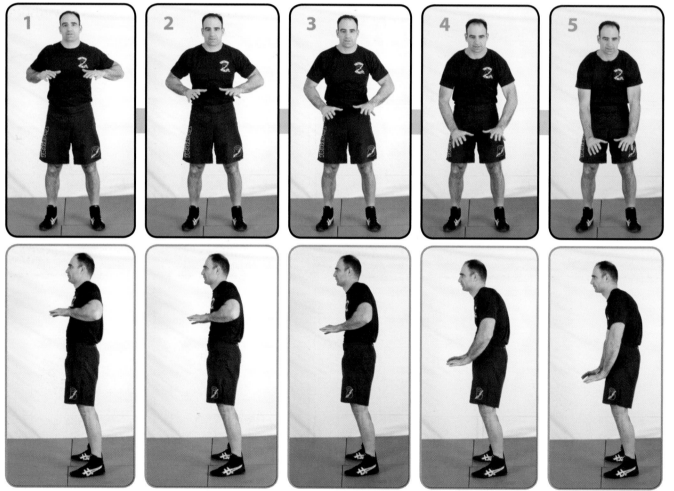

1) Stand upright with your feet between hip and shoulder width apart and your hands at chest level, palms facing down.
2) Inhale deeply through your nose, tighten the muscles of your pelvic floor, and then begin to exhale a thin stream of air out through your clenched teeth, tightening your entire midsection.
3) As you exhale, push your hands downward, creating dynamic tension throughout your body.
4) Continue to exhale, pushing your hands downward and shortening your abs, as if you were performing a "crunch."
5) Simultaneously your arms should reach full extension, your midsection maximally contracts, and you run out of air to exhale. At this point, your abdominals should be near cramping. If they do cramp, just ignore it; it will eventually go away.

Application: TGU Sit-Up:

· Follow steps 1–5 for the TGU Sit-up.
· Before you attempt to sit up, take a second; inhale, tighten your abs, and begin to exhale through your teeth; then slowly sit up, matching your breath with the movement.
· Note: You should feel a strong contraction across your abdomen as you sit up and the foot that was popping up in the previous set should now feel like it's glued to the ground.
· Alternate sets between the standing crunch drill and TGU sit-up.

Turkish Get-Up Rx:

Strength: 3–5 sets of 1–5 reps per side (medium-heavy weight).

TGU Part 2: Transition to Kneeling

It is critical to smoothly transition to and from the kneeling position when holding a kettlebell overhead. Study the sequence below to get the right idea of what's happening. However, be sure to practice a few reps without the kettlebell first. Some folks will find this challenging enough even without the weight. Don't rush the results. You want consistency before intensity.

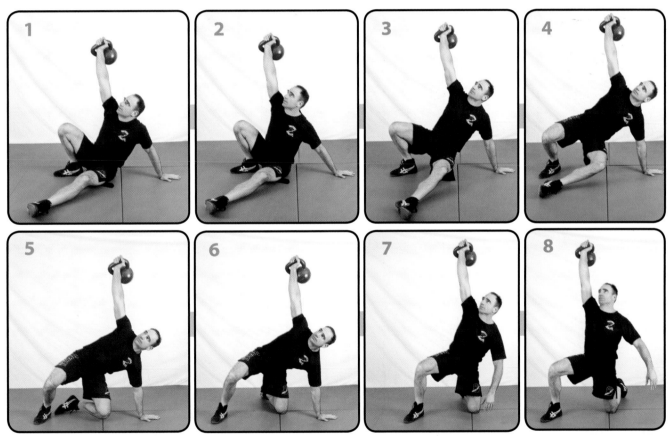

1) It is common to relax the tension in the lats and shoulder of the posted hand when pausing in the sitting position. This puts the shoulder closer to the ear, which is not optimal for performance or safety. 2) Begin by pressing the shoulder of your support hand (the hand that is on the ground) away from your ear. This is an important but often overlooked step. It puts your shoulder in a strong position. It keeps the shoulder "active," as when you are performing dips on parallel bars. 3) Simultaneously press off your hand and your posted foot, lifting your hips off the floor. 4) This will create the space necessary to bring your left leg underneath you. 5) Continue pulling your bottom leg through until your knee is directly beneath your hip. 6) Note the finish position of the knee and how it relates to your posted hand. 7) Begin to straighten your torso. 8) Once your torso is completely upright, ensure that your right foot is directly under your knee, your shin is near vertical, your shoulder is "active" near the ear, and your hand position is at a 45-degree angle.

TGU: Kneeling to Supine

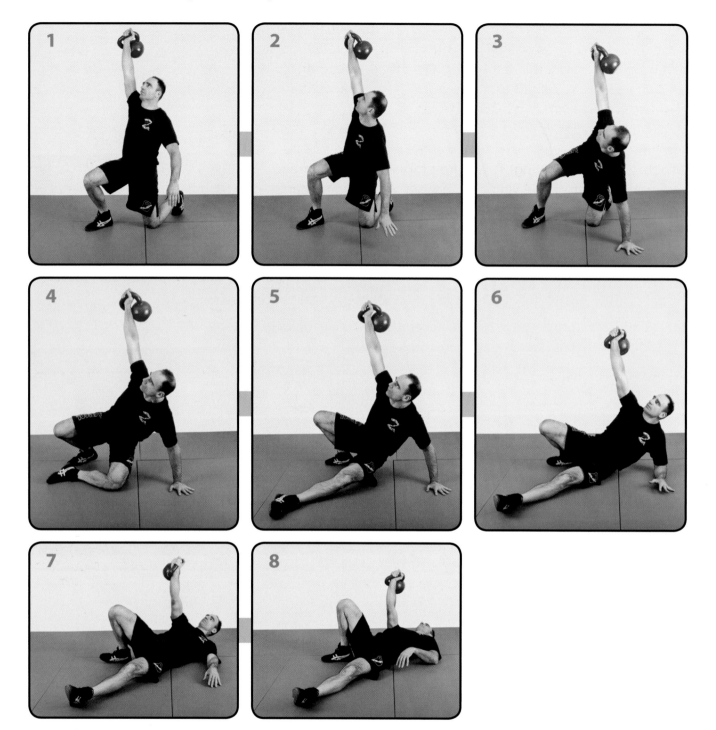

1) From the kneeling position:
2) Slightly rotate your torso in a clockwise direction. Note: Remember the "thumb points the way." In other words, the thumb of your free hand points toward the direction you should rotate your upper body (i.e., toward the instep of the posted foot).
3) Continue folding your hip backward and place your free hand 45 degrees off the corner of your knee. This is an extremely strong and stable position to attain.
4) Pressing off your posted hand and foot, slide your bottom leg through; keep your shin in light contact with the ground all the way through the movement.
5) Continue sliding through until your bottom leg is fully extended and corresponding glute is in full contact with the ground.
6) Slowly lower yourself back to your forearm.
7) Lower yourself down to your side.
8) Keep lowering yourself until you are lying flat on your back.

✕ Common Error: Reaching Back

Reaching back is, by far, the most common error when transitioning from the kneeling position. It is also potentially the most dangerous because it puts you in a mechanically disadvantaged position. It is interesting that under stress, this is what most people default to. I liken it to the natural reaction of outstretching a stiff arm behind you when you suddenly slip or fall backward, resulting in a broken wrist or separated shoulder. Although this reflex is natural, we can reprogram a better response through training. To ensure proper hand placement and movement from the very first rep, get your training partner and practice the "dry fire drill" below.

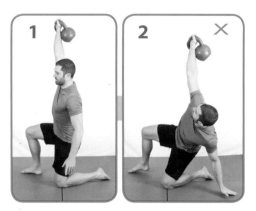

√ Corrective Action: Dry Fire Drill

I cannot overemphasize the importance of this exercise. People need to be physically manipulated into the correct position for reps to establish correct movement patterns.

From the kneeling position:

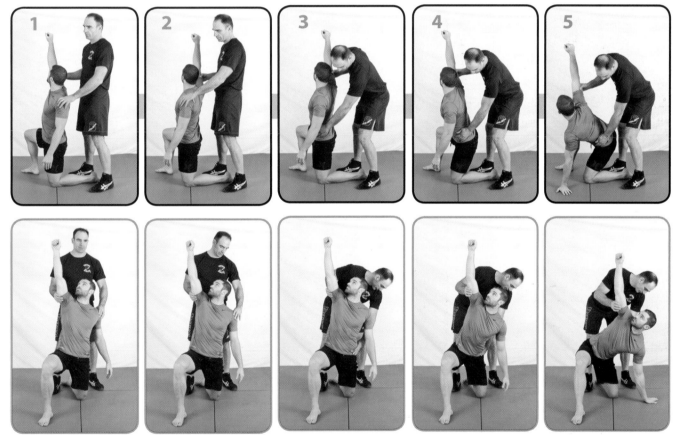

1) Place your hands on your training partner's shoulders.
2) Physically rotate his shoulders so that his free arm moves forward and toward the instep of his posted foot.
3) Move your left hand from his shoulder to the front of his hip.
4) Pull his hip straight back toward his heel, keeping his free arm completely relaxed.
5) Continue pulling his hip backward until his free hand lands on the floor, approximately 45 degrees off the outside corner of his knee. Assist your partner back to the kneeling position and repeat steps 1–5 for 5 repetitions for each side.

Application: TGU to the Kneeling Position

Be a good spotter/coach to your training partner as he practices the sit-up, the transition to kneeling, then back to the sitting then supine position. Repeat for 3–5 repetitions per side.

TGU Part 3: Transition to Standing

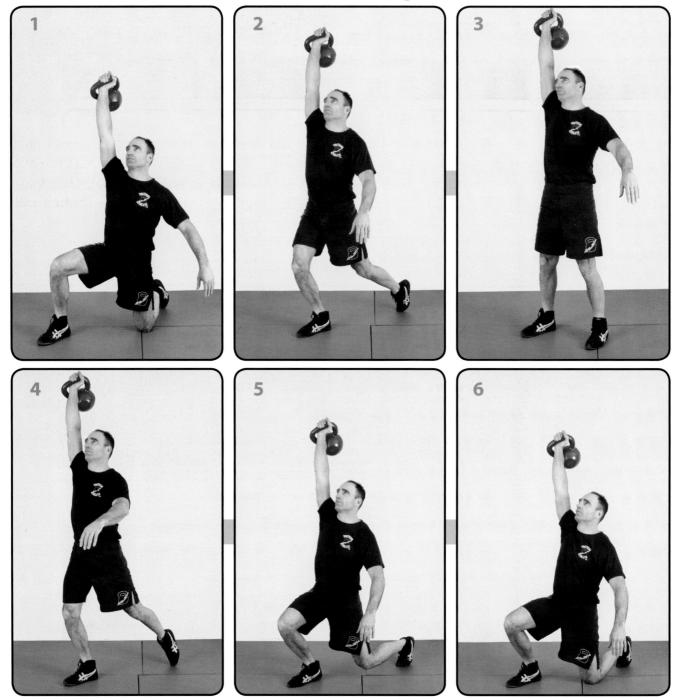

1) From the kneeling position, shift your gaze from looking up to out, keeping a neutral neck position. Make sure your foot is directly beneath your knee.
2) Keeping your right shin vertical, load your weight onto your heel, contract your outside glute, and stand up.
3) Complete the top position by stepping up with your back leg. Congratulations! You just successfully completed the first half of the tactical TGU. Pause for a moment; gather your thoughts and breathe.
4) Now it's time to carefully reverse the steps to lower yourself to the floor and back into the starting position. Shift your weight to the foot under the kettlebell and step backward with your free leg. Pretend your feet are on railroad tracks, not a tight rope, when you step back.
5–6) Lower yourself to the kneeling position. Repeat for 3–5 reps per side.

Caution:

Stay tight, move slowly, keep your elbow locked, and remain focused on the kettlebell. This is especially important when transitioning from standing to kneeling, kneeling to sitting, and sitting to supine. The combination of a bent elbow, a little momentum, and the sudden jolt could cause the kettlebell to come crashing down. Take your time, and be smooth.

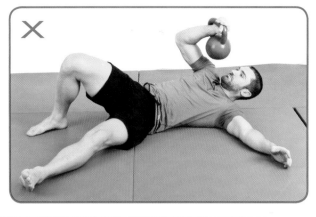

✗ Common Error for Women:

There is one common error I see predominately with women. When transitioning from sitting to kneeling or from kneeling to sitting their foot will get stuck. Compare these photos and note the bottom knee and shin angles. Women have a natural tendency to keep their knees closer together. Make a conscious effort to open the hip angle and keep the entire length of your shin in close contact with the ground.

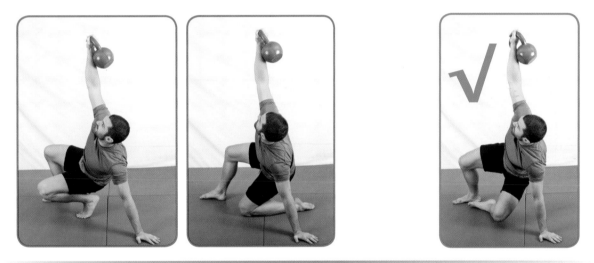

Pop Quiz: What's wrong with these pictures?

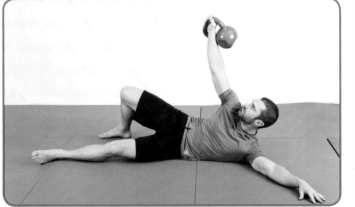
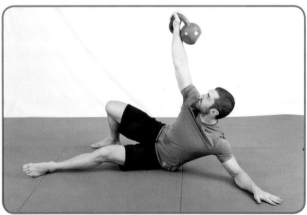

Answer: Bottom arm position is not 45 degrees off the hip. Glenn's being a "big fat cheater" because he's keeping his bottom arm on the mat, making it way easier to sit up.

Pop Quiz: What's wrong with these pictures?

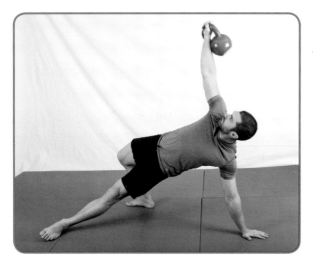

Answer:
Inefficient. Hip extended too high prior to pulling the bottom leg through. Waste of motion.

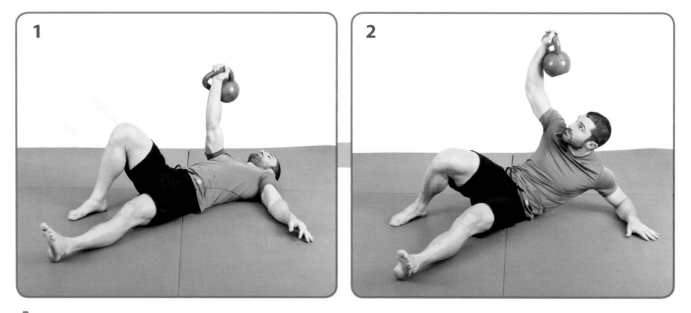

Answer: Hand rotates during sit-up causing the elbow to unlock and weight to crash.

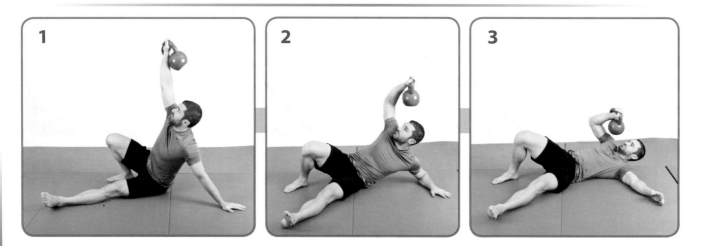

Answer: Allows hand to rotate while moving from the sitting to supine. Rotation causes elbow to unlock and the bell to crash.

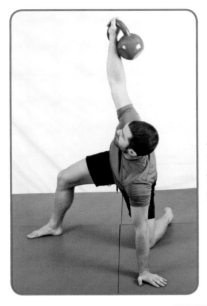

Answer:

Slight over-rotation, hand is in front of knee. The hand is also too far from the knee. This happens when the hips don't move rearward, controlling the descent.

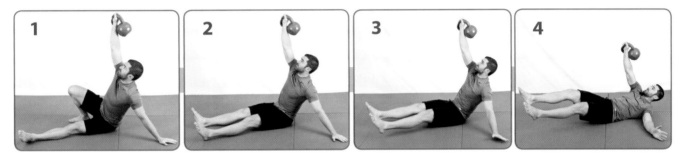

Answer:

Not keeping foot posted. Don't do a reverse sit-up!

Rx for Success:

- Keep your reps low—3–5 with moderate weight, say, or singles with heavy weight. This exercise is best practiced in parts or with a spotter until all the motions are mastered.
- My favorite way to practice the tactical TGU, especially when I'm short on time, is to set a timer for 10 minutes and perform singles (i.e., 1 rep consists of once up and once down), alternating sides after every rep. I've found this to be a safe and productive way to train tactical TGUs.

Mastering the TGU is an excellent investment of your time and effort. My personal success story has been repeated many times with the clients I train. Boxers, grapplers, no-holds-barred fighters, police officers, military personnel, and the average "Joe" or "Jane" all have reaped the benefits of the TGU. Whether you have a history of shoulder problems or are trying to prevent them, please heed my advice: Just say "no" to the bench press and "Hello" to the TGU.

TGU: Kettlebell Substitutions

Common Question: Can I TGU something other than a kettlebell?

Answer: Yes, you can. However, just because you can do something doesn't me you always should!

Implement variations

Let's explore a few alternatives for when kettlebells aren't readily available. If you travel a lot, there is a chance you may find yourself one day without your kettlebell (Oh no!). If this happens, do not fear. With a little imagination, you can adapt and overcome. TGUs are beneficial regardless of the implement you practice with. 1) Dumbbells are economical and plentiful, and they will work in a pinch. Unfortunately, a dumbbell doesn't have the benefit of an offset center of gravity, but it's better than doing nothing. 2) Short, thick-handled barbells and 3) full-sized Olympic barbells also lack the offset center of gravity but make up for it by the requirement of having to balance the longer and/or thicker bar. Be careful that the barbell doesn't twirl in your hand, stressing your shoulder or eventually unlocking your elbow. (Old-time strongman and stunt man Joe Bonomo demonstrates the use of the barbell for this exercise in his classic book *Barbell Training Routines*.) 4) Sandbags and 5) rucksacks are great options, especially in austere training environments. They both have an offset center of gravity, which strengthens and stretches the shoulder throughout the entire exercise. Whatever you "get up" with, be sure to keep your wrist straight.

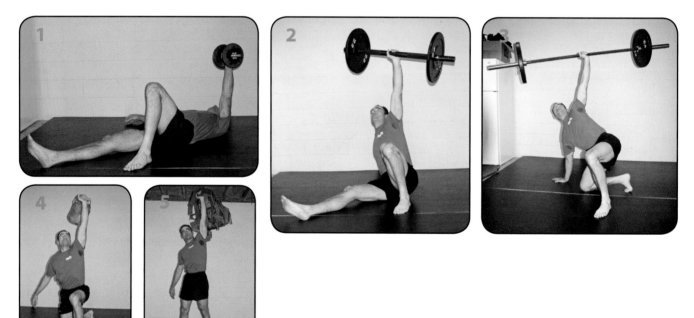

Lifting People

Several years ago, a friend photocopied and mailed me an article written by Sigmund Klein, an old-school strongman and hand balancer. In the article Sigmund demonstrated various people lifts he performed during his exhibitions. One lift caught my eye. He clean and jerked a person who was balled up. It looked achievable, but I needed a volunteer to try it out on. I was outside training at the time when my two little volunteers ran past me. My kids were about seven and nine at the time. I chose my daughter even though she was older and a few pounds heavier than my son. Kristina always felt lighter because she would naturally cling on to you, whenever you picked her up, like a little koala bear. Michael, on the other hand, always felt like a sack of potatoes, no assistance whatsoever.

I quickly briefed Kristina on what to expect then tried the C&J. The lift was successful, but I tweaked my shoulder a little. That was a bit disappointing. I studied the pictures some more, and then I realized that I could use the same setup for the TGU. I gave Kristina a second briefing, emphasizing the importance of staying calm and not panicking when she reached the top position. I calmly explained the consequences if she panicked: (1) it would probably dislocate Dad's shoulder (2) that would result in her rapidly impacting the ground and (3) worst of all . . . Mom will be mad when she finds out! Understanding that nothing good will come from panicking, Kristina did a great job staying calm and remained curled a tight little ball. The lift was easy and fun.

For years I practiced TGUs with my kids, since they weighed only sixty pounds. My strength gains kept up with their weight gains pretty well up until their mid- to late teens. My wife is now the littlest person in the house and serves as a good warm-up. My son's so big now it won't be long before he starts lifting me!

Before you go out and attempt to lift children overhead, I strongly recommend that you consider the following:

- Completely master the movements of the TGU. Your technique must be flawless.
- Develop a reserve of strength, by lifting heavy inanimate objects (KBs, DBs, BBs, sandbags, etc.) above the weight of the person you plan to lift.
- Don't lift nervous, weak, or injured people.
- Always use a spotter.
- Don't attempt any lifts under the influence of drugs or alcohol!

Detail Analysis of the Human TGU

People never seem to get tired of a live demonstration of the human TGU. Regardless if I say "don't try this at home," guys don't listen. If you're going to do it anyway, you might as well learn how to do it right.

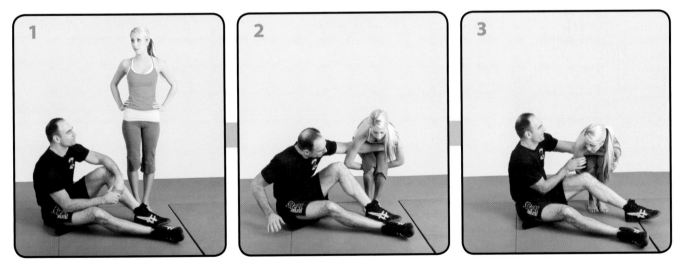

1) Sit on the floor and have your lifting partner stand next to you, feet together, on the side of your working arm.
2) Have your partner bend at the waist and put her forearms under her knees, lightly gripping her wrists. Insert your hand, thumb up, between the upper arm and chest, securing your grip on the far arm, above the biceps and close to the armpit.
3) Your partner now prepares to be lifted by further crossing her arms under her legs until she securely grips her elbows with her hands. As your partner tightens up, place the palm of your free hand on her elbow closest to you.

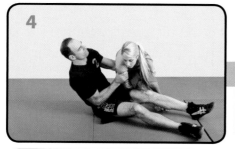

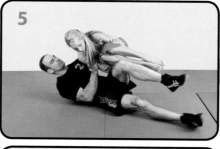

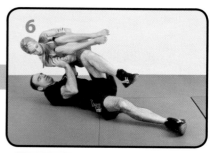

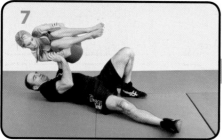

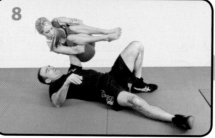

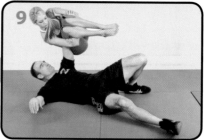

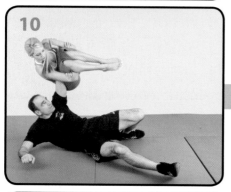

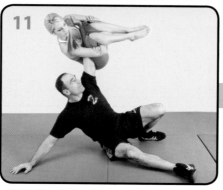

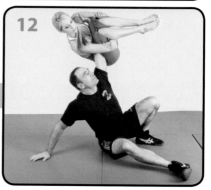

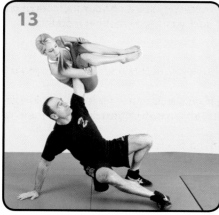

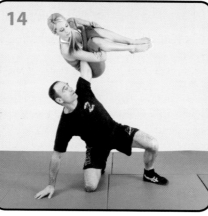

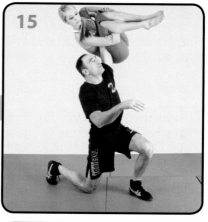

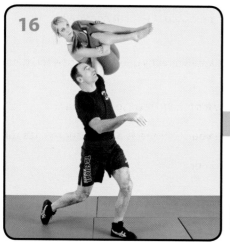

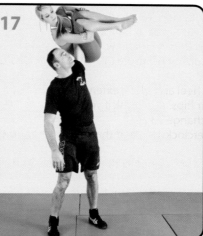

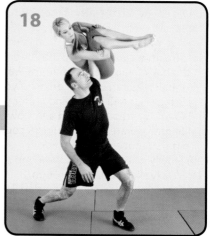

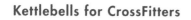

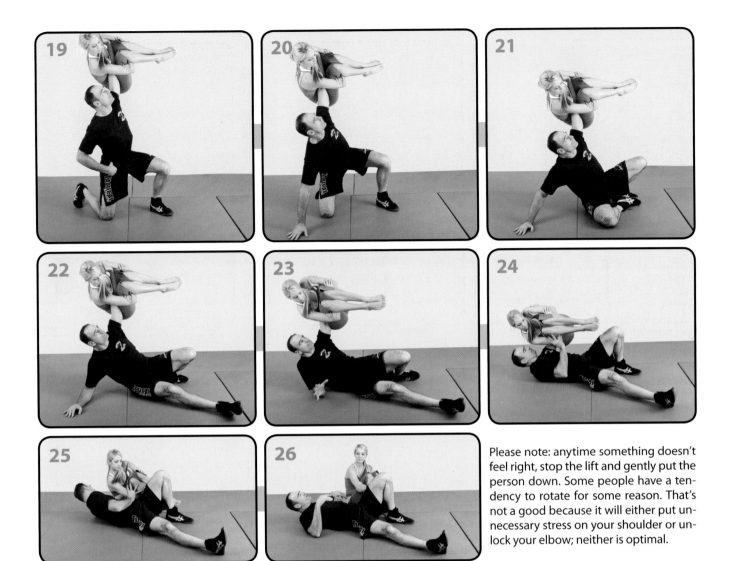

Please note: anytime something doesn't feel right, stop the lift and gently put the person down. Some people have a tendency to rotate for some reason. That's not a good because it will either put unnecessary stress on your shoulder or unlock your elbow; neither is optimal.

4) In one motion, sit back and pull your partner toward you.
5) As you roll backward, pull your partner onto your chest. Be sure to bend and lift your leg closest to your partner as you roll backward. This helps cushion and control her landing.
6) Continue rolling backward until you're flat on your back. Press your partner with both hands until your left arm is locked. **Note: the hand on the elbow and your bent knee helps stabilize your partner while you're adjusting your hand or grip position. You must make sure your wrist and elbow are straight!**
7) Remove your knee and post your heel close to your butt. Continue using your off-hand as a stabilizer.
8) Remove your stabilizing hand and lay it out to the side. Ask your partner "Are you OK?" or "Do you feel alright?" If the answer is "yes," proceed. If "no," then immediately put her down.
9) Inhale, tighten up, then exhale through your teeth and drive off your heel and attempt to sit up.
10) Continue driving off your heel and forearm.
11) Continue sitting up, moving from your forearm to hand.
12) As you reach the top of the sit-up, ask again; "Are you OK." If "yes," proceed to the next step, if no, put her down.
13) Pressing off your heel and hand, lift your hip up off the ground.
14) Pull your leg through until you knee is directly under your working arm.
15) Straighten your torso to the kneeling position. Ensure the foot of your lead leg is planted directly under your knee and press the ball of your trail leg into the floor.
16) Inhale, tighten up, and drive off your heel and glute, extending your legs.
17) Bring your trail leg up and under your hips. Again, ask if your partner is "OK." Now it's time to reverse directions.
18) Carefully step backward and slowly change levels.
19) Slightly rotate your shoulders counterclockwise, and then put your fingertips on your hipbone as a reminder that it's the hip that moves straight back.
20) Slowly move your hips back and place your hand 45 degrees off the front of your knee.
21) Slowly slide your leg through.
22) Once your leg is fully extended, lower yourself to your forearm.
23) Lower yourself to the back of your arm and side.
24) Lower yourself to your back and place your free hand on the side of your partner's leg, near the knee, to control the descent.
25) Slowly place your partner next to you.
26) Celebrate!

Turkish Get-Up Series

Section 4
Clean Series

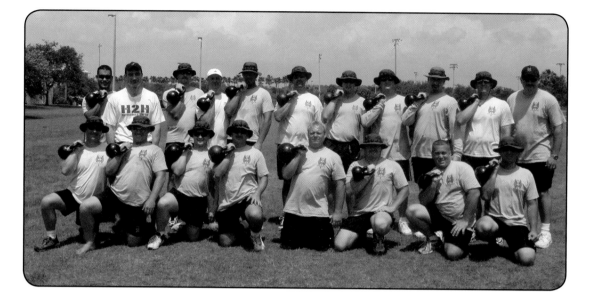

In this section, you will learn a variety of methods to effectively clean your kettlebells to the rack position. Clean, in this context, does not mean to wash, and rack isn't a place to let it air dry. In weightlifting terminology, to "clean" a weight is to move it, in one motion, from the floor (or below the hips) to chest/shoulder height (aka rack position) without touching any other part of your body. The clean is an efficient means of setting the kettlebells in the correct position for overhead lifts. It's the precursor for the military press, push press, jerk, and others.

In this section, you will learn how to perform the:

- **Rack position**

- **Dead clean**

- **(Swing) clean**

- **Bottoms-up clean**

- **Double clean**

- **Front squat**

Benefits

The kettlebell clean is a great alternative to the barbell clean, especially if you have wrist flexibility issues. It teaches your body to generate power from the hip and to absorb impact and decelerate force. The benefits of these skills transfer to many sports and occupations. The clean can be practiced by itself or in combination with body weight exercises or other kettlebell exercises like the push press or jerk. Many combination exercises will be addressed in later portions of this book. As with all foundational lifts, invest extra time learning the basics, and you'll soon be ready for the many variations.

Contrary to the belief of many beginners, the KB clean is not supposed to be a forearm-toughening exercise! It actually serves as a valuable assistance exercise for the snatch. How your hand inserts into the handle during the clean is exactly how it inserts when performing the snatch. Properly executed, the bell should land as light as a feather and cause no bruising or pain to the wrist, forearm, or shoulder. If you feel pain, stop and make a "note-to-self": Something is wrong! Access the situation, identify the problem, make the necessary corrections, and then move on.

I. Rack Position

An effective teaching strategy is to begin with the end in mind. We'll start at the finish position (aka the rack position) and then work our way down. To avoid confusion, let's address some of the similarities and differences of the kettlebell rack position verses the barbell rack.

Similarities:
1) Weight rests high on the chest.
2) Thumbs are near the collarbones.

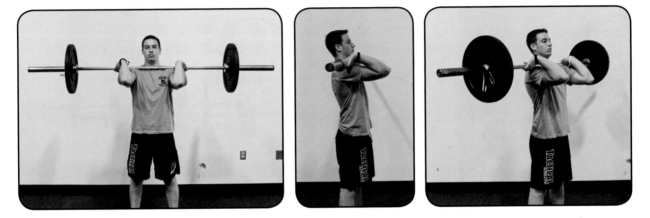

Distinct Differences:
1) BB: Wrists bent, palms away, elbows high vs. KB: Wrists straight, palm facing opposite shoulder, elbow attached to torso.
2) BB: bar rests on front of delts to support weight, kettlebell rests in "pocket" (forearm, biceps, delts,) and the entire arm is attached to your body, in some cases elbow rests on top of iliac crest (i.e., top of the hip bone).

The Kettlebell Rack: What It Is . . .

- The wrists are straight, the back of my upper arm is tight against my ribcage, lats are flexed.
- The bell is resting on three points of contact: forearm, biceps, and shoulder. The knuckle of my thumb is in contact with my collarbone, and there's no space between my triceps and torso.
- The kettlebell is directly over the hip, knee, and center of foot.

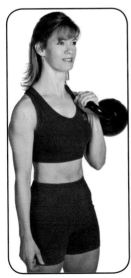

Note: Hand position, thumb on or inside bra strap.

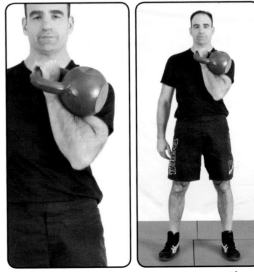

Clean Series

The Kettlebell Rack: What It's Not . . .

✕ Common Rack Errors:

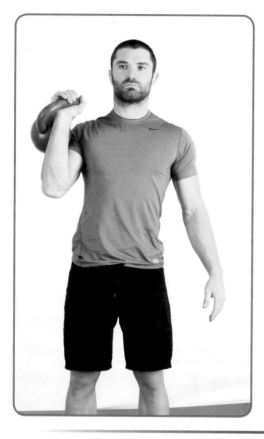

1. Too Wide, Vertical Forearm, Elbow Drift:

The hand is not connected to the upper chest, the elbow is disconnected from the torso, and the forearm is vertical. This is a very compromising and dangerous position for the shoulder. The offset center of gravity of the kettlebell resting on your vertical, unattached, and unstable forearm creates leverage that will crank your hand back behind your shoulder. This will cause your elbow to rise, resulting in the BJJ submission called the Americana. The problem is that you can tap, but the kettlebell will won't stop. Once in motion, it will finish the movement and the kettlebell will always win!

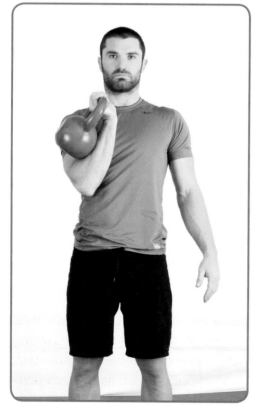

2. Bent Wrist:

The wrist must be straight when cleaning a kettlebell. There's an old saying in boxing "a bent wrist is a broken wrist." You probably won't break your wrist cleaning a kettlebell, but you sure will cause unnecessary strain and jack it up in short order.

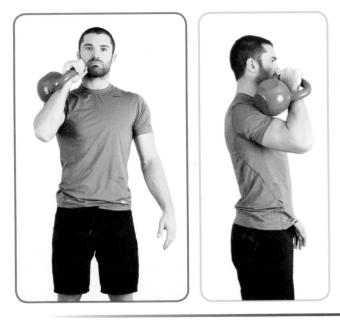

3. Elbow not attached to torso:

Elbow must be attached for shoulder safety and efficient power transfer later on when you perform presses, push presses, and thrusters.

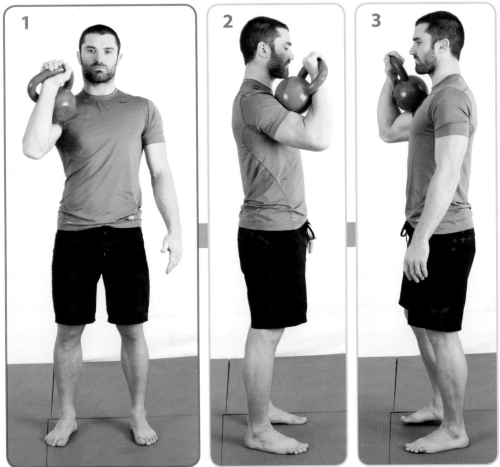

4. Palms away, elbow detached:

This is a serious problem that needs to be addressed ASAP. It is pretty common with some folks who have thousands of reps of barbell cleans. With a bar, it's essential to have your elbows up, palms facing forward, wrists bent, with the bar resting on the front of your shoulders; with a kettlebell, not so much.

An effective teaching strategy is to start at the finish position, commonly known as the rack position, and then work our way down.

1. Rack Hold Drill

This drill is the easiest, safest, least dynamic way to get the kettlebell to the rack position. Two hands are used to lift and set the kettlebell in the rack position, adjustments are made to ensure proper position, and then two hands are used to put it back down.

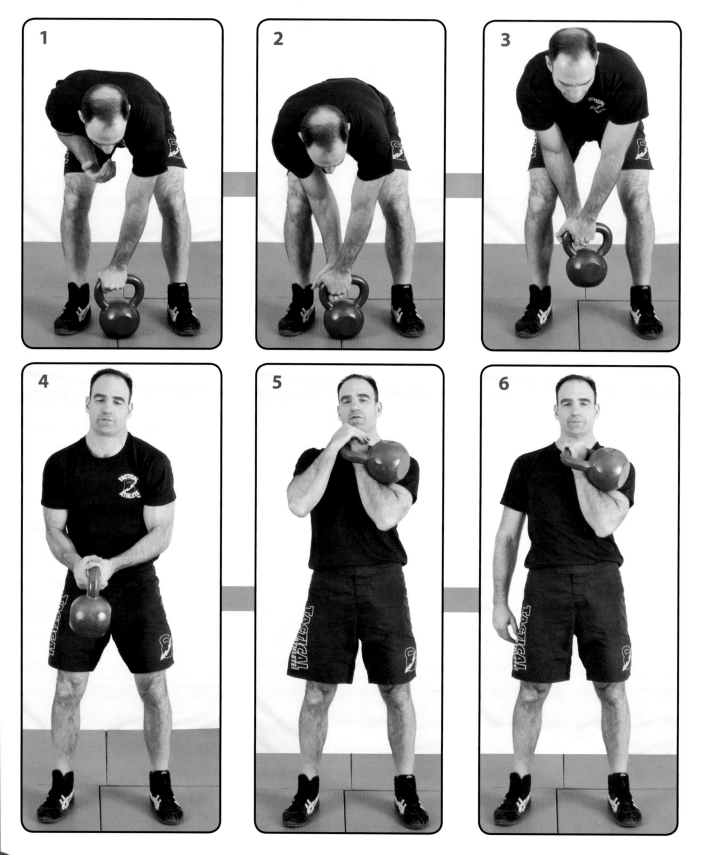

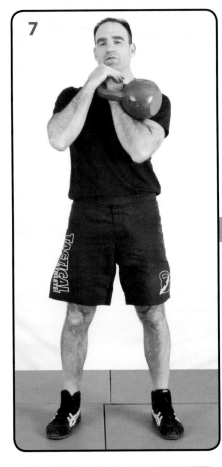

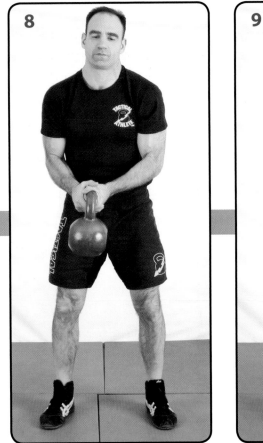

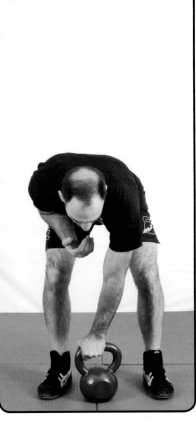

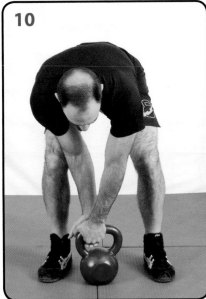

1) Start position:
   • Feet between hip and shoulder width apart, toes pointing in the direction you're facing.
   • Kettlebell is centered between your feet, handle in line with the base of your toes.
   • Keep your chest open, shoulders back and down.
   • Fold at the hips (i.e., sit back and down), shift your weight to your heels, and keep your neck in a neutral position.
   • Establish a one-handed grip; left hand goes into the corner closest to your thumb and forefinger (i.e., right corner).
2) Use your right hand as an assist, gripping directly over the knuckles of your left hand.
3) Inhale through your nose, tighten up, and drive through your heels, deadlifting the kettlebell off the ground.
4) Once fully upright, curl the kettlebell toward your chest with both arms.
5) Continue curling until your hands are under your chin and the knuckles of both thumbs are touching your collarbone. Make sure your wrist is straight, thumb rests on your collarbone, and the back of your arm is Velcroed to your side.
6) Release your right hand (assist hand). This is the rack position. Hold the rack position for 30 seconds to 1 minute.
7–10) Use two hands to put it down, then repeat sequence with the other arm.

Clean Series

2. Two Hands Up, One Hand Down Drill

This drill emphasizes the proper timing and coordination of the arm, body, and kettlebell as it unwinds and descends from the rack position. Pay attention to the kettlebell position and path on which it moves out of the rack position.

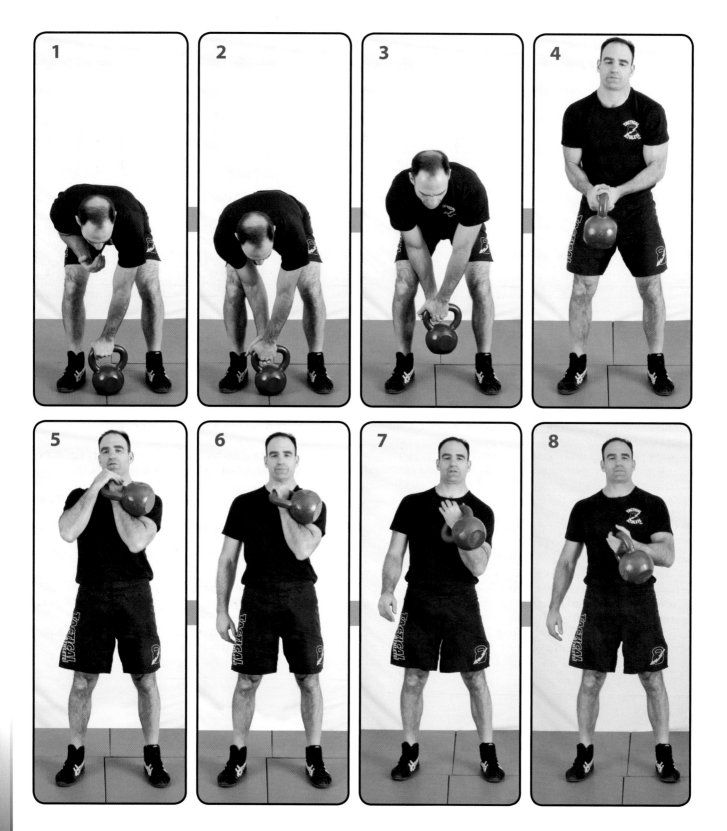

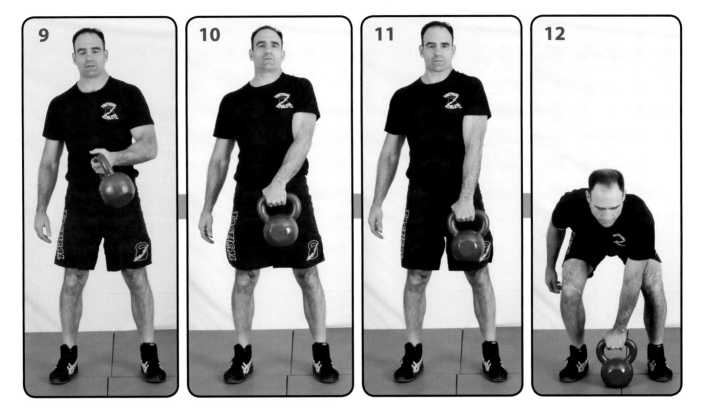

1) Start position:
   - Feet between hip and shoulder width apart, toes pointing in the direction you're facing.
   - Kettlebell is centered, between your feet, handle in line with the base of your toes.
   - Keep your chest open, shoulders back and down.
   - Fold at the hips (i.e., sit back and down), shift your weight to your heels, and keep your neck in a neutral position.
   - Establish a one-handed grip; left hand goes into the corner closest to your thumb and forefinger (i.e., right corner).
2) Use your right hand as an assist, gripping directly over the knuckles of your left hand.
3) Inhale through your nose, tighten up, and drive through your heels, deadlifting the kettlebell off the ground.
4) Once fully upright, curl the kettlebell toward your chest with both arms.
5) Continue curling until your hands are under your chin and the knuckles of both thumbs are touching your collarbone. Make sure your wrist is straight, your thumb rests on your collarbone, and the back of your arm is Velcroed to your side.
6) Release your right hand (assist hand). Pause in the rack position.
7) Keeping your armpit tight, move your elbow rearward, relax your biceps, and allow your hand to begin its descent. Note: Elbow stays in contact with your torso.
8) Allow your thumb to externally rotate as your hand comes off your chest, moving down your centerline.
9) Internally rotate your thumb as your hand approaches your belt line.
10) Your palm should be facing your body by the time your arm is straight.
11) Immediately engage your hip flexors, pulling your hips back as your arm straightens, guiding the kettlebell back to the starting point. The timing of bringing your hips back is critical. If you unhinge your hips too early, the kettlebell will jerk you forward, pulling you out of position and causing unnecessary stress on your back. If you unhinge too late, your wrist, elbow and shoulder will absorb the shock.
12) Practice the above sequence with a light kettlebell, concentrating on your timing. Note: You are guiding the kettlebell to the ground. It's more of a controlled fall. You are not trying to slow it down, nor are you performing a reverse curl.

Clean Series

II. Dead Clean

Once you feel comfortable guiding the kettlebell from the rack position to the floor, it's time to move it from the floor to the rack position. In weightlifting, the act of moving a weight from the floor to your chest is called a clean. In kettlebell lifting, the clean usually begins from the back swing. For our purposes, we will start with the dead clean, where each rep begins and ends from the floor. It reinforces good lifting mechanics, it's similar to the barbell clean, and can be easily combined with other body weight exercises.

Dead Clean

It's a good idea to practice a few air drills (without the weight) first to ensure that you get the consistency of the movement first before adding intensity.

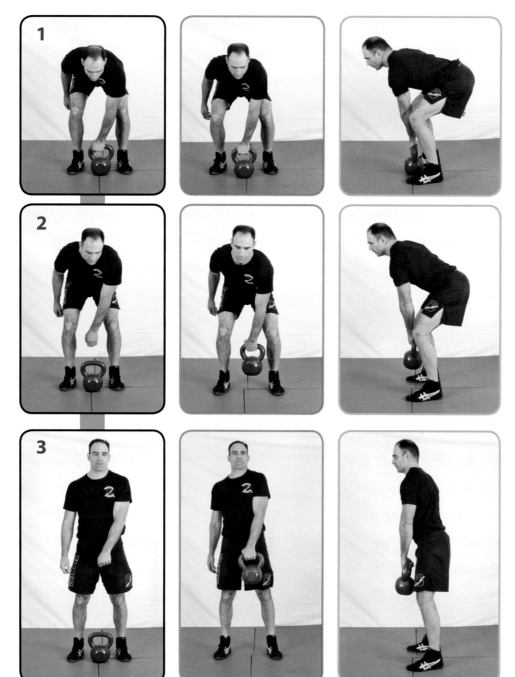

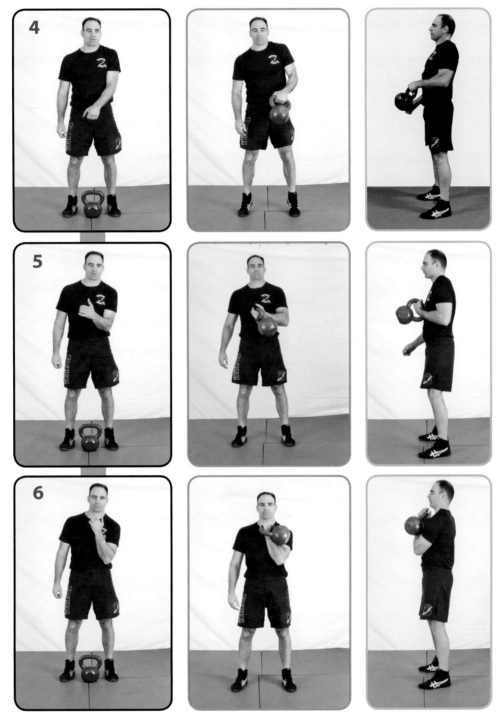

1) Start position:
   - Feet between hip and shoulder width apart, toes pointing in the direction you're facing.
   - Kettlebell is centered, between your feet, handle in line with the base of your toes.
   - Keep your chest open, shoulders back and down.
   - Fold at the hips (i.e., sit back and down), shift your weight to your heels, and keep your neck in a neutral position.
   - Establish a one-handed grip with your left hand. Elbow must be straight. Actively flex your triceps to ensure that you keep your arm straight.
2) Keeping your back straight, neutral head position, drive off your heels, extending your hips and legs.
3) Continue driving through your heels until you are completely upright. Upon extension, you will feel the kettlebell begin to drive your arm and shoulder up.
4) As soon as you feel your shoulder begin to rise, immediately allow your elbow to bend.
5) Quickly drop your elbow toward the front of your hip.
6) Finish in the rack position. Reverse the motion, returning the kettlebell to the floor (starting point). Repeat for desired reps or time on each side, or alternate hands after every rep.

Clean Series

Dead Clean Common Errors

✕ Common Error #1: Elbow Not Connected:

As the kettlebell moves up and down, the elbow must stay connected to your torso.

√ Corrective Action:

Engage your lats by squeezing an imaginary tennis ball in your armpit.

✕ Common Error #2: Hinging Hips Too Early

This will cause unnecessary stress to your lower back and elbow. Timing is everything.

√ Corrective Action:

Go back and practice the two hands up/one hand down drill. Focus on pulling your hips back at the last possible moment.

Dead Clean Rx

The combination drills listed below are very demanding full-body exercises. They are presented from easiest to hardest. Make sure that you have perfected the dead clean before attempting the first combination. Pay particular attention to the breathing sequence and back position. Once you've mastered all three combinations, reverse the order for maximum benefit. Start with the hardest combination first. As you get tired, scale to the next easiest variation, and so on. The key is to keep moving and use good form.

Note: These drills are best performed on a flat, level surface with a kettlebell that has a flat and even bottom.

Combo Drill #1: Squat Thrust and Dead Clean

By inserting a squat thrust between the reps, you'll dramatically increase the intensity.

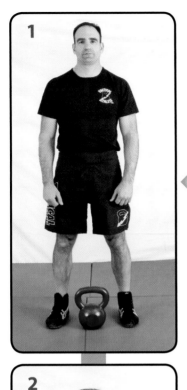

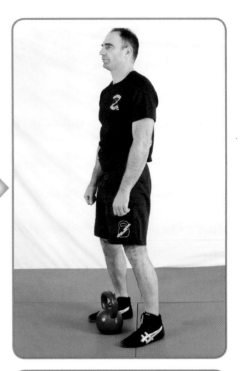

1

Begin by placing the kettlebell in between your feet.

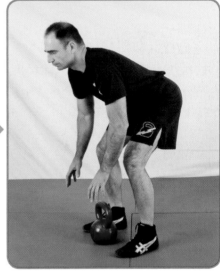

2

Perform a squat thrust over the kettlebell. Initiate the movement by folding at the hips, keeping your back straight.

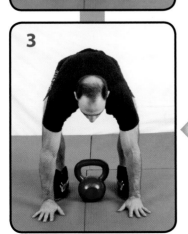

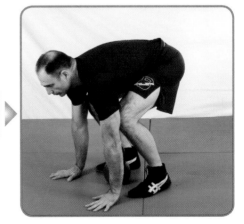

3

Bend your knees and place your hands on the ground slightly in front of your feet.

Clean Series

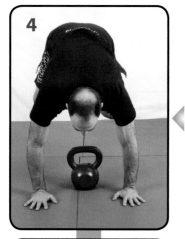

4

Kick your feet backward, keeping them shoulder width apart.

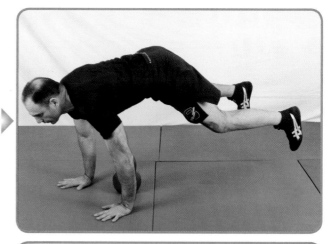

5

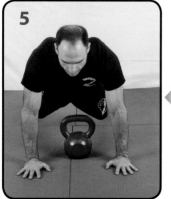

Continue extending your legs and hips until you are in the push-up or front-leaning rest position. Resist the urge to perform a push-up in this position. Keep your abs and butt tight . . . no sagging!

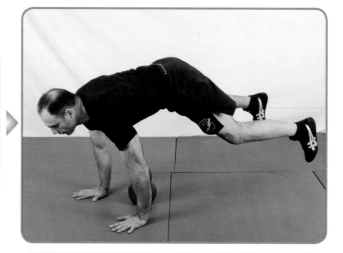

6

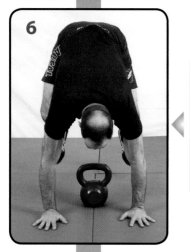

Inhale deeply through your nose as you move back into the squatting position. It is essential to pressurize your abdominal cavity by breathing "into the belly" and bearing down with the diaphragm.

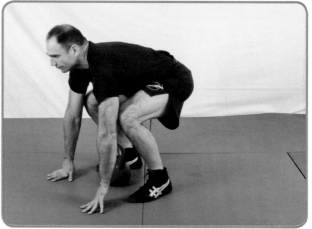

7

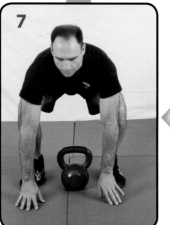

It is important that you bring your feet up enough where the kettlebell is in between your feet, not in front of them. Be sure you put yourself in position for a straight pull.

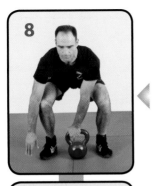

8 Trace your left hand from the floor to the bell, up to the handle, securing your grip on the handle. Keep your butt low, arm straight, back straight, and neck neutral.

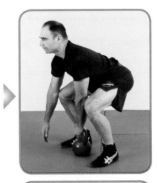

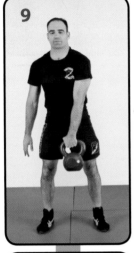

9 Drive off your heels, rapidly extending your legs and hips.

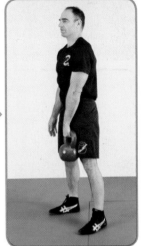

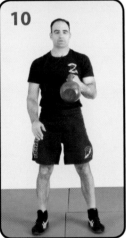

10 As the kettlebell floats up, drop your elbow.

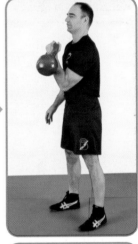

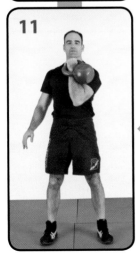

11 Continue dropping the elbow until you are in the rack position. Return the kettlebell to the starting position. Alternate hands after each squat thrust rep. Perform for time or reps.

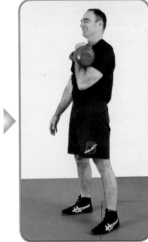

Clean Series

Combo Drill #2: Squat Thrust/Offset Push-Up/Dead Clean

Now it's time to add the push-up and increase the intensity!

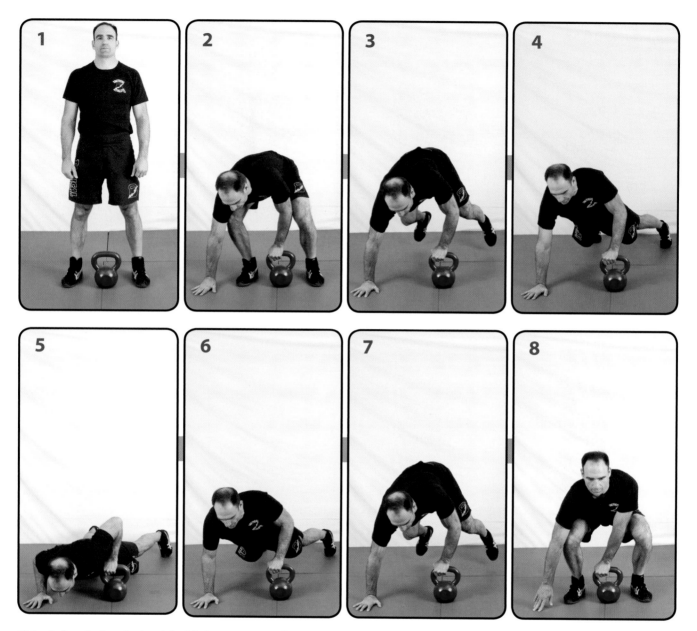

1) Begin by placing the kettlebell in between your feet.
2) Perform a squat thrust. Place your left hand on the KB handle and your right hand on the floor to the right of the kettlebell.
3) Kick your feet backward, keeping them shoulder width apart.
4) Continue extending your legs and hips until you are in the push-up. Keep your abs and butt tight!
5-6) Perform an offset push-up, loading most of your weight onto your right arm.
7) Explode out of the push-up position and inhale through your nose as you move back into the squatting position. It is essential to pressurize your abdominal cavity by breathing "into the belly" and bearing down with the diaphragm.
8) Ensure the kettlebell is between your feet, your weight is on your heels, butt low, back and arm straight.

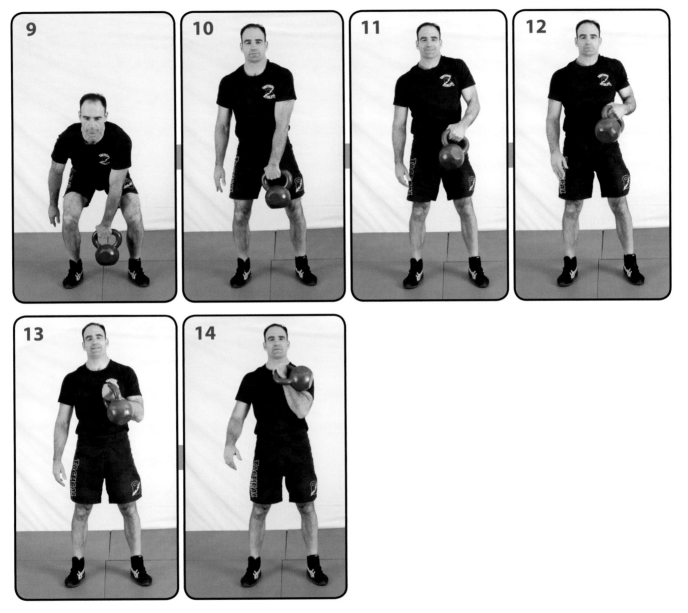

9) Drive off your heels, rapidly extending your legs and hips.
10) Continue extension until you are in the upright position.
11) As the kettlebell floats up, drop your elbow.
12–14) Continue dropping the elbow until you are in the rack position.
From there, Place the KB back on the floor, switch hand positions, and repeat on the other side.

Clean Series

Combination Drill #3: Explosive Push-Up Dead Clean

This is the most demanding of the three combinations. The key is to keep it explosive. As soon as you lose your explosiveness, whether it's after 1 rep or 10, immediately switch to the previous variation.

Note: This drill is best performed on a flat, level surface with a larger kettlebell that has a flat and even bottom.

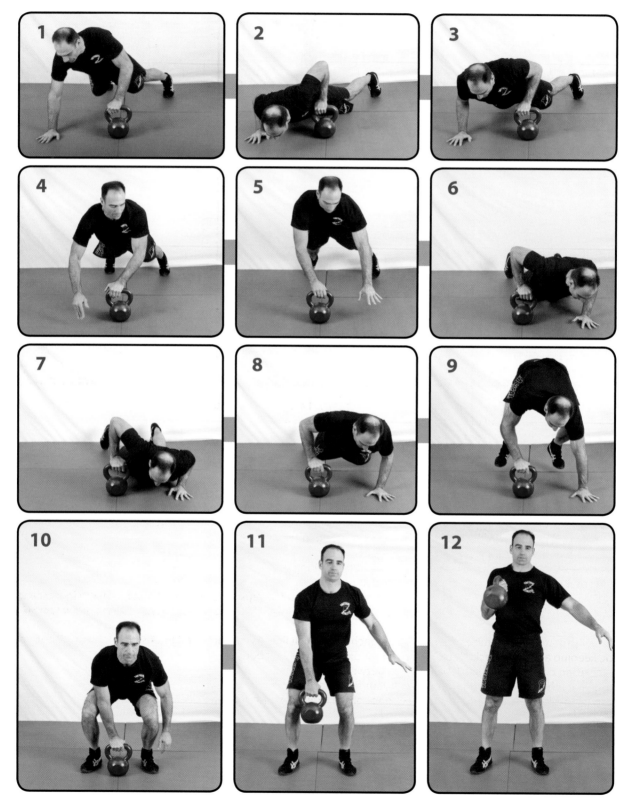

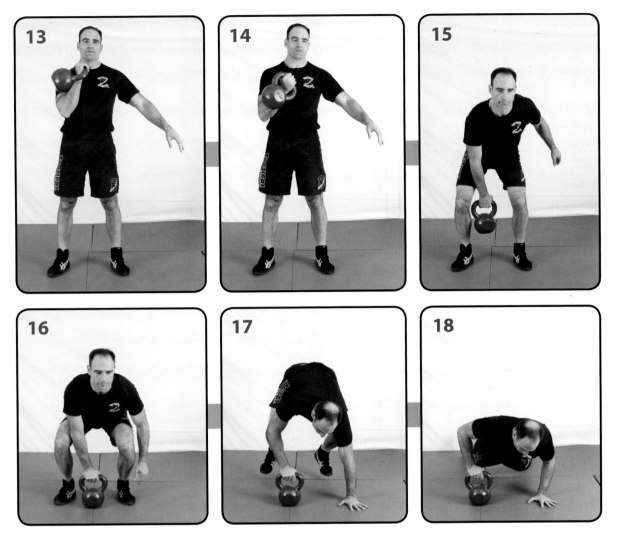

1) Start from the offset push-up position (left hand on the handle, right hand on the floor).
2) Perform a push-up, loading most of your weight onto your right arm.
3) Explode out of the push-up position.
4) Fully extend both arms, pushing your upper body up and to the left.
5) Quickly and swiftly switch your hand position on the KB handle by releasing your left hand and replacing it with your right.
6) Decelerate into the bottom of the offset push-up position.
7) Load your left arm as you reach the bottom position.
8) Explosively push off both hands.
9) As your arms extend, inhale through your nose as you bring your knees and feet toward your chest.
10) Finish in a proper deadlift position (back straight, chest open, arm straight, etc.).
11) Drive off your heels, rapidly extending your legs and hips.
12) Drop your elbow, allowing the kettlebell to float upward along your centerline.
13) The kettlebell should land softly in the rack position.
14) Keeping your armpit tight, move your elbow rearward, relax your biceps, and allow your hand to begin its descent. Allow your thumb to externally rotate as your hand comes off your chest. Note: Elbow slides back staying in contact with your torso.
15) Internally rotate your thumb as your hand approaches your belt line. As your arm straightens, simultaneously pull your hips back, keeping a straight back. Note: Your palm should be facing your body.
16) Keep sitting back until the kettlebell lands in between your feet.
17) Place your left hand on the ground and kick your feet back.
18) From the push-up position, repeat the sequence of the explosive push-up/dead clean combination.

Clean Series

Kettlebell Clean: Standard

If there is one exercise with the potential for beating up your forearms during the learning curve, it is this one. The purpose of the clean is not to toughen your forearms. The clean, properly executed, should land as soft as a feather. Proper technique is the key. I sometimes refer to the KB clean as the swing-clean during my seminars to emphasize the back swing portion of the clean. Otherwise many people turn it into a hang clean. Nevertheless, the clean is an important assistance exercise for learning the snatch.

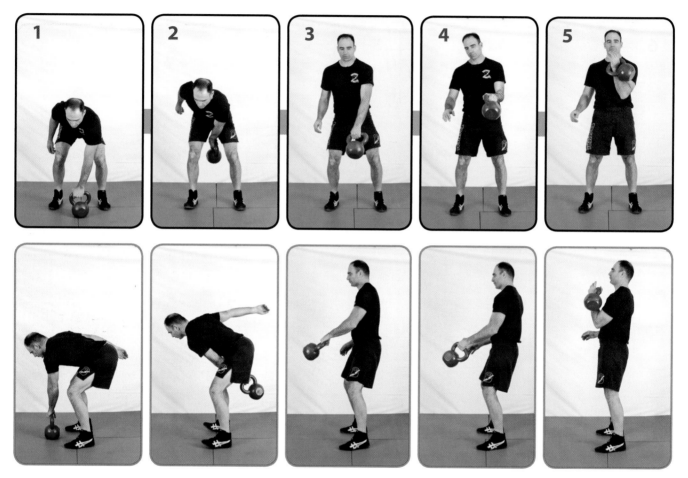

1) Start position:
   • Feet between hip and shoulder width apart, toes pointing in the direction you're facing.
   • Kettlebell is centered, 3–6 inches in front of your toes.
   • Keep your chest open, shoulders back and down.
   • Fold at the hips (i.e., sit back and down), shift your weight to your heels, and keep your neck in a neutral position.
   • Establish a one-handed grip on the kettlebell.
2) Perform the back swing:
   • Inhale through your nose, tighten your abs and glutes.
   • Keeping your weight on your heels, slightly extend your legs and back angle, contract your lats, and hike the kettlebell back between your legs.
   • As the kettlebell reaches the end of the back swing, press through your heels and extend your legs and hips.
3) As your hips and torso become upright, pull your left shoulder back (squaring your shoulders).
4) The shoulder must be pressed down; armpit squeezed tightly, triceps resting on the ribcage, but your elbow is relaxed to allow the kettlebell to rise. As it rises, begin to externally rotate your thumb. Avoid the tendency to curl the KB. If you feel a "pump" on your biceps, you're doing it wrong! The arm must stay loose. The combination of hip extension and shoulder retraction does all the work of driving the kettlebell upward.
5) As the kettlebell floats up toward the rack position, loosen your grip. Loosening your grip is important because it decreases friction in your hand and allows you to keep a straight wrist as your hand inserts into the kettlebell handle. The handle should set diagonally across the palm of your hand; wrist neutral; no flexion! Note: The kettlebell should travel the shortest distance possible, following a vertical path, rather than a big arc.

6) As the kettlebell lands between your forearm and shoulder, immediately tighten the abs and let out a little bit of air (similar to a boxer exhaling with a punch). The KB, arm, and torso must become one solid unit at the top of the clean. Do not allow the kettlebell to flip up and "crash" on your forearm.

7) Keeping your armpit tight, relax your biceps and allow your hand to begin its descent. Allow your thumb to externally rotate as your hand comes off your chest and slightly lean back to counterbalance and shorten the arc of the descending kettlebell. Note: Elbow stays in contact with your torso and the kettlebell rolls off your forearm.

8) As your hand approaches your belt line, internally rotate your thumb so that your palm is facing your body.

9) Just before your forearm crashes into your pelvic area, fold at the hips (i.e., sit back and down) and shift your weight to your heels.

10) Allow the kettlebell to reach the end of the back swing. Repeat for desired time or reps.

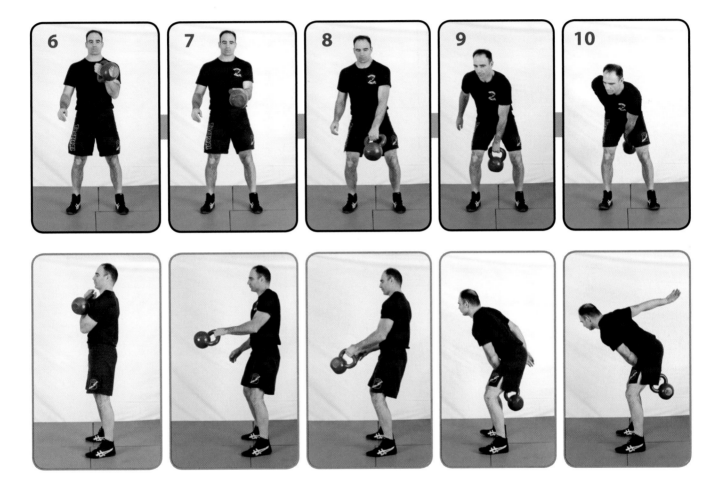

Kettlebell Clean Common Errors

It's amazing how many common errors can rear their ugly head when practicing the clean. Take your time, identify and iron out each error. Consider the clean as you would the one-arm swing—a foundation and assistance exercise for the snatch. Any errors left unchecked during the clean will only be magnified when you take the kettlebell overhead in the snatch. Be patient and focus on solving one problem at a time.

✕ Common Error #1: Hand on Thigh

People have a tendency to put their hand on their thigh to help stabilize their movement, usually compensating for a weak core and back.

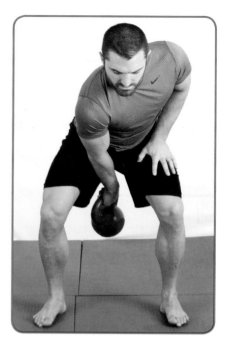

√ Corrective Action: Burpees . . . Just Kidding!

- Awareness and verbal correction is usually all that is needed. Be sure to keep your nonworking hand off your body. It only leads to poor form.
- Be sure the trainee is properly pressurizing and stabilizing his core. Review the breathing sequence taught in the swing series: inhaling through his nose when descending, and exhaling through his teeth upon extension.

✕ Common Error #2: Curling

Curling is common when there is a lack of hip drive or the weight is too light. The arm must be relaxed. We are not trying to increase the "peak" on our biceps. If you are feeling a "pump," you're doing it wrong!

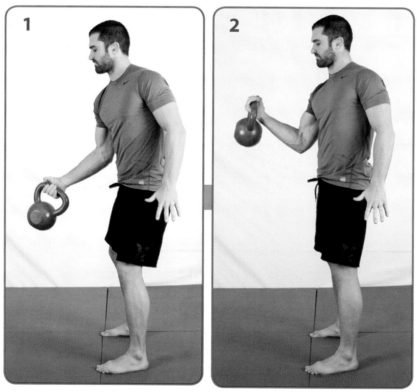

√ Corrective Action:

- Review the standing vertical jump drills from Section 1, Part 2.
- Use a heavier kettlebell (a size that the trainee cannot curl). This will force him to use his hip drive.

✗ Common Error #3: Elbow Detached from Torso

This error could be a carryover from practicing a lot of barbell cleans. Regardless, when cleaning a kettlebell, the elbow needs to be attached to the torso. It protects the shoulder.

√ Corrective Action: Cloth-in-the-Armpit Drill

Place a sock, washcloth, or small towel in your armpit and then perform a few kettlebell cleans. Squeeze your lats and press your upper arm against the ribcage. A properly executed clean will not disturb the resting place of the cloth. As soon as your arm moves out of position, the cloth will drop to the ground. If this happens, you might as well put your kettlebell down and start "pushing." Yeah burpees!

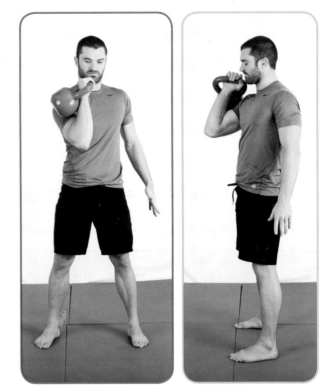

✗ Common Error #4: Bent Wrist

Keeping too tight of a grip on the KB handle causes this error. People erroneously think that the tighter they grip the handle the better because it will slow down the rotation and land softer. All this will do is tear up the callous on your hands and cause your wrist to flex, creating unnecessary strain.

√ Corrective Action: Open Your Hand

It's counterintuitive but it works. As the kettlebell floats up toward the rack position, loosen your grip or open your hand. This allows your hand to insert deep into the kettlebell handle. The handle should set diagonally across the palm of your hand, similar to a false grip on gymnastic rings. Always keep your wrist straight and neutral. There's an old saying in the sport of boxing: "a bent wrist is a broken wrist." In kettlebell lifting, we always keep the wrists straight. Timing is the key to a soft landing!

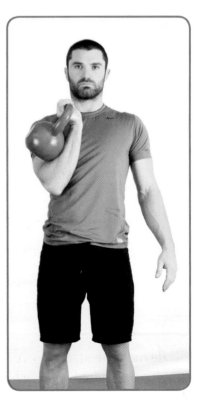

✕ Common Error #5:
Wide Rack, Vertical Forearm, Elbow Drift

This is a recipe for disaster and must be fixed ASAP. Your hand is not connected to upper chest, your elbow is disconnected from your torso, and your forearm is vertical. As stated earlier, this is a very compromising and dangerous position for the shoulder. The dynamic nature of the clean, the offset center of gravity of the kettlebell, and incorrect arm position will result in the BJJ submission called the Americana. You can tap but the kettlebell won't stop. Once in motion, it will finish the movement and the kettlebell will win!

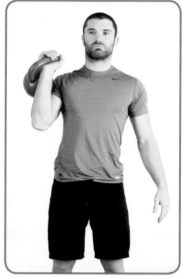

√ Corrective Action:
Review Proper Rack Position

- Practice rack holds for time.
- Practice wall drill left/right.

Wall Drills-Left/Right

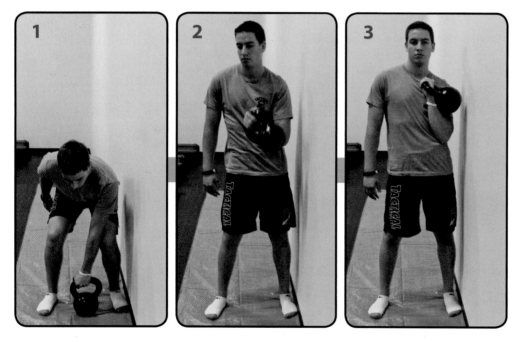

- Assume the starting position standing next to a wall. Side of your foot must touch the wall. Establish your grip with the hand that corresponds to the foot touching the wall.
- Perform the back swing.
- Drive off your heels, extending your hips and knees. Keep your upper arm tight against your side and your elbow relaxed.
- As you square up (i.e., retract) your shoulder the kettlebell will float up landing in the rack position.

✕ Common Error #6: KB Crashes on the Forearm

The kettlebell should not crash on your forearm. It's a timing and technique issue. Oftentimes the elbow disconnects from the torso, creating a bigger arc and harder landing. To soften the impact, practice the following drills.

√ Corrective Action #1: Less Power

Use slightly less power in your hip drive. That doesn't mean short stroke. Continue full hip extension, but just employ less power.

√ Corrective Action #2: Master the Clean in Reverse

- Using two hands, set the kettlebell in the "rack" position.
- Perform only the negative portion of the clean. Allow the kettlebell to roll off your forearm, hinge at your hips, and allow the KB to swing between your legs. It is important to internally rotate the thumb during the back swing, so that it points 45–90 degrees behind by the time it reaches the end of the pendulum.
- Repeat for 5–10 reps.

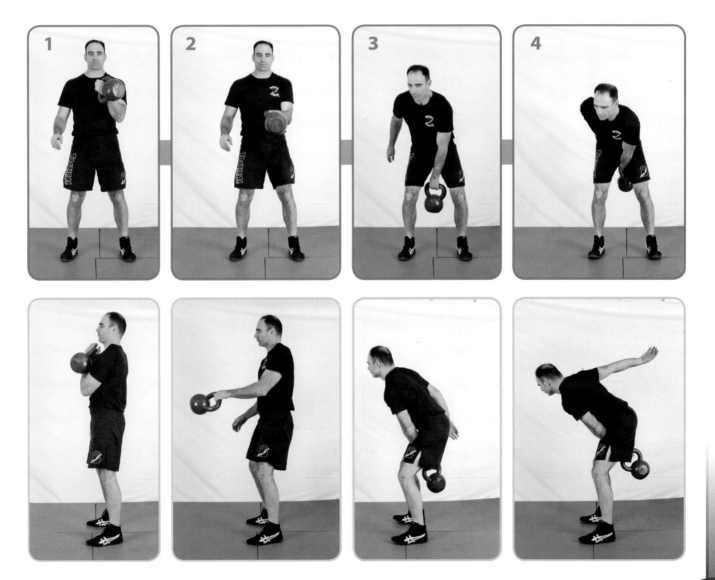

√ Corrective Action #3: Wall Drill, Front

The kettlebell should travel the shortest distance possible—straight up, rather than arcing out.

- Stand facing a wall while performing cleans. Your toes should be about six inches from the wall.)
- Perform a distance check by standing in front of the wall and assuming the start position. To ensure correct distance, your forehead should be a fist's width plus your thumb's distance away from the wall.

  Caution: If you are too far from the wall, you won't get the desired training effect. If you're too close, your forehead will smack the wall. Hopefully, it will only take a rep or two for you to make the proper adjustment!

- Perform cleans facing the wall. This drill forces you to pull your shoulder back at the right time and keep your elbow in tight, which will result in efficient movement and softer landings.
- Remember: No pain IS gain!

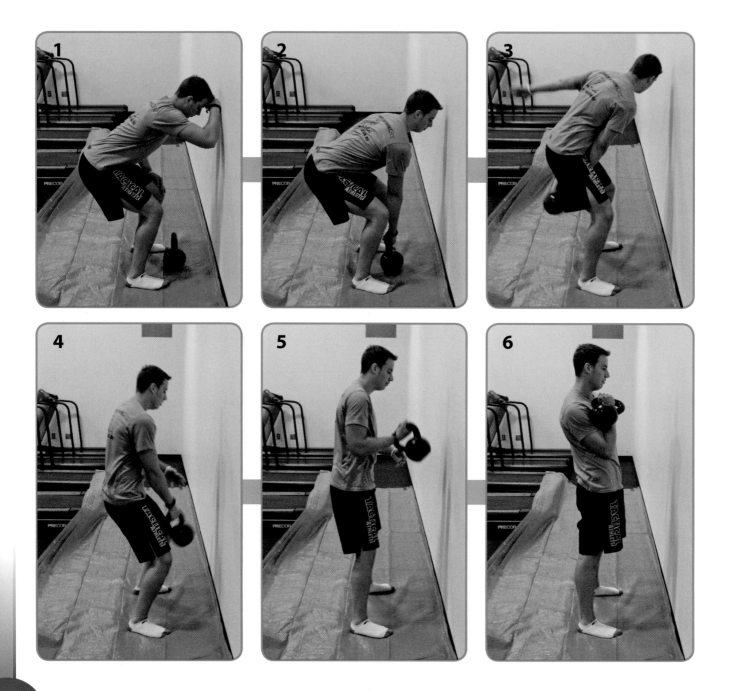

✗ Common Error #7: Knees Forward

This error results when people drop their hips straight down, instead of back and down. In addition, the knees move forward in front of the feet, weight shifts to the balls of the feet, and the back swing is muted to the hang position. The poor body mechanics result in sore knees and lower backs.

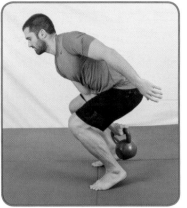 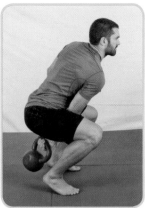

√ Corrective Action: Knee Check

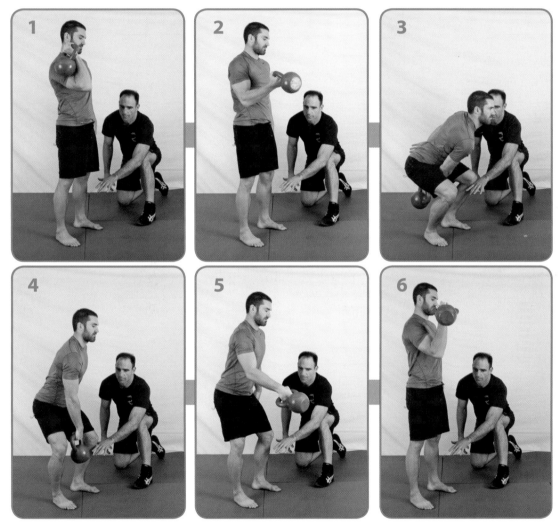

1) Have your training partner assume the rack position. Kneel off to one side, open your hand and place the web of your hand at his knee height (just below the patella) directly above the front of his toes. Place the back of your arm against the inside of your knee to brace for impact.
2) Keep your hand in position as your training partner begins the drop phase of the clean from the rack position.
3) As he completes the back swing, be sure to hold firm and don't let his knee push your hand away.
4) Keep your hand in position as he begins hips and leg extension.
5) Maintain your position as he continues hip, leg, and back extension.
6) Once he returns to the rack position, repeat the above sequence until he makes the appropriate adjustment to where his knee is no longer hitting your hand. Note: Initially, his knee may push your hand out of position. And once he makes the adjustment, his balance may be a bit shaky for a few more reps. But eventually he will establish the body mechanics.

✕ Common Error #8: Casting

Casting occurs when you extend your arm away from your body, throwing the kettlebell off your forearm.

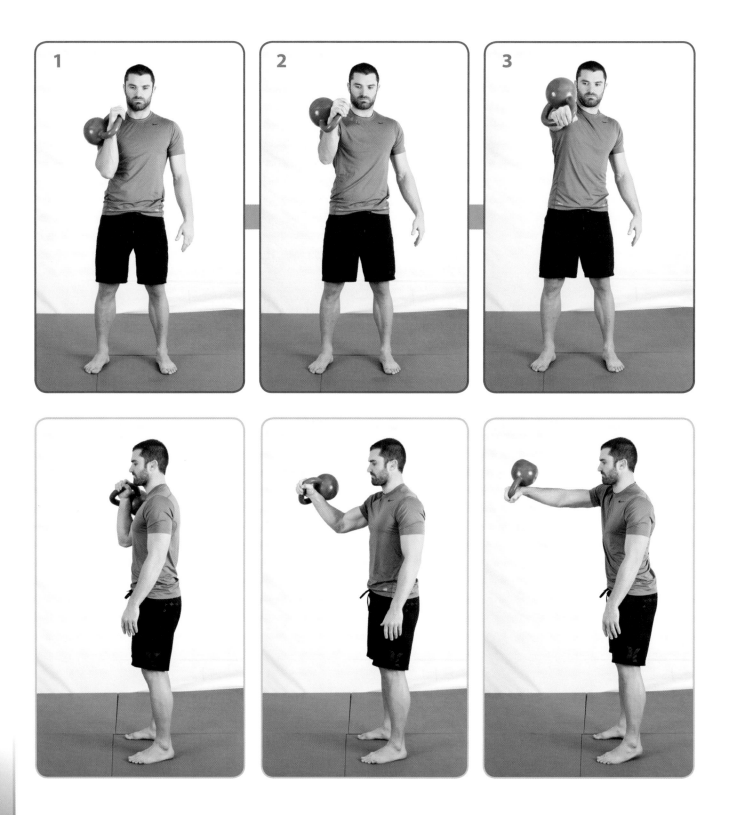

√ Corrective Action#1: Wall Drill, Front

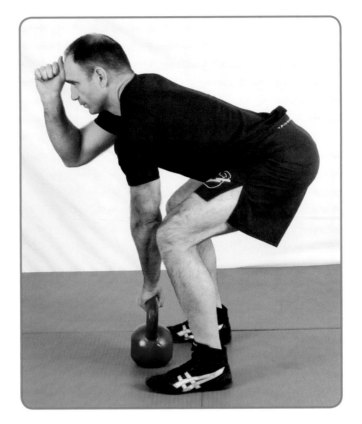

√ Corrective Action#2: Master the Clean in Reverse

See pg 191.

Bottoms-Up Clean

The bottoms-up clean is a great grip and wrist strengthener. It is also a great exercise when your forearms are sore from the learning curve of the kettlebell clean and dead clean, or the calluses on your hand start acting up.

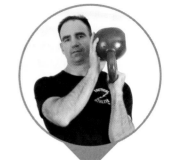

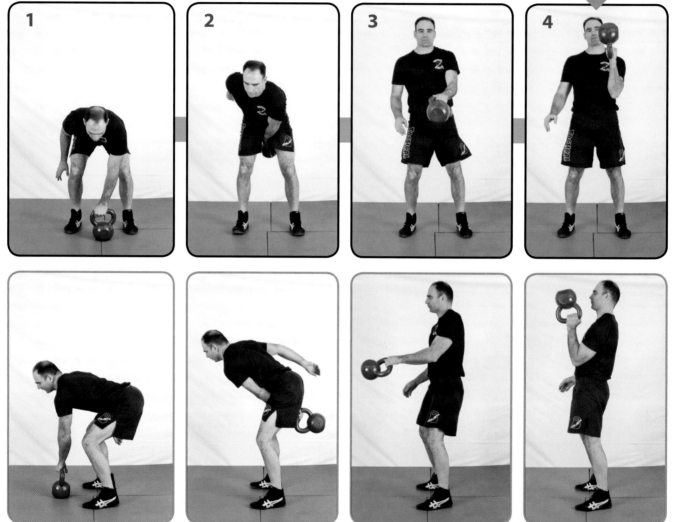

1) Start position:
   - Feet between hip and shoulder width apart, toes pointing in the direction you're facing.
   - Kettlebell is centered, 3–6 inches in front of your toes.
   - Keep your chest open, shoulders back and down.
   - Fold at the hips (i.e., sit back and down), shift your weight to your heels, and keep your neck in a neutral position.
   - Establish a one-handed grip in the corner of the kettlebell handle, nearest the thumb and forefinger.
2) Perform the back swing:
   - Inhale through your nose, tighten your abs and glutes.
   - Keeping your weight on your heels, slightly extend your legs and back angle, contract your lats, and hike the kettlebell back between your legs.
   - As the kettlebell reaches the end of the back swing, press through your heels and extend your legs and hips
3) As your hips and torso become upright, pull your left shoulder back (squaring your shoulders). Make sure you are pressing your shoulder down, squeezing your armpit tightly, your triceps is resting on your ribcage, and your elbow is relaxed so that the kettlebell can rise. As it rises, begin to externally rotate your thumb until it's in the "thumbs up" position.

4) As the kettlebell floats up, keep your forearm vertical, armpit tight, and apply a death grip on the handle. Stabilize the kettlebell in the "bottoms up" position for a 1 second count. Note: If at any time the kettlebell drifts toward your face, for any reason, feel free to intercept and check it with the palm of your free hand. I've seen more than one person fail to effectively stabilize the kettlebell, resulting in kettlebell to face contact. Thankfully, nobody ever got hurt, just embarrassed. The funny thing about each incident was that they all actually watched the bell move slowly closer and closer to their face with their eyes getting bigger and wider right until the moment of impact. Amazingly, not one person ever thought to bring the other hand up to protect their face.

5) Keeping your armpit tight, relax your biceps and slightly lean back to counterbalance and shorten the arc of the descending kettlebell. Note: Elbow stays in contact with your torso.

6) As your hand approaches your belt line, internally rotate your thumb so that your palm is facing your body.

7) Just before your forearm crashes into your pelvic area, fold at the hips (i.e., sit back and down), shift your weight to your heels, and allow the kettlebell to reach the end of the back swing. Repeat for desired time or reps, or you can hold for time and reps.

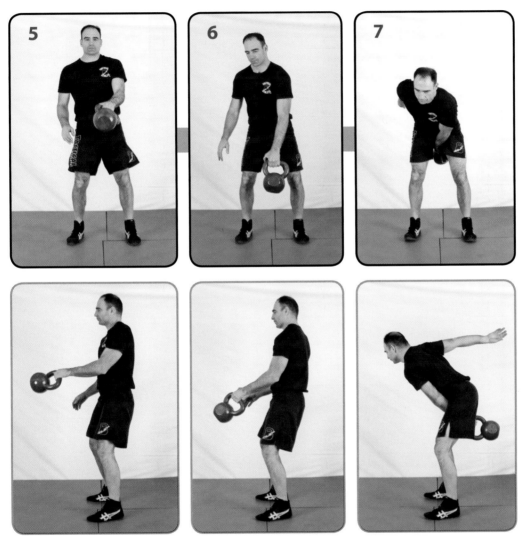

Tips for Stabilizing the Bottoms-Up Clean

- It is critical to instantly and simultaneously tighten your entire body, especially your grip, glutes, and the armpit of your working arm the moment the kettlebell reaches the "bottoms-up" position.
- It is also helpful to keep the kettlebell handle loosely gripped during the back swing. Then, as your elbow begins to bend and the kettlebell begins to rise, tighten your grip. This movement is similar to how a hockey player would grab the jersey of an opposing team member, pull him in, and then hit him with the free hand.
- Simultaneously make a tight fist with the free hand. Better yet, put a pair of grippers in your free hand and squeeze it at the same time that you reach the top position.

Double Clean

It is important to learn how to safely and effectively clean two kettlebells to the chest. This will open up a full spectrum of two-handed kettlebell lifts that will add variety and intensity to your workouts. The double clean sets the stage for the kettlebell thruster, front squats, double kettlebell military press, and many more.

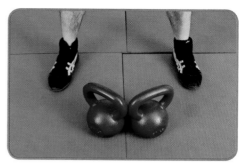

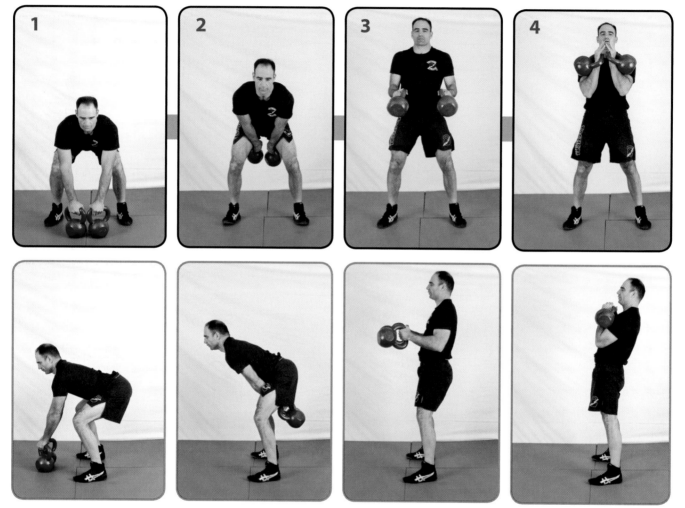

1) Start position:
   - Feet about shoulder width apart, toes pointing in the direction you're facing.
   - Kettlebells are centered, 3–6 inches in front of your toes, handles angled at approx 45 degrees toward each other.
   - Keep your chest open, shoulders back and down.
   - Fold at the hips (i.e., sit back and down), shift your weight to your heels, and keep your neck in a neutral position.
   - Grip toward the inside handle of each kettlebell.
   - Hand position is an important first step for the safety of your fingers.
2) Perform the back swing:
   - Inhale through your nose, tighten your abs and glutes.
   - Keeping your weight on your heels, slightly extend your legs and back angle, contract your lats, and hike the kettlebell back between your legs.
   - As the kettlebell reaches the end of the back swing, your palms should be rotated so that your thumbs are pointing backward.
3) Press through your heels, extending your legs, hips, and back. As your torso becomes upright, keep your armpits tight and pull your elbows slightly backward. This will help accelerate the kettlebells up toward your chest.
4) The moment you feel your arms free of load, relax your grip and insert your hands into the kettlebell handles. As the kettlebell lands between your forearm and shoulder, immediately tighten the abs and let out a little bit of air (similar to a boxer exhaling with a punch). The handles should set diagonally across the palms of your hands; wrist straight and neutral; no flexion!

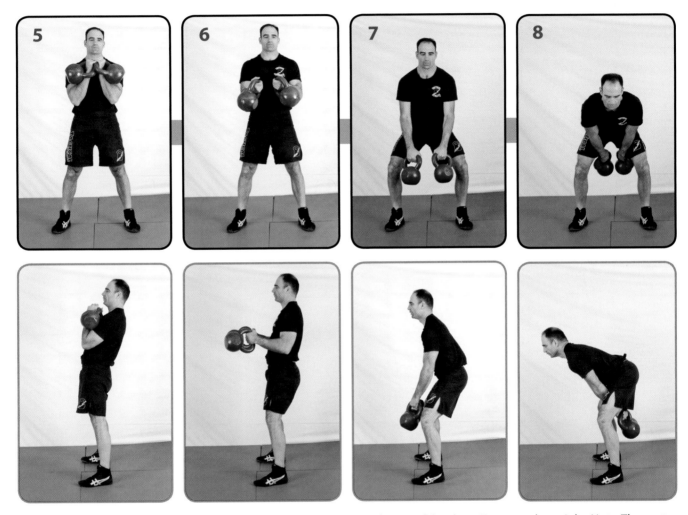

5) The KBs, your arms, and your torso must become one solid unit at the top of the clean. Keep your butt tight. Note: The center of the kettlebell is directly over the center of the foot.

6) Keeping your armpits tight, relax your biceps and allow your arms to move off your chest to begin their descent. Note: Elbows stay in contact with your torso.

7) As your hand approaches your belt line, internally rotate your thumbs so that your palms are facing your body. Keep your weight on your heels.

8) Fold at the hips (i.e., sit back and down) and allow the kettlebells to decelerate to the end of the back swing. Repeat for desired time or reps.

Clean Series

Rack Position with Two Kettlebells

When cleaning two kettlebells, it is always a good idea to move your fingers out of the way as the kettlebells move into the rack position. It's never a question of "if" the kettlebell handles will collide together but "when." And when they do, you don't want any of your digits to be caught between them. Here are two techniques to keep your fingers safe:

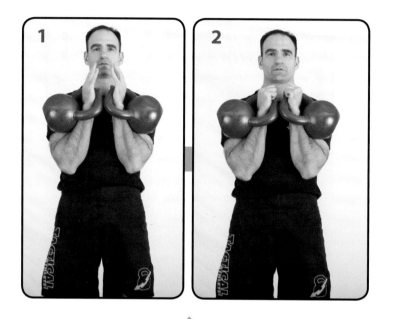

1) As your hands insert into the KB handles, extend your fingers.
2) As your hands insert into the KB handles, maintain grip with thumb and forefinger, but immediately tuck your last three digits (i.e., middle, ring, and little fingers) safely behind the handles.

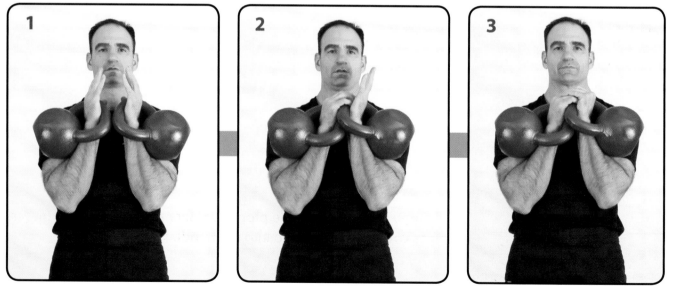

Men may overlap their grip if desired; women must keep the KB's to the sides of breasts.

(Rack Position for Women)

Depending on build, most women may have to adjust their rack position. Note: Thumbs stay inside or in line with bra or crop top straps. Do not allow them to drift any wider. Be sure to keep the armpits tight.

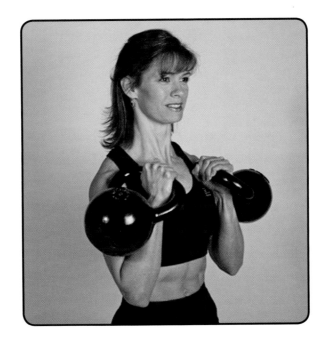

Double Rack Common Errors

✕ Common Error #1:
Smashing Fingers between Kettlebells

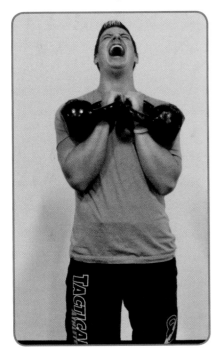

√ Corrective Action:
Keep your hands in the proper corners and extend your fingers as you insert your hand into the handles.

✕ Common Error #2: Elbows Disconnected from Torso

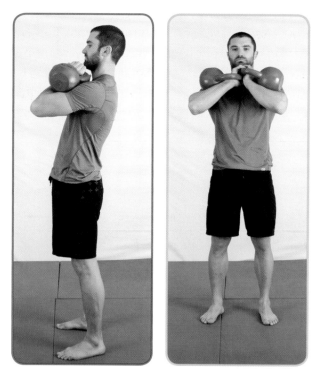

√ Corrective Action:

Verbal correction, rack holds, double sock drill.

✕ Common Error #3: Resting Kettlebells on Shoulders

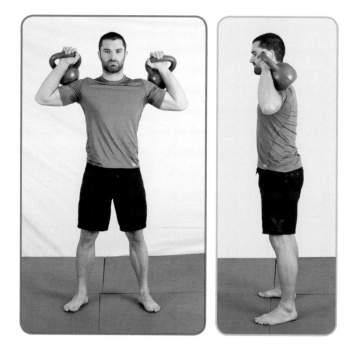

√ Corrective Action:

Verbal correction and rack holds for time.

The Front Squat

The front squat is an outstanding squatting exercise for sprinting athletes or athletes who sprint in their sport (i.e., football, rugby, lacrosse, or soccer). The front squat can be performed with one or two kettlebells. Front squats with two kettlebells are particularly demanding because the weight rests on your ribcage, which makes breathing more difficult. It also builds strength endurance in the shoulders and reinforces the ability to keep your hands up and elbows tight against your torso. All of which are particularly important skills for wrestlers, BJJ, and MMA athletes.

Front Squat: Standard

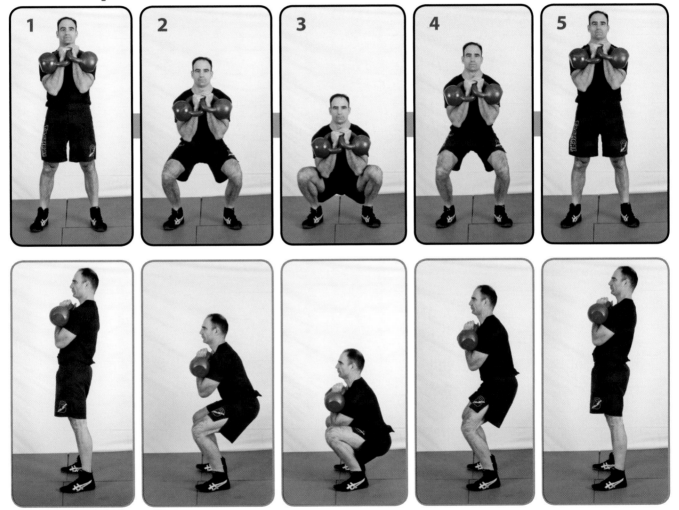

1) Clean two kettlebells to the rack position, elbows attached to torso. Adjust your stance (if necessary) where your heels are hip width or slightly wider. Toes point straight ahead or slightly to the outside and your weight is on your heels.
2) Start the descent by sticking your butt back while keeping your chest lifted up. Descend through your heels and fight the tendency to lean forward too much. Note: As your hips move back, your torso will break contact with your elbows. This is an important distinction. Do not lift your elbows up!
3) Continue to descend into the full squat position, hips below the knees. The descent should be slowed and stopped by the tightening of the glutes. Be sure your knees track in the direction that your feet are pointing.
4) Contract your glutes and drive off the heels to start the ascent. As you rise, try to extend your torso near vertical, reattaching your elbows to your torso.
5) Continue hip and leg extension, actively exhaling during the last half of the assent, until you're standing vertical with knees completely straight. Repeat for 3–5 reps. The value of kettlebell front squats is gained by doing reps, not singles.

Clean Series

Mobility Drills:

If your squats stink becEause you lack mobility in your ankles, knees, and hips, then you're not alone. Here are a few drills that will increase your ROM (range of motion):

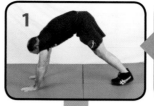
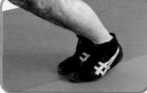
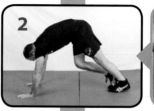
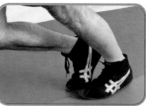
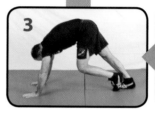
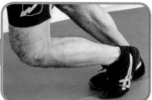

a. Ankle Flexion

1) Begin in a neutral stance, feet together. Bend over and place your palms on the ground. Walk your feet back until your legs are straight and you feel a slight stretch in your calf. Your weight is on your hands and the balls of your feet.

2–3) Alternate pressing your heels into the mat. As your ROM increases, slightly move your hands away from your feet. Repeat for desired number of reps.

b. Knee Extension/Flexion

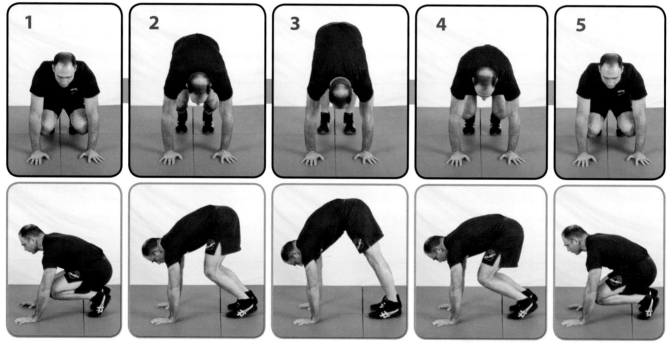

1) Begin in a neutral stance, feet together. Bend over and place your hands on the floor in front of your feet, knees flexed, weight on the balls of your feet.

2–3) Fully extend your legs until your knees are straight. If you can't straighten your legs, move your hands away from your toes until you can.

4–5) Rebend your knees to full flexion. Repeat for desired number of reps.

c. Knee Extension/Flexion (feet apart)

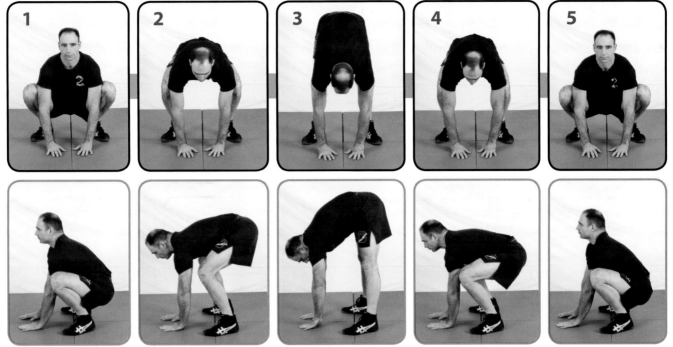

1) Stand erect, heels between hip and shoulder width apart, toes slightly pointed out. Keep your chest open, back straight, then squat down, placing the palms of your hands on the ground between your feet. As you squat be sure to open your hips and shift your weight to your heels. Ensure that your knees track in the same direction as your toes. Do not allow your knees to collapse inward; rather press them slightly outward when you squat.

2-3) Keeping your hands on the ground, fully extend your legs.

4-5) Return to the squat position (full flexion). Repeat for desired number of reps.

PNF Squat:

If the mobility drills aren't getting you as low as you desire, try the following exercise.

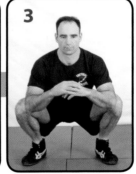

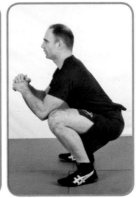

1) Perform a squat to your bottom position. Keep your chest up, back straight, weight on heels, and then place your elbows inside your knees. Inhale, contract your glutes, and press your knees against your elbows. Hold for 5–10 seconds.

2) Passively exhale (through your mouth), relax and allow your butt to drop toward your heels. Inhale, contract your glutes, and press your knees against your elbows. Hold for 5–10 seconds.

3) Passively exhale (through your mouth), relax and allow your butt to drop toward your heels. Inhale, contract your glutes, and press your knees against your elbows. Hold for 5–10 seconds. Repeat until you stop making ROM gains. Stand up and shake out any residual tension in your muscles.

Clean Series

Shoes:

Olympic weightlifting shoes, or a cheap pair of low-cut work boots that have a heel higher than the sole, can make a dramatic difference in the depth and efficiency of your squat. It's not a good idea to lift in a running shoe with a lifted heel. In kettlebell lifting, your feet don't move as much as in O'lifting. Sometimes when training in flats or barefoot, I place a piece of ¼-inch–½-inch thick hard rubber matting, plywood, or even 5-pound plates under my heels. It works in a pinch. A good quality pair of O'lifting shoes is ideal.

Single Kettlebell Front Squat

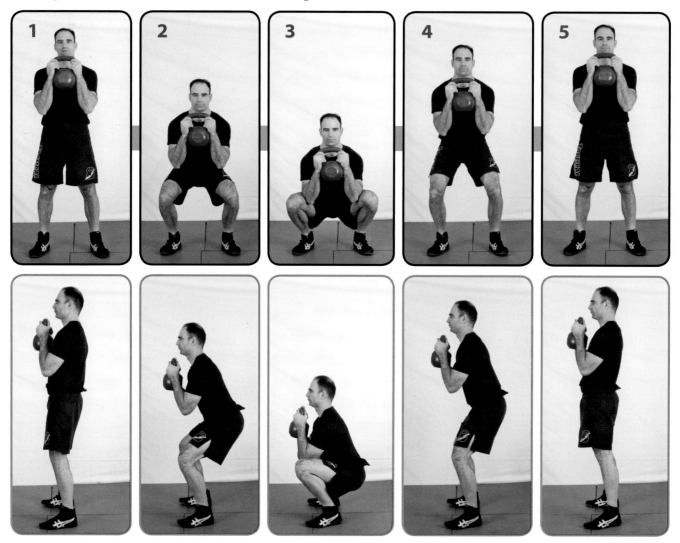

1) Hold a light kettlebell by the horns in front of your chest. Adjust your stance (if necessary) where your heels are hip width or slightly wider. Toes point straight ahead or slightly to the outside and your weight is on your heels.
2) Inhale through your nose, breathe deep into your lower abs, then begin the descent by sticking your butt back while keeping your chest lifted up. Descend through your heels and fight the tendency to lean forward too much. Note: As your hips move back, your torso will break contact with your elbows. Do not lift your elbows up!
3) Continue to descend into the full squat position, hips below the knees. The descent should be slowed and stopped by the tightening of the glutes. Be sure your knees track in the direction that your feet are pointing.
4) Contract your glutes and drive off your heels to start the assent. As you rise, try to extend your torso near vertical, reattaching your elbows to your torso.
5) Continue hip and leg extension, actively exhaling during the last half the assent, until you're standing vertical with knees completely straight. Repeat for 5–15 reps. The value of the kettlebell front squats is gained by doing reps.

Front Squat Common Errors

✕ Common Error #1:
Knees Forward, Weight on Balls of Feet

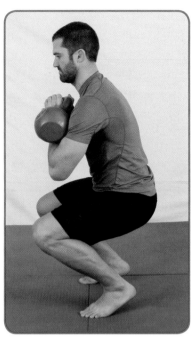

√ Corrective Action:
Wall Squats, Good Mornings, Box Squats.

✕ Common Error #2: Round Back
If your profile looks like a dog pooping in a field, it's wrong!

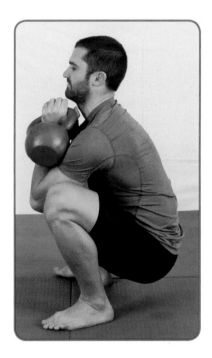

√ Corrective Action:
Wall Squats, Good mornings, box squats

✕ Common Error #3: Wide Rack, KBs on Shoulders

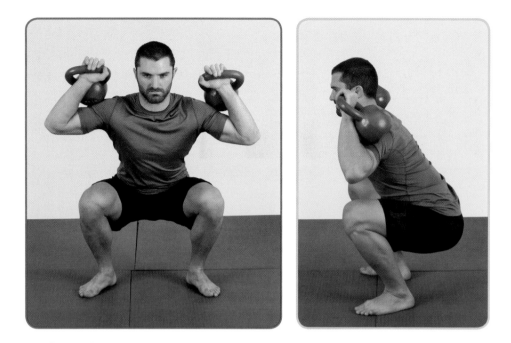

√ Corrective Action: Rack holds, stacking the handles.

Rx: Kettlebell Clean Combinations

The following drills will hone your skills and coordination as well as increase your metabolic conditioning.

Combo Drill #1: Dead Clean/Swing/Clean

This simple, yet demanding, combination of the dead clean, the one-arm swing, and (swing) clean will challenge your cardiovascular system.

1. Perform a dead clean.
2. Allow the kettlebell to swing between your legs, and then perform a one-arm swing.
3. Allow the kettlebell to swing between your legs again, and then immediately perform a traditional clean. Be sure to "dial down" the power for the traditional clean (you don't need as much power for the clean as for the swing), but make sure that you still extend your hips fully.
4. Place the kettlebell on the floor between your feet.
5. Switch hands and repeat the sequence.
6. Alternate hands after every combination.
7. Perform for sets or time.

Combo Drill #2: Squat Thrust/Clean/Swing/Clean

We're going to add one more element to pick up the pace for this combo.

1. Place a moderate-weight KB between your feet. Perform a squat thrust and then, keeping your arms straight from the squat thrust, inhale and pressurize your midsection.
2. Grab the KB handle with your right hand, drive it from the floor, and perform a dead clean, followed by a one-arm swing, and then a traditional clean. Return the KB to the floor between your feet.
3. Perform another squat thrust and repeat the dead clean/swing/clean sequence with your left hand.
4. Completing the combo with both hands equals 1 repetition. Perform 1 repetition every 30 seconds for 10 minutes.

Mastery of even just these few moves opens the door to a number of combinations you can do. Your goal should be to become "brilliant in the basics" and then begin to mix them up.

But there's nothing sacred about these particular groupings. Be creative about putting together new complexes of KB moves and about constructing varied workouts by combining them with other exercises in couplets, triplets, chippers, or any number of functional groupings. If thinking up new routines gives you a headache, then I would recommend my wife's Busy Woman Workout DVD Series. There are hundreds of routines that are in follow-along format with excellent coaching cues. No thinking is required, just plug and play!

Section 5
Overhead Series

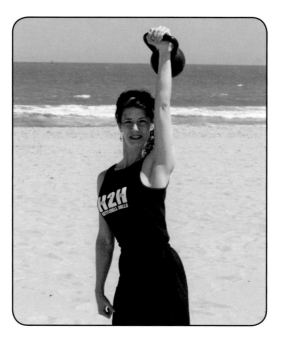

Overview

Typically people are weak when it comes to moving and stabilizing loads overhead. When I was first introduced to kettlebell training I was abnormally weak in this area. If my shoulder was going to dislocate, it would be when my arm was extended overhead. My range of motion was also pathetic. I can tell you from personal and professional experience: Kettlebells are the best shoulder rehab tool on the planet. If you did nothing but overhead kettlebell static holds, your shoulder strength, stability, and range of motion would improve dramatically. In addition to the TGU series, the overhead series is an essential part injury-proofing your shoulders.

In this section, you will learn how to perform the following kettlebell exercises:

Military press
Push-press
Thruster
Snatch

If you have any shoulder issues, be sure to build up your strength and flexibility practicing the military press. Do not be in a rush to perform the KB snatch. Take it one step at a time. There's solid reasoning why I left the snatch for last.

I. Military Press

Throughout history, the military press has been a classic test of strength. More importantly, the major benefit of pressing kettlebells is that it builds underlying muscular strength, stability, and flexibility needed for safely receiving the kettlebell overhead during more dynamic exercises such as the snatch.

The military press movement demonstrated below is the most efficient because the vertical path of the kettlebell is identical to that of the push press and jerk. The hand angle of the finish, or top, position is the same as finish position of the TGU, push press, jerk, and snatch. This is a full-range of motion exercise, similar to performing a handstand push-up on a set of parallel bars.

Begin with a light kettlebell and practice the following movement.

I. Military Press

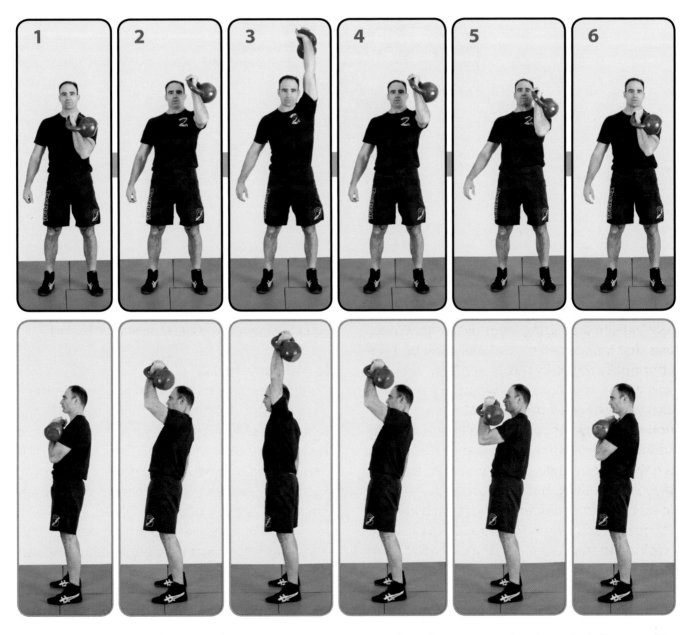

1) Clean the kettlebell to the rack position. The press starts and stops in the rack position. Your hand must be below your chin, upper arm attached to your torso, and your thumb attached to your collarbone.
2) Keeping the same hand angle, begin to press the kettlebell up and off your chest. Keep your forearm vertical and thumb pointing toward your body.
3) Continue pressing in a vertical path straight overhead. Note side view KB path (between toe/heel) and hand position.
4) Reverse the motion, pulling your elbow straight down. Note slight counterbalance (i.e., lean) on initial descent.
5) Continue pulling your elbow down toward your side.
6) Reestablish the rack position.

Key Points of Top Position

The following key points are important for safe and effective training. Repetition establishes habit. The top position of the military press is the same top position of the TGU, push press, and snatch. It is important to get it correct, stable, and comfortable in this position.

- Arm is straight (elbow locked)
- Wrist is straight
- Thumb points toward the rear (not the side)
- Handle 45 degrees across palm, low on wrist

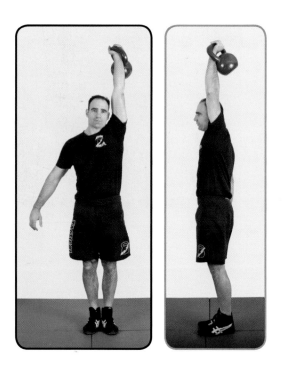

A good strategy for developing a solid top position is to practice static holds. Static holds will safely and effectively build tremendous amounts of shoulder strength, endurance, and flexibility. Vary your time and intensity. Start with a light weight and hold overhead for 30–60 seconds. Do one or two sets as a warm-up prior to any overhead training. This is time well invested. Your shoulders will thank you for it later.

Common Errors at the Top Position
What's wrong with these pictures?

Palm is facing out. Notice how the kettlebell is directly over Glenn's head. This position puts a lot of load on the triceps and will eventually cause muscle failure and the elbow to unlock.

√ Corrective Action:

Externally rotate your thumb more toward the rear. A 45-degree angle is about right. It reduces muscular stress on the triceps and provides better mechanical alignment and bone support.

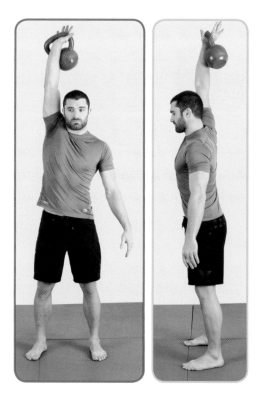

✕ Common Error #1: Too Wide

Arm is angled out to the side. This may be due to an old injury or lack of flexibility.

√ Corrective Action:

Static holds will strengthen and increase flexibility over time. Don't rush the result.

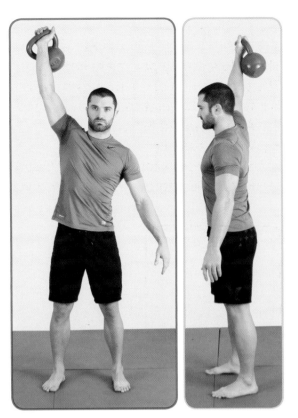

✕ Common Error #2: Bent Wrist

Handle is high in the hand, causing the wrist to bend—not good!

√ Corrective Action:

Adjust kettlebell in the rack position so that it lies diagonally across the palm of your hand.

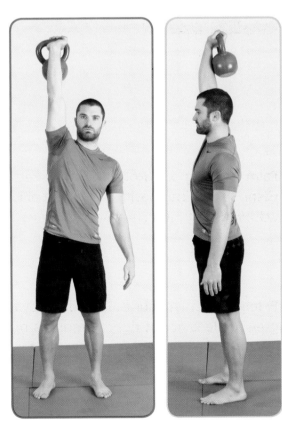

Overhead Series

Now that you have fixed the top position common errors, let's go back and practice the military press with a light weight until you have consistency of movement. Once your movement is consistently correct, it's time to introduce the high-tension techniques.

High-Tension Techniques

The following high-tension drills will dramatically increase the safety, stability, and effectiveness of your military press. The principles of neuromuscular recruitment as outlined below can be effectively transferred to a multitude of strength exercises such as: weighted pull-ups, handstand presses, deadlifts, and so on. Correctly implemented, these techniques should result in new PRs (personal records). Equally important, it's a very safe way to train during near maximal efforts.

I am convinced that whoever came up with the "no pain, no gain" slogan was a twenty-year-old. Now that I'm in my mid-forties with the mileage of an eighty-five-year-old, if I can train with no pain, that's gain in my book. I first learned these techniques from Pavel Tsatsouline in late 1999. At that time, I was contemplating changing careers. My shoulders were trashed from three surgeries and over thirty dislocations, I had meniscus removed twice from my right knee, ACL reconstructed on my left, and a whacky fall on concrete left my lower back a bit unstable. The fact of the matter is, as I began to practice and apply these high-tension muscle-recruitment techniques to the military press, then later to the deadlift and pull-up, I would notice the pain disappear. Interestingly enough, just by focusing on generating maximum tension I would end up lifting more weight with less or no pain.

If you take the time to learn and apply these techniques, the absolute "worst" thing that can happen to you when you are lifting near-maximum loads is that you will hit a "sticking point," stall, then put the weight down. That's it . . . a sticking point, a failed lift. Not a catastrophic injury!

Adding Tension

The best way to practice is to find a kettlebell that you can military press for no more than 4 or 5 reps. You want a weight that's heavy enough so that you have to struggle to get that fifth rep. Once you find that weight, perform 2 military presses for each arm, to establish a baseline, then put the weight down and rest for 1 minute. Then perform 2 more reps, following the instructions of Drill #1. Rest 1 minute. Then follow Drill #2, rest 1 minute and repeat this cycle until you've finished every drill. Pay attention and notice how your body is responding and your exertion from drill to drill. There should be a noticeable difference from Drill #1 to Drill #5. Remember, it's the details that make the difference. Engage your mind and engage your muscles!

Baseline: Clean the Kettlebell to the Rack Position
- Perform two military presses per arm, then place the kettlebell on the floor.
- Rest 1 minute.

Note: While you're resting, reflect on what you are doing and why. Make sure your pressing mechanics are correct, analyze how your body feels, and note the perceived exertion of the lift.

Tension Drill #1:
From the Rack Position (tight fists and armpit)

- Simultaneously squeeze the handle of the kettlebell, make a tight (i.e., white knuckle) fist with your free hand, then crush an imaginary tennis ball in the armpit of your free arm. This action will actively recruit the muscles of the lats, pecs, and shoulder, making the lift easier and safer.
- Once tight, immediately press the kettlebell overhead and then return to the rack, relax for a second, then tighten back up and press for your second rep. Keep in mind, you are practicing the skill of generating tension.
- Repeat sequence with the kettlebell in your other hand.
- Rest 1 minute.

Tension Drill #2:
From the Rack Position (tighten your base)

- Grip the floor with your toes, and contract your quads, hamstrings, and glutes.
- Simultaneously squeeze the KB handle, make a tight fist with your free hand, and squeeze an imaginary tennis ball or clip book in the armpit of your free arm.
- Once you're tight, immediately press the kettlebell overhead and then return to the rack, relax for a second, then tighten back up and press for your second rep.
- Repeat sequence with your other hand.
- Rest 1 minute

Note: Tightening your glutes is key! It's the biggest muscle group in your body and will always carry over to a positive strength gain.

Drill #3:
From the Rack Position (tighten pelvic floor and actively exhale)

- Grip the floor with your toes, contract your quads, hamstrings, and glutes, and contract the muscles of the pelvic floor. Women would know this maneuver as the Kegal exercise.
- Simultaneously squeeze the KB handle, make a tight fist with your free hand, and squeeze an imaginary tennis ball or clip book in the armpit of your free arm.
- Once you're tight, actively exhale through your teeth and shorten your abs as you press the kettlebell overhead. Abs and glutes must be tight! Return to the rack, relax for a second, then tighten back up and press for your second rep.
- Repeat sequence with your other hand.
- Rest 1 minute.

Note: The combination of "pulling up" the muscles of the pelvic floor, actively exhaling, and shortening the abs results in greater neuromuscular stimulation and force production.

Drill #4: From the Rack Position (heels together)

- Place your heels together, assuming the position of attention.
- Grip the floor with your toes; press your heels together, contracting the muscles of your inner thighs; contract your quads, hamstrings, and glutes; and contract the muscles of the pelvic floor.
- Simultaneously squeeze the KB handle, make a tight fist with your free hand, and squeeze an imaginary tennis ball or clip book in the armpit of your free arm.
- Once you're tight, actively exhale, shorten your abs as you press the kettlebell overhead, and then return to the rack. Relax for a second, then tighten back up and press for your second rep.
- Safety: Be sure to widen your stance back to hip width when you switch the kettlebell from one hand to the other. You'll only forget once; it's a self-correcting error.

Note: Did you notice the weight went up straighter and easier? If not, do it again. Your balance should have improved, also.

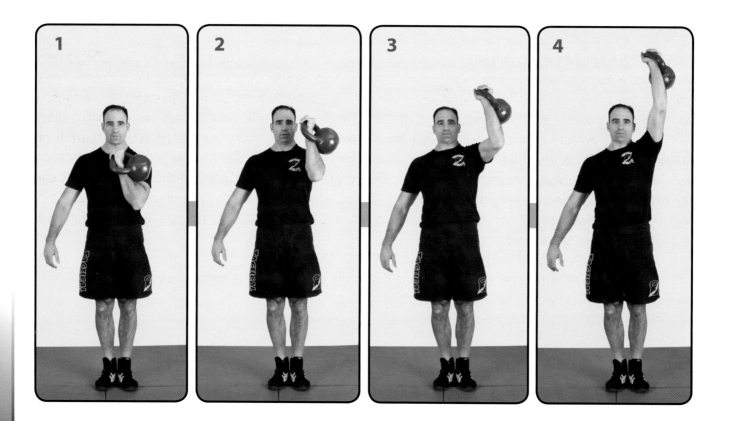

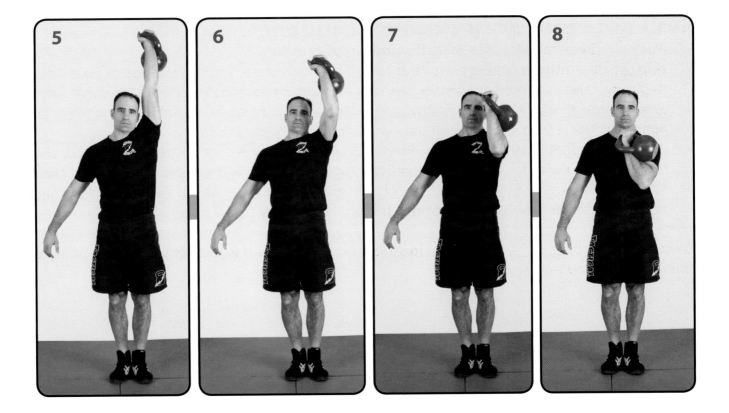

Skill Transfer

One of the biggest reasons for practicing the MP from the position of attention, besides safely pressing more weight, is skill transfer. Watch gymnasts when they perform handstands, L-sits, levers, muscle-ups, and so on. Notice how they keep their feet together, point their toes (recruits more muscle besides being aesthetically pleasing), and tighten their abs and butt, i.e., the "hollow position." There is not a loose muscle on their body. They know how to turn it on (maximally contract) and turn it off (maximally relax) at exactly the right time.

The body position, arm movements, and tension techniques executed in the military press can be effectively applied to weighted pull-ups. As a matter of fact, I would go so far as to say that every time you practice the military press, you should practice your weighted pull-ups. Together they create optimum muscle balance.

Drill #5: From Rack Position (gripper)

- Place a gripper in you free hand (a tennis ball would work also).
- Grip the floor with your toes; press your heels together, contracting the muscles of your inner thighs; contract your quads, hamstrings, and glutes; and contract the muscles of the pelvic floor.
- Simultaneously squeeze the KB handle; make a tight fist with your free hand, crushing the gripper; and squeeze an imaginary tennis ball or clip book in the armpit of your free arm.
- Once you're tight, actively exhale, shorten your abs as you press the kettlebell overhead, and then return to the rack. Relax for a second, then tighten back up and press for your second rep.

Note: Using a gripper is a good way to overcome a sticking point. Use it every once in a while, you don't need to make it a crutch.

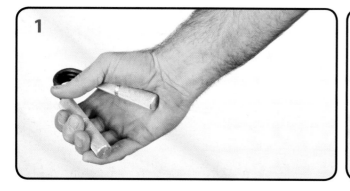
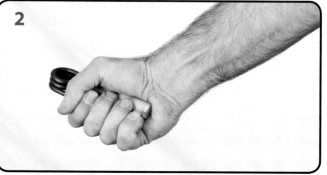

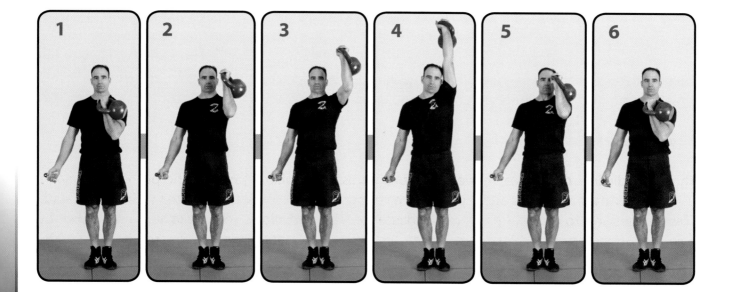

Military Press Rx

Here are two simple yet effective strength routines. Perform the warm-up, and then practice the exercises in a circuit-training format.

Routine #1

Warm-up: One-arm overhead static hold 30–60 seconds (light-medium weight)

3–5 rounds of 3–5 reps:
- Deadlift (barbell, bands, KB)
- One-arm military press (right, then left)
- Weighted pull-ups, palms facing away (scale up or down to get your reps)
- Rest 1–2 minutes, and then repeat for desired number of rounds

Routine #2

Warm-up: Double KB overhead static hold 30–60 seconds (light-medium)

3–5 rounds of 3–5 reps:
- Double KB front squat, pause, military press (no momentum)
- Weighted pull-ups (scale up or down to get your reps)
- Rest 3–5 minutes, and then repeat

Remember: The goal is not muscle fatigue. Lift as heavy as possible, staying as fresh as possible, as often as possible.

II. Push Press

There is a distinct difference between the push press and military press. In the push press, you're using power from your legs and hips, not the strength of your arms, to move the weight overhead. This enables you to move heavier weight overhead. This also allows you to move the same weight overhead more times, building muscular endurance and increasing metabolic conditioning. Endurance is defined as the ability to bear fatigue, working as long as possible at a given intensity. This is where the kettlebell really shines, because it is a strength endurance tool.

Push Press

Get a moderate to heavy kettlebell and practice the following movement.

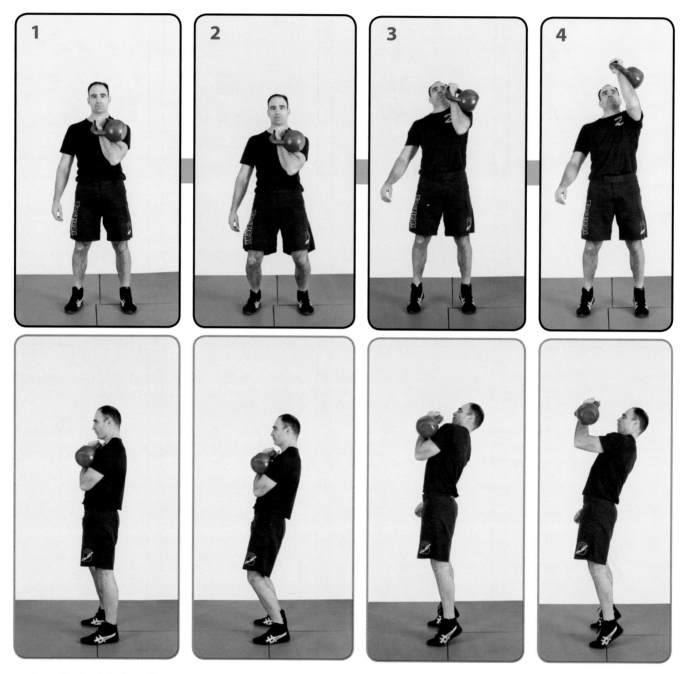

1) Clean the kettlebell to the rack position. The push press starts and stops in the rack position. Your hand must be below your chin, your upper arm attached to your torso, and your thumb attached to your collarbone.

2) Perform a slight knee dip. The knees unlock, dropping the hips straight down, weight stays on your heels, and arms stay connected to your torso.

3-4) Drive off your heels, rapidly straightening your legs and leading with your chest. This is what gives the kettlebell the upward acceleration, not your arms. Keep your arms as relaxed as possible. Note: The hand angle stays the same as the kettlebell lifts up and off your chest.

5) Your forearm remains vertical and your thumb is still pointing toward your body.

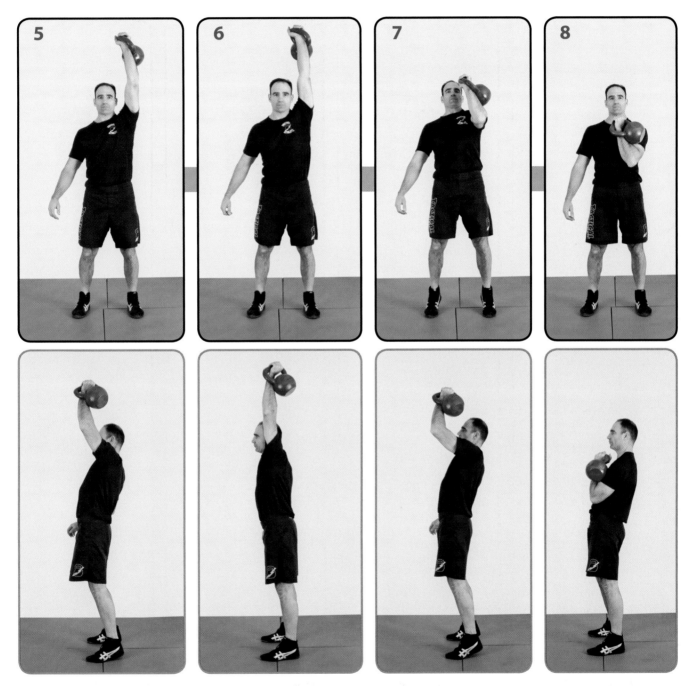

6) As the kettlebell passes your head, push your chest through to the upright position, straightening your arm and locking the kettlebell overhead. Note: The vertical path of the kettlebell is straight overhead.

7) Lower the kettlebell to rack position by simultaneously unlocking your elbow and leaning your torso slightly backward. As the kettlebell begins to descend, rise up on your toes to meet the bell halfway.

8) As the kettlebell touches your upper chest, slightly flex your knees to soften the impact. Repeat for desired time or reps.

Overhead Series

Skills and Drills

Dip and Drive Drill

Initially, one of the hardest things to learn in the push press is to relax your arms and to actually drive the weight up overhead with your legs, through your heels, instead of your arms. Here's how the drill works:

- Clean one KB to the rack position.
- Perform a quick dip and drive, keeping your arm totally relaxed. Just see how high you can get the kettlebell. Don't try to lock overhead at this point.
- Repeat the dip and drive sequence a second time. Trying to drive the kettlebell higher.
- Repeat one more time, but this time when the kettlebell reaches its apex, push your chest forward and straighten your arm, locking the KB overhead.
- Repeat entire drill for as many reps as you can in good form. Think: "Dip-drive, dip-drive, dip-drive then lock it out."
- Change arms and do it again.

Practice this drill first with one then two kettlebells. Stay focused on keeping the arms relaxed. Don't try to push the weight up or decelerate it on the way down. Use your legs like shock absorbers. Think "though your heels." Quickly exhale when you dip and quickly inhale as you extend. Inhaling as you extend helps expand your chest, which in turn helps launch the bells off your torso. When the kettlebells come back down, you exhale on contact, allowing your knees to bend followed by a quick inhale and extension, repeating the cycle again.

Push Press Rx

The push press can be used with one or two kettlebells. To keep it simple for now, we'll use just one.

Routine #1

3 rounds of:

One-arm military press (right) as many reps in perfect form, stopping 1 or 2 reps before muscle failure. Immediately followed by:

One-arm push press (right), as many reps as possible.

One-arm military press (left), as many reps in perfect form as possible, stopping 1 or 2 reps before muscle failure. Immediately followed by:

One-arm push press (left) as many reps as possible.

Rest 1–2 minutes, repeat.

Routine #2

For Time:

10 clean and push press (right), (i.e., each clean and push press = 1 rep)

10 clean and push press (left)

Repeat 10 times (100 reps per arm)

III. Thruster

The thruster is a combination of the front squat and push press, and it is a beloved exercise in Cross-Fit. It is normally performed with a barbell. However, use two kettlebells as a substituted for a barbell if a barbell is not available or just for variation. If you only have one kettlebell then you can perform one-arm thrusters, switching hands every 10 reps.

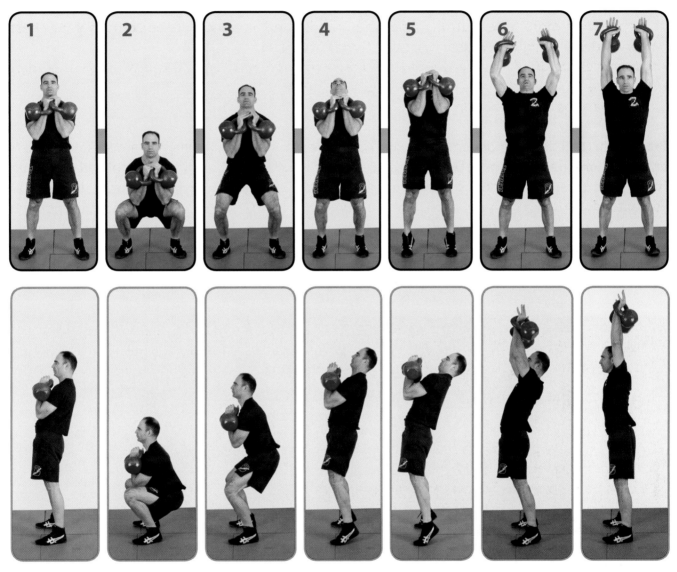

1) Perform a double kettlebell clean. Stack the handles in the rack position, and then adjust your feet to a proper width for squatting.
2) Inhale, then perform a front squat. Make sure your weight stays over your heels and you open your hips and knees as you descend. Tighten your abs and glutes as you reach the bottom position.
3) Immediately drive off your heels, extending your legs and hips.
4) Be sure to reattach your elbows by the time you reach the quarter squat position.
5) At this point, switch to a high gear and explode off your heels, fully extending your hips and legs as you lead with your chest. This action will propel the weight off your chest.
6) As the weight launches above your head, slightly lean forward.
7) Continue pushing your chest forward and lock your arms straight overhead. Be sure your palms are not flat but rather pointing behind you at approx 45 degrees. Perform for time or reps.

Avoid this silliness . . .

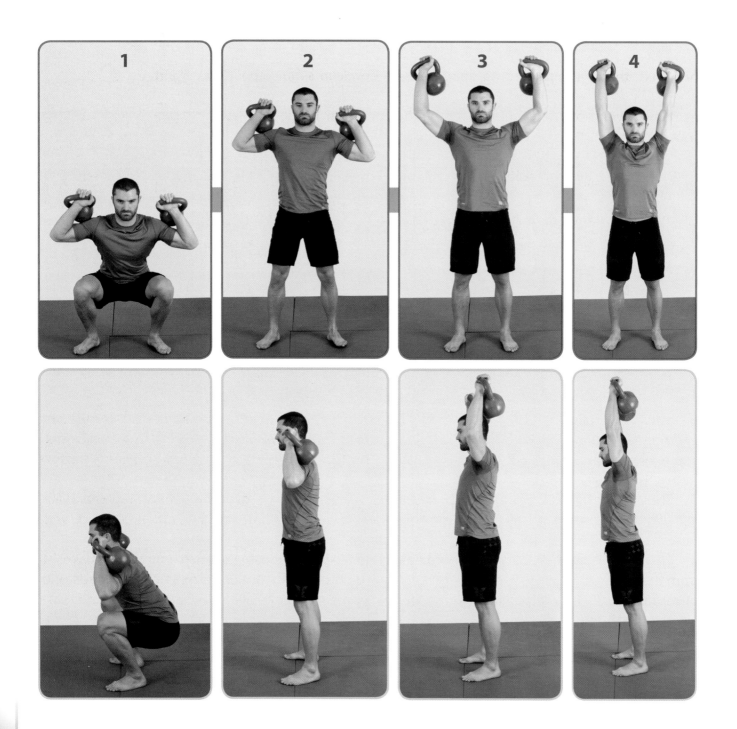

Thruster Rx

"Fran" is one of CrossFit's benchmark workouts. It's normally performed with 95 pounds on a barbell. Kettlebell Fran is performed with two 36-pound kettlebells. Even though it's 23 pounds lighter than the prescribed weight, your times should be about the same. On the other hand, Fran performed with two 53-pound kettlebells is only 11 pounds heavier than the prescribed barbell weight, but it will about double your normal Fran time. Give it a try and remember the definition of CrossFit: "constantly varied, functional movement, executed at high intensity."

KB Fran

21-15-9 for time:
Kettlebell thrusters (two 16 kg kettlebells)
Pull-ups
(Exercise sequence = 21 KB thrusters, 21 pull-ups, 15 KB thrusters, 15 pull-ups, 9 KB thrusters, 9 pull-ups)
(Do as many reps in good form as possible; if needed, break sets down into digestible parts, time stops when all numbers are completed.)

IV. Snatch

The snatch is a graceful total-body exercise that builds outstanding muscular and cardio-respiratory endurance. It builds resiliency in the entire posterior chain (i.e., abdominal muscles, trunk extensors, and hip joint muscles) as well as the shoulders, forearms, and fingers. It basically works every muscle from your nose to your toes.

The athleticism developed in practicing the snatch has positive carryover to most sports and life activities. It is interesting to note that in the former Soviet armed forces, the kettlebell snatch was tested instead of push-ups.

The kettlebell snatch is a highly coordinated and technical movement where you take the weight from the end of the back swing to overhead in one uninterrupted motion. The snatch is the capstone of kettlebell exercises. It is built upon the solid foundation of movements we have learned and mastered up to this point.

- The one-arm swing is a major assistance exercise to get the kettlebell to the proper height and angle for the hand insertion.
- The method of hand insertion is practiced when performing kettlebell cleans.
- The arm movement of the two-hand swing release and H2H switch applies to the arm movement of the snatch.
- The top position of the military press and push press, is the same finish position of the snatch.

This is why I consider the snatch the capstone of kettlebell exercises. It's a coordinated summary of all these skills. That is also why I choose to teach it last.

Snatch (Standard)

Let's take a look at the entire movement, and then we'll break it down and practice one element at a time.

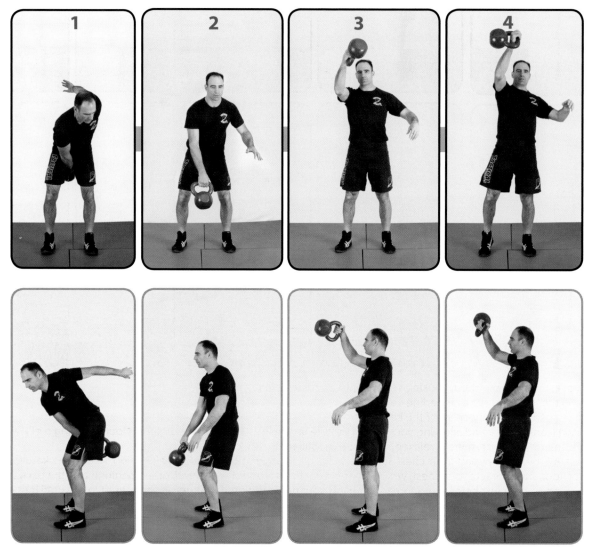

1) Assume a good starting position and perform a back swing.
2) Drive off your heels and extend your legs and torso. At this point the kettlebell is just below waist level. To add acceleration to the KB, pull the working shoulder quickly backward.
3) As the kettlebell accelerates upward, make sure your hand rotates to a 45-degree angle (thumbs up) and relax your grip. The kettlebell should continue to accelerate up above head height. At this point:
4) Quickly straighten your arm, inserting your hand deep into the KB handle. This action pushes the kettlebell onto your arm. It should land soft like a feather.
5) Do not change your hand angle when you straighten your arm! All movement must cease when the kettlebell reaches the top position. Wrist should be straight, thumb pointing back. There should be absolutely no hand turning or twisting in the top position.
6) Pause for a second, assess the situation. To lower the kettlebell:
7) Turn the hand holding the bell so that the thumb rotates away from the free arm as you simultaneously turn your torso and lean backward. The benefits of this combined action are:

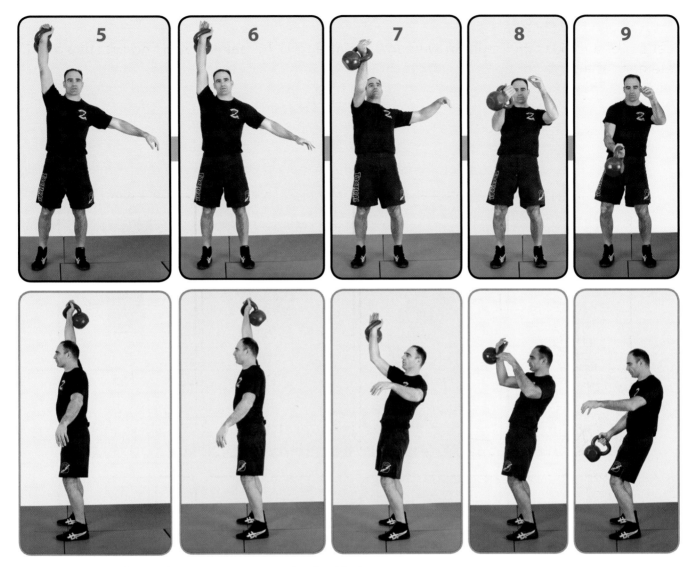

- It unlocks the elbow without causing stress on the shoulder joint.
- Orients the kettlebell for a centerline descent.
- Decreases the trajectory or arc of the kettlebell.

8) Continue leaning back and allowing your hand to rotate until you're looking at your palm. Notice the angle of the elbow is greater than 90 degrees, hand is relaxed, and handle is still set low across the palm.

9) As the kettlebell moves past your chest, allow your hand to rotate to the thumbs-up position. Regrip the kettlebell as the back of your arm contacts your chest, which is when your hand is about waist level, or the beginning of the back swing.

10) Pull your hips back just before your forearm impacts your pelvic region. The thumb continues to rotate until it points backward at the end of the back swing.

11) From the back swing, repeat. To facilitate learning and coordination, it's better to practice multiple sets of low reps with light weight (8–12 kg). This will prevent fatigue and bad habits.

Part 1: Lowering the Kettlebell (aka the drop)

At this point, everybody should be comfortable pressing or push-pressing the kettlebell overhead and holding the top position. From this point we'll focus on the technique of lowering the kettlebell into the back swing. Essentially, we'll learn how to snatch from the top down. Once that is mastered, we'll learn it from the bottom up. Be sure to use a light kettlebell (8–12 kg) to master the movements and to get the proper timing. Strive for mechanical competency and consistency before adding intensity.

There are various ways to lower the kettlebell from the top position. I've experimented with different methods throughout my ten-plus years of kettlebell lifting. I have come to the conclusion that the method presented below is one of the most efficient and causes the least amount of trauma to the body. This method of lowering the kettlebell closely resembles the technique used by most Russian professional kettlebell lifters.

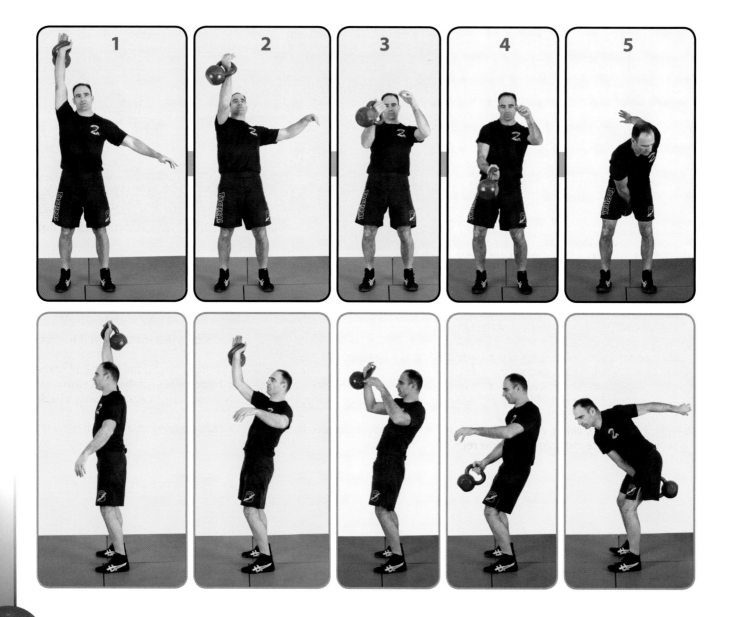

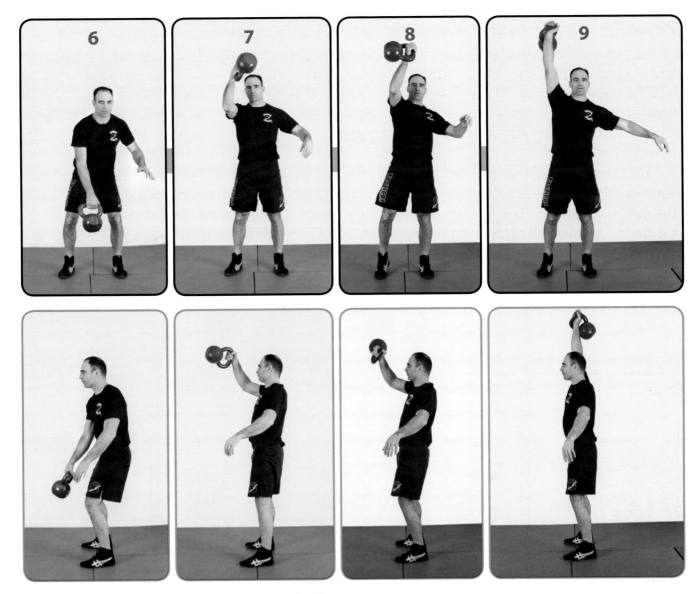

1) Choose a light kettlebell, clean it and press it overhead.
2) Turn the hand holding the bell so that the thumb rotates away from the free arm as you simultaneously turn your torso and lean backward. The benefits of this combined action are:
   • It unlocks the elbow without causing stress on the shoulder joint.
   • Orients the kettlebell for a centerline descent.
   • Decreases the trajectory or arc of the kettlebell.
3) Continue leaning back and allowing your hand to rotate until you're looking at your palm. Notice that the angle of the elbow is greater than 90 degrees, hand is relaxed, and handle is still set low across the palm.
4) As the kettlebell moves past your chest, allow your hand to rotate to the thumbs-up position. Regrip the kettlebell as the back of your arm contacts your chest, which is when your hand is about waist level, or the beginning of the back swing.
5) Pull your hips back just before your forearm impacts your pelvic region. The thumb continues to rotate until it points backward at the end of the back swing.
6–9) From the back swing, clean and press, and then repeat practicing the drop. To facilitate learning and coordination, it's better to practice multiple sets of low reps to prevent fatigue.

Overhead Series

Lowering the Kettlebell: Common Errors

✕ Common Error #1: Pitching

Pitching is caused by keeping the arm locked straight and allowing the kettlebell to be thrown over the top of the forearm. It's inefficient and can cause unnecessary stress to the shoulder, elbow, and back. This error is usually a result of learning it wrong the first time.

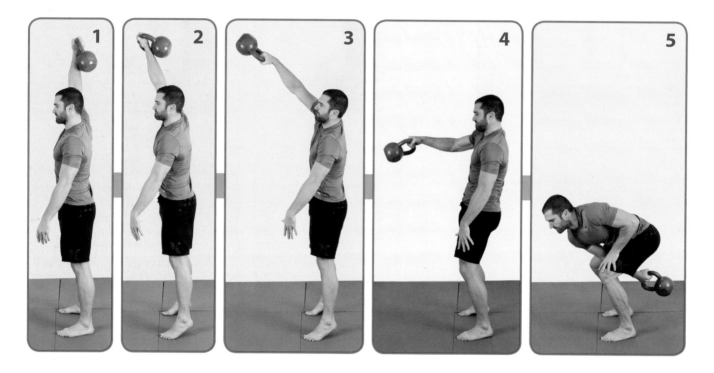

√ Corrective Action:

1) Dry fire drill (i.e., without the weight). Review the photos and go through the steps, one by one, without a kettlebell. Concentrate on getting the hand motion, arm angle, backward lean and timing of the hips correct.

2) Face-the-wall drill:
Practice the lowering drill with a kettlebell while standing in front of a solid wall. The wall is an awesome training tool. It forces you to do the right thing to avoid smacking it with the kettlebell. Be sure to practice with both arms, keep the reps low and switch arms before getting tired.
 1) Distance check from wall: one arm's length
 2) Clean and press the KB overhead,
 3) Slight turn, unlock arm, slightly lean back
 4) Keep elbow at 90 degrees or greater
 5) Regrip the handle as your hand internally rotates
 6) Pull your hips back at the last second and transition to a nice smooth (not jerky) back swing. Repeat sequence for a few reps

Face The Wall Drill

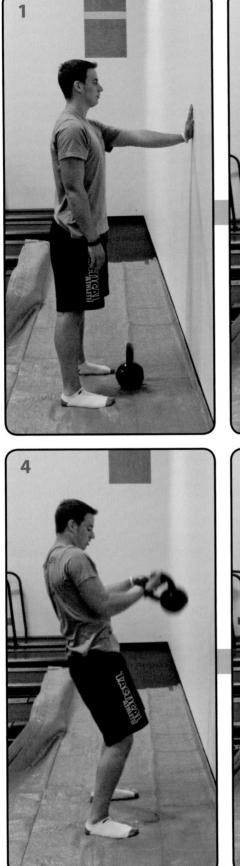

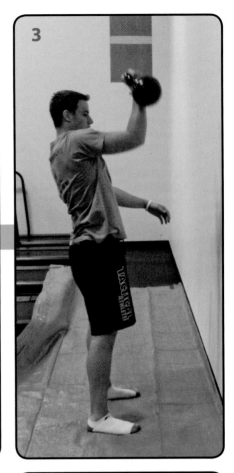

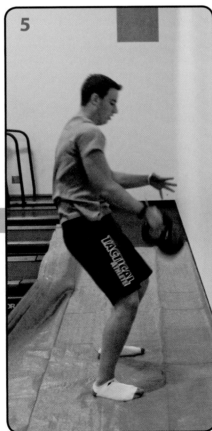

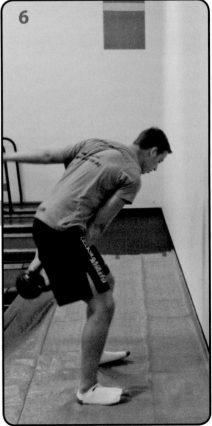

✗ Common Error #2: Around the World

Instead of guiding the kettlebell down the centerline, the kettlebell moves out to the side. This action puts your shoulder in an undesirable position and increases the chances of the bell clipping the inside of your knee . . . ouch!

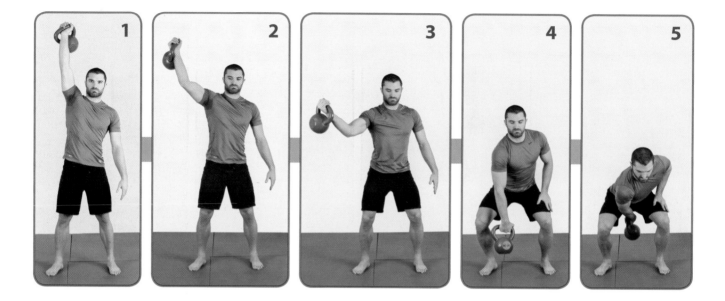

√ Corrective Actions:

1) Practice in front of a full-length mirror. You will see for yourself exactly where your alignment is or isn't. Tip: Stand several feet from the mirror.

Wall Drill: Left/Right

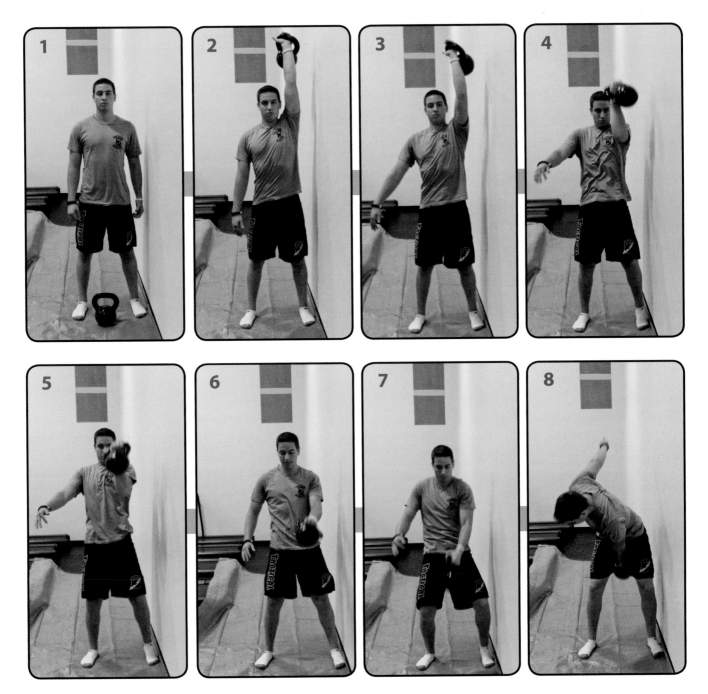

Wall drill: left/right

1) Stand next to a solid wall. The side of the foot closest to the wall needs to be touching the wall.

2) Grip the kettlebell with the hand that corresponds with the foot touching the wall, then clean and press it overhead.

3) Slightly turn, unlock arm, slightly lean back.

4) Keep elbow at 90 degrees or greater, palm facing you.

5) Guide the kettlebell down your centerline.

6) Regrip the handle as your hand internally rotates.

7) Wait until the last second to pull your hips back.

8) Transition to a nice smooth (not jerky) back swing.

The wall is a great motivation tool and incentive to keep the kettlebell in line.

Overhead Series

Part 2: Accelerating the KB Overhead

Acceleration is the name of the game to get the correct height for the snatch. Establish a solid foundation in the one-arm swing. Mastering the snatch is only a matter of minutes once a student has mastered the one-arm swing.

Let's do a quick review of the one-arm swing and then take it to the finish position.

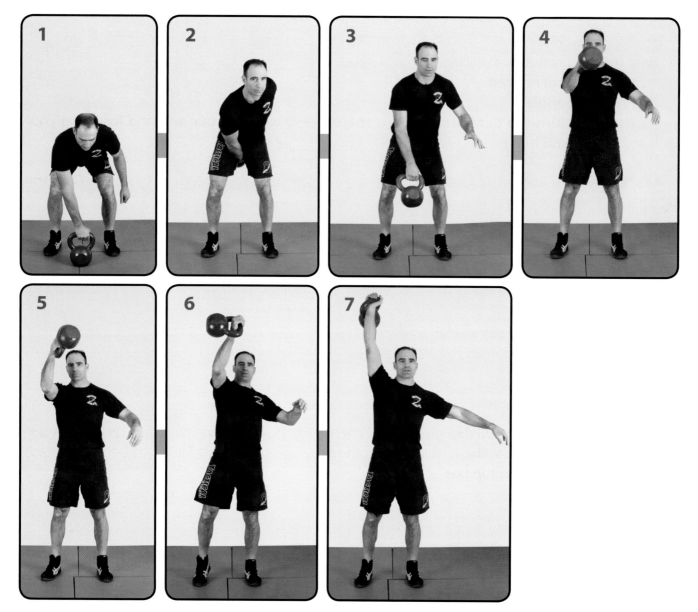

1) Assume a good starting position.
2) Perform a back swing.
3) Drive off your heels, extending your legs and torso. At this point the kettlebell is just below waist level. To add acceleration to the KB, pull the working shoulder quickly backward.
4) As the kettlebell accelerates upward, make sure your hand rotates to a 45-degree angle (thumbs up) and relax your grip. That's your swing review! Now let's follow through to the overhead position:
5) The kettlebell should continue to accelerate up above head height. At this point:
6) Quickly straighten your arm, inserting your hand deep into the KB handle. This action pushes the kettlebell onto your arm. It should land soft like a feather.
7) Do not change your hand angle when you straighten your arm! All movement must cease when the kettlebell reaches the top position. Wrist should be straight, thumb pointing back. There should be absolutely no hand turning or twisting in the top position. Pause for a second, assess the situation, and then lower the kettlebell. Repeat for desired time or reps.

Drills and Skills:

Timing and sequencing is the key. The following exercises show different practice combinations to reinforce the mechanics of accelerating the kettlebell to the optimum height and angle, making for an easier "hand insertion," softer landing, and minimal stress on your shoulder.

Drill #1: One-arm swings (high): It is very helpful at this stage to practice a series of 2–3 one-arm swings to maximum height, just above your head. Focus on:
- **The acceleration pull**
- **Keeping the kettlebell centerline**
- **Keeping the arm relaxed**
- **Correct hand angle**
- **Immediately turn the third swing into a snatch by extending your arm and inserting your hand into the KB handle**

Drill #2: One-arm swing (high), then snatch. Alternate one-arm high swing, then snatch. One-arm high swing, then snatch.

Drill #3: Practice in succession 1 one-arm low swing (just below waist level), 1 one-arm high swing, and then 1 snatch to lockout over head.

Common Acceleration Errors:

✗ Common Error #1: Pulling High Right/Left

Pulling with the elbow will pull the trajectory of the kettlebell off the centerline axis. This was a common method of teaching the "high-pull" back in the day. It's inefficient and not best because it leads to a wide, out-of-alignment top position.

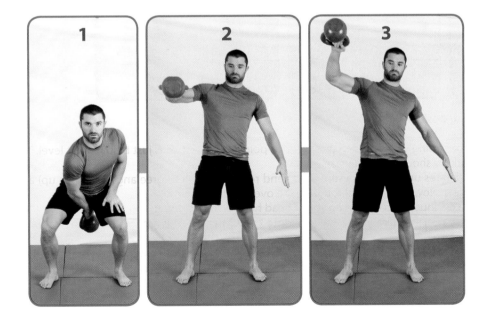

√ Corrective Action:

1) Pull the shoulder back, instead of your elbow. Keep your arm relaxed.

2) Perform snatches standing next to the wall

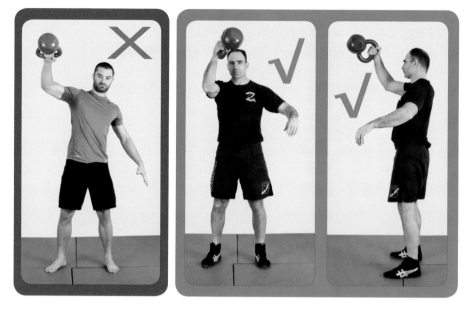

✗ Common Error #2: Curling and Pressing

To make up for lack of power and acceleration; some folks tend to turn the snatch into an awkward combination of a half-swing and half curl and press overhead.

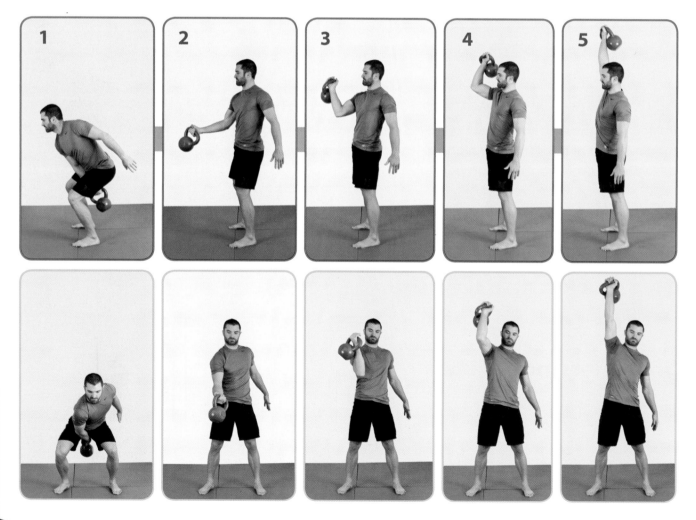

√ Corrective Actions:

1) Practice one-arm swings.
2) Practice one-arm high swings.
3) Practice one-arm high swing–snatch combination.
4) Practice low swing–high swing–snatch combination.

Snatch Top Position Common Errors:
What's wrong with these pictures?

Thumb pointed sideways not back

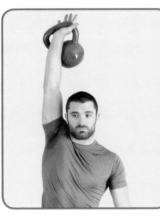 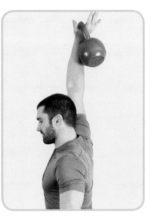

Wide top position

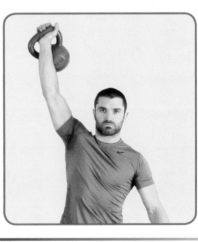 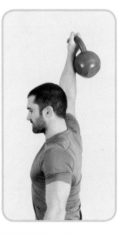

Shoulders not squared

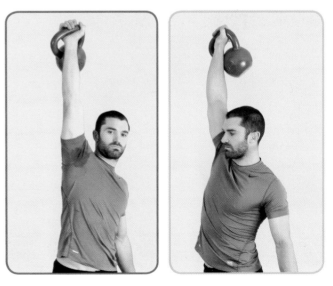

Bent wrist

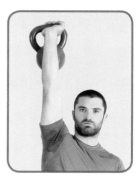

Snatch Rx

Personally, I wouldn't be in a big rush to snatch heavy kettlebells. Keep your training light and happy. Concentrate on proper technique and all will be right in your world. As part of your warm-up, after joint mobility drills, you can work in a few sets of light and easy snatches. Start with at least one set of overhead static holds, then 3 sets of 10 snatches each arm with a light weight. You can finish with one set of 5–10 reps of a medium weight, then move on to your real workout.

Listed below are three simple snatch routines. Feel free to scale as needed.

Routine #1:

10 rounds x 10 reps (each arm) for time:
10 snatches right, switch, 10 snatches left = 1 set

Routine #2:

AMRAP (as many reps as possible) in 10 minutes

Routine #3:

50, 40, 30, 20, 10 (each arm) for time with a 1-minute rest in between sets
Note: the key to building work capacity is work. A strategy to increase your work capacity and reduce the chance of injury is to switch to an easier exercise and keep moving. For example: If you are starting to struggle with the snatch, shorten the movement and turn it into a clean. If your clean gets ugly, change it to a one-arm low swing. If your grip starts to fail, then switch hands every rep. If that becomes too tiring, try a two-arm swing. If you're too smoked, just put the bell down and finish your numbers with jumping jacks.

Section 6
Kettlebell Rx
Program Design

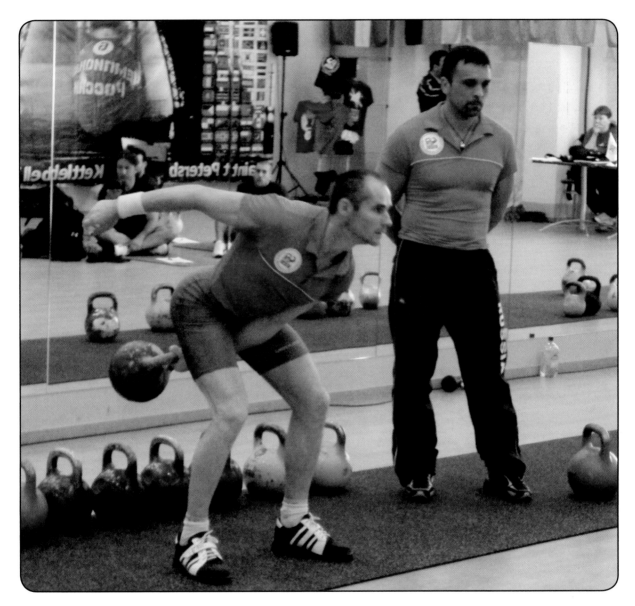

There's a fine line between training optimally and overtraining. Most people tend to set high fitness goals then proceed to crush themselves daily trying to accomplish them. The consequences of this approach are predictable: Overuse injuries will begin to increase and performance will decrease. If you are in your twenties and biomechanically sound, the process may take longer, but you are still vulnerable to overtraining. Many people thirty-five or over stop training all together because of chronic and acute overuse injuries suffered from years of bad programming and exercise selection. In this section, I show you a more excellent way to train yourself and others.

I. Ideas Have Consequences

"As a man thinks within himself, so he is."

—Proverbs 23:7

Modern behavioral scientists agree: How you think effects how you feel. How you feel effects your behavior. Your behavior influences your choices (i.e., strategy). Your choices affect your performance (i.e., results). It's a domino effect that begins in your mind. If you think it's important to keep a high level of fitness, then you will. If you don't, you won't. Likewise, if you don't think or consider yourself an athlete, chances are you're probably not training like one. Most people don't train for events they believe will never happen to them. Most people are also generally weak. An underlying theme of CrossFit is to train for the unknown or unknowable. The Tactical Athlete motto is to be "Ready, In Season and Out of Season" because there is no off-season. When I worked at Direct Action Resource Center (DARC), they had a promotional video that ended with a question: "If you *knew* you were going to fight for your life tomorrow, would you change the way you train today?"

A paradigm is the way an individual perceives, understands, and interprets the surrounding world. Our success as an athlete or coach depends on how accurately our mental map (i.e., worldview) matches reality. Principles are natural laws or fundamental truths that are universal and timeless. They operate with or without our acceptance, and the outcomes are predictable and self-evident. We can control our choices, but the consequences of those choices are controlled by principles. Every failure is an opportunity to ensure that we never make it again, especially when future consequences can be much more disastrous. Common sense is recognizing patterns. The three leading causes of injury in the weight room are (1) poor technique, (2) accidental injury and (3) inappropriate program design.

1) Poor Technique—there is no excuse for it. Strive for perfection and the result will be excellence. **Great programming + poor technique = poor results**.

2) Accidental Injury—most "accidents" are preventable and a direct result of violating safety procedures, lack of situational awareness, lack of common sense, or any combination of all three.

3) Inappropriate Program Design—more isn't always better. **Perfect technique + inappropriate program design = poor results**.

Perfect technique + great programming = optimum results.

A Person Must Know His or Her Limitations

You may choose to crush yourself on a daily basis by adding more weight, reps, speed, and volume. But at around the 8-week mark, you'll eventually "hit the wall." This is a very real biological limitation. If you choose to ignore these limitations, put your head down and attempt to blast through "the wall," you'll soon be singing the "overtraining blues." The results (i.e., pattern) are as predictable as attempting to drive your vehicle without oil. You'll make some progress toward your destination, but there will be a catastrophic breakdown before you arrive.

According to Lodge and Crowley's *Younger Next Year*:
- Platelets regenerate every 10 days.
- Blood cells regenerate every 3 months.
- Muscle cells regenerate every 4 months.
- Bone cells regenerate every 2–3 years.

Your body improves on its own biological schedule. Exceeding your body's limitations leads to overtraining. When developing or implementing any strength and conditioning program, always consider the overall training volume of any given time period relative to the demands of your sport, vocation, or lifestyle. If you listen to your body when it whispers, you don't have to hear it scream!

Reality Check

Weaker Athletes

In 1974, Gene Hooks wrote *Weight Training for Athletics* and in a chapter entitled "Strength: The-Forgotten-Key," he said, "[Coaches] must realize that they are today working with a weaker athlete. The mechanization of modern life has robbed our youth of the many manual chores that once developed strong bodies. Unless something is done to change our way of life, further athletes will be increasingly weak." Almost forty years later, nothing has been done; the increasingly technological modern life is making our youth weaker still. Generally speaking, normal people are normally weak.

Older Athletes

"The problem with getting old is that your mind writes checks that your body can't cash."

—Rich Easdown, Vietnam Veteran, Australian SAS

–Care is needed when coaching athletes over the age of thirty-five.
–With age, ligaments, cartilages, and muscles lose their elastic properties.
–More attention should be paid to warm-ups at the beginning of training sessions.
–Metabolism slows down with age.
–Ability to recover worsens.
–Duration of rest after competition and peaking sessions should be increased.

Avoiding the Overtraining Blues

"It's easy to be hard, but it's hard to be smart."

—Paul Ferarris, Sgt Major, USMC (retired)

Here's a quick list of symptoms (i.e., patterns or red flags) that may indicate you might be overtraining.

- *A compulsive need to exercise*
- *Lack of energy*
- *Sudden drop in performance*
- *Lack of coordination*
- *Decrease in training capacity/intensity*
- *Mild leg soreness*
- *Pain in muscles and joints*
- *Increased incidence of injuries*
- *Headaches, insomnia, depression*
- *Decreased appetite*
- *Decreased immunity (increased number of colds and sore throats)*
- *Moodiness and irritability*
- *Loss of enthusiasm for the sport*

Here's the irony of overtraining/under-recovery. People who subscribe to the "no pain, no gain" or "pain is only weakness leaving the body" paradigm fail to see the overtraining indicators for what they are. Instead, they perceive them as evidence that they must not be training hard or long enough. So they convince themselves to do more positive self-talk then double their efforts to train harder and longer. It's a vicious cycle. If this is where your current (mental) map has been taking you, then it's time to throw it out and get a more accurate one. Recovery is why you get better, not more training!

The principles outlined below will help you avoid the pitfalls of overtraining and lead you to a path of steady progress and optimal performance.

Training Journal

Successful athletes and coaches keep training journals. It's a key component to improving an athlete's performance because it provides an objective means of evaluating progress. It's been said, "Those who ignore history are doomed to repeat it." The same holds true in your training. If you do not keep track of what works and what does not, how can you improve? This is especially true when working with many athletes at one time. Use a spiral-bound notebook and a pen. It doesn't have to be fancy.

- Keep accurate training logs!
- Set specific goals (both long term and short term).
- Goals must be: observable, measurable, and repeatable.
- Follow a periodized approach to training; change focus every few weeks.
  - Change only one training parameter at a time.
  - Continue doing what works.
  - Discontinue what does not . . . it's that simple.
- Always consider overall training volume relative to the athlete's particular sport or vocation.
- Keep in mind: Competition is your ultimate test!

General Training Guidelines

- Never sacrifice form for time or reps. Always stress *quality over quantity.*
  Everyone has a competitive spirit but it's imperative you check your ego at the door. If you are performing a workout, lead by example. If you are running a workout, take responsibility for the safety of your athletes. If someone lacks the self-discipline to maintain acceptable form, then step up and look out for that person's best interest.
- Perform as many reps as possible in strict form. Terminate all sets *before* form deteriorates.
- Instead of risking injury by forcing more reps, incorporate longer active rests (i.e., jogging, jumping rope, walking stairs, etc.).
- Low-rep strength practice *before* sport-specific skill work.
- High-repetition kettlebell lifts/metabolic conditioning should be done *after* all sport-specific skill work or after low-rep strength training.

These Three Things . . .

Many years ago there was a comedian whose routine was imitating a former boxer who was sharing his tips for success in the boxing world. He said, "You only need to do three things to be a good boxer: train every day, get a good nickname, and train every day . . . these *three* things."

For physical conditioning, you should focus on developing the three basic physical qualities of *strength, endurance,* and *flexibility.* They are the foundation for the development of high levels of neuromuscular coordination, balance, speed, reaction and movement time, power, and agility, which in turn are the basis for skill learning and successful athletic performance. The goal is to improve the three basic physical qualities to the highest levels with minimum time and effort. To achieve this goal, we must train optimally.

II. Foundation of Strength

> "Strong people are harder to kill
> than weak people and more useful in general."
>
> —Mark Rippetoe

Strength underlies all other factors when one considers the total functioning of the body. There is no shortcut to strength development, as there is none for the development of skill, agility, or endurance in an athlete. There is no substitute for a long-term program of hard work to develop the quality of strength needed by an athlete for optimum performance in any specialty. Without sufficient strength, other factors such as endurance, flexibility, agility, and skill cannot be used effectively.

It is important for many athletes and fitness enthusiasts to learn how to build strength without gaining weight, while minimizing soreness and recovery time. Unless you're a sumo wrestler or football lineman, your goal should be to get as strong as possible, while remaining at the lowest possible body weight. This is achieved by "high-tension," low-repetition training. This will increase your "reserve of strength" and establish a solid foundation where endurance can be built upon. A high ratio of strength to body weight will make you quicker and faster.

The 3–5 Strength Building Plan

The 3–5 strength program is a simple, safe, time-efficient, and effective means to build strength. I first learned these high-tension/low-rep strength principles back in late 1999 (see section 5 for more info). I've trained countless athletes, coaches, and non-athletes with equal success. If your body is breaking down from years of overtraining and hard living, or you want to keep your body from breaking down, then this is the program for you.

3–5 exercises (performed in a circuit)
3–5 repetitions (lift slow and tight, stop a rep or two short of failure)
3–5 sets (shake out all tension between sets)
3–5 minutes of rest between the sets
3–5 workouts per week

Criteria for an Effective Strength Program:

1. Develop a high level of strength with a minimal increase in muscle mass.
2. If strength is built through muscle hypertrophy rather than neural adaptations, the weight gain outruns the strength gain. Anyone who has competed in sports that have weight classes knows that moving up to a higher weight class, due to an increase in body weight (i.e., muscle or not), usually doesn't lead to better performance.
3. Eliminate or minimize post-workout soreness and fatigue.
4. A bodybuilder can afford to limp around for five days following his squat workout; athletes cannot.
5. Maximize training safety.
6. All of the above requirements can be met by heavy (80–90 percent 1RM), low rep (3–5), lifting not to failure. Striving for maximum muscular tension, not muscular fatigue. It is the natural way for the body to protect itself and is the opposite of isolation.

5 Basic Laws of Strength Training

(Excerpted from *Periodization Training for Sports* by Tudor O. Bomba PhD)
- Develop Joint Flexibility
- Develop Tendon Strength
- Develop Core Strength
- Develop Stabilizers
- Train movement not individual muscles

Minimalist Strength Circuit

Choose 3 exercises:
- Deadlift (barbell, bands, or KB)
- One-arm military press (right, then left)
- Weighted pull-up, palms facing away (scale up or down to get your reps)

Perform 3–5 rounds of 3–5 reps:

– Rest 1–2 minutes in between rounds.

– Gradually build up training loads until you are working with a weight you can perform 2 strict reps with.

– When you reach 5 reps for 4–6 consecutive workouts, then increase the weight and repeat the training cycle.

Principles of Progressive Overload
(overload, load, underload)

1. Increase load.
2. Increase number of reps against a constant load.
3. Increase speed of performance or movement.
4. Increase time for a given position or load to be maintained (static holds).
   - Do not rush the results.
   - The load should be increased gradually.

Coach Sommers, author of the excellent book *Building the Gymnastic Body*, is spot-on when he says:

*In my opinion, the most common and yet serious flaw in **thinking** of most coaches, trainers and athletes is that they neglect to allow enough time in the under-load, or recovery stage, where the level of effort is physically perceived as being relatively easy. This is actually a crucial part of any training cycle, allowing the current gains to be solidified and the musculature/joints/connective tissue/central nervous system (CNS) and the psyche to completely heal and recover in preparation for the next steady state cycle of perceived over-load, load and under-load.*

Beginners often mistake the rapid improvements that they make in load/rep increases as increases in strength when in reality their untrained physique is simply becoming more neurologically efficient through practice. In reality, it takes a minimum of 6 weeks to see actual physical improvements in basic strength.

The body improves on its own biological schedule. If you listen to your body carefully and respect its limitations while challenging it appropriately, you will be able to enjoy an almost completely pain-free and injury-free training experience; and while continuing to make excellent gains in strength. Remember that Coach Sakamoto built his incredible record of 163 freestanding Handstand Push-ups over the course of years with consistent patient effort, and not while engaging in a mad dash to the finish.

Tips: Maximum Results, Minimum Time

- Perform exercises in a continuous circuit.
- Follow the 3–5 Strength Building Plan principles.
- Apply high-tension techniques, one at a time, for each lift. Take the time to feel the desired effects of each tension technique. Repeat this sequence for each of the above exercises.
- Practice the skill of generating tension (see Military Press).
- Lift as heavy as possible, staying as fresh as possible, as often as possible.
- Strength is technique.
- Think "perfect practice"—"practice makes permanent."

"When other factors are equal, the athlete with the most strength and stamina will be successful."

—**Coach Van Vliet, UBC 1939**

Kettlebell Rx Program Design

III. Increase Fitness Levels—Less Is More

"It is important to not only be faster, but to maintain that speed through time. This endurance is made possible through physical and mental fitness. Physical fitness develops not only speed, energy, and agility to move faster, but it also develops the endurance to maintain that speed for longer durations. With endurance, we not only outpace the enemy but maintain a higher tempo longer than he can. Mental fitness builds the ability to concentrate for longer periods of time and to penetrate below the surface of the problem."

—Warfighting, USMC

What Is Fitness?

CrossFit defines fitness as increased work capacity across broad times (short/medium/long) and modal domains (variety of activity). Work capacity is measured by power output. It's the ability to move large loads over long distances quickly.

Power = Force x Distance (work) / time.

Endurance is defined in *Science and Practice of Strength Training* by Zatsiorsky and Kraemer as "the ability to bear fatigue. Human activity is varied, and as the character and mechanism of fatigue are different in every instance, so is endurance."

Circuit training was originally developed in England, during the mid-1950s, by Morgan and Adamson as a physical fitness conditioning system for use with low-fitness students. It was designed to simultaneously develop the four aspects of general fitness: strength, power, muscular endurance, and circulo-respiratory endurance. It was designed for large groups, emphasizing competition against oneself with minimum time expenditure. (*Wrestling Physical Conditioning Encyclopedia* by John Jesse)

Circuit training uses three variables (loads, repetitions, and time) at submaximal levels. The principles of progressive overload still apply. The original concept placed emphasis on decreasing the time required for performing the exercise or the circuit (doing more work in less time), rather than increasing the resistance load or time. Training can be undermined if speed takes precedence over correct performance.

Exercise Selection Principles

Consider the following criteria for exercise selection.

- Exercise must be safe
    - Multi-joint compound movements
- Exercise must be easy to learn
    - Co-opting universal motor recruitment patterns
- Exercise should not require elaborate equipment—"just say no" to all machines
    - Kettlebell, pull-up bar, rings, and such
- Exercise and equipment must be effective
    - Increase human performance (i.e., sport, job, life)
- Overall program must be short so as not to burn the athlete out
    - High-output functional movement—high intensity, low duration

5 Variables of Circuit Training

(all 5 are interrelated, do not remain constant)

- Duration (time, distance) of work effort
- Intensity (speed, resistance) of work effort
- Number of stimuli (reps) of work effort
- Duration of recovery (intervals)
- Nature of recovery (active/passive)

Intensity is an independent variable and can be measured by heart rate.

Training LoadHeart Rate
5–10 seconds after the set

Training Load	Heart Rate
Low	up to 130–140
Moderate	140–160
High	160–180
Sub-maximal	180–190
Maximal	More than 190

You can't build work capacity without work. In the same regard, you don't have to crush yourself on a daily basis to see results. Focus on technique. Here's a quick rule of thumb for deciding when it's appropriate to put the kettlebell down and take a rest: As soon as a repetition doesn't feel like the first rep then it's time to put it down. Sounds simple, but it works!

When in Doubt:

– Master the basic lifts (virtuosity).
– Beginners: stress technique not intensity.
– Everything is scalable; if necessary, perform multiple sets of lower reps.
– Terminate sets before form starts to deteriorate.
– Avoid going to failure.
– Treat each workout as a practice session.
– Limit yourself to one or two crushing workouts a week.
– Strive for perfection, the result will be excellence.

IV. Kettlebell Only Circuits

The following kettlebell circuits are simple, short, intense, and effective. The first nine circuits require only one "medium-size" kettlebell. The prescribed load (weight) is based on your perception of what feels light, medium, or heavy for you. It will vary from person to person. As your conditioning levels increase, the weight that was initially in the "medium" category will slide down to the "light" category. These circuits are very versatile. Each circuit stands alone. Depending on your conditioning level, you can do the long circuit only, short circuit only, a combination of long and short circuits, or multiple rounds. The "total time" displayed for each circuit gives you an idea of how long it should take. These circuits can be performed up to six days per week as your "cardio" or metabolic conditioning. Since they are brief, it is easy to incorporate them into your training program. You can perform them immediately after your strength training or on separate days as the entire workout.

# Reps	# Reps	Swing Variation (med. KB)
Swing Only		
8	4	2-Arm Swing—or—Power Swing
8	4	1-Arm Swing—right
8	4	1-Arm Swing—Left
8	4	H2H Swing—switch hands each rep (aka: DARC Swing)
1 set = 32 reps 4 sets = 128 reps	1 set = 16 reps 4 sets = 64 reps	

+ Long Circuit: 4 sets of 8 reps = 3:30
Short Circuit: 4 sets of 4 reps = 1:45
Total Time: Long + Short Circuit = 5:15 (long circuit followed by short circuit)
Total Volume: 192 swings

# Reps	# Reps	Swing Variation (med. KB)
Clean Only		
8	4	1-Arm Clean—right
8	4	1-Arm Clean—Left
16	8	Alternating Dead Clean
1 set = 32 reps 4 sets = 128 reps	1 set = 16 reps 4 sets = 64 reps	

+ Long Circuit: 4 sets = 3:05
Short Circuit: 4 sets = 1:30
Total Time: 8 sets = 4:35 (long circuit followed by short circuit)
Total Volume: 192 cleans

Snatch Only

# Reps	# Reps	Swing Variation (med. KB)
8	4	Snatch—right (med. KB)
8	4	Snatch—left (med. KB)
16	8	Alternating Dead Snatch (light KB)
1 set = 32 reps 4 sets = 128 reps	1 set = 16 reps 4 sets = 64 reps	

+ Long Circuit: 4 sets =5:20
Short Circuit: 4 sets =3:00
Total Time: 8 sets = 8:20 (long circuit followed by short circuit)
Total Volume: 192 snatches

Descending Swings

Set	# Reps Left	# Reps Right	Size KB
1	10	10	Med.
2	8	8	Med.
3	6	6	Med.
4	4	4	Med.
5	2	2	Med.
Total	30	30	
4 rounds=	120 reps	120 reps	

4 rounds of Descending Swings = 240 reps = 6:20 time

Do *not* put the KB down. Switch hands using **H2H Switch** or **Half-Rotation Switch.**

Descending Cleans

Set	# Reps Left	# Reps Right	Size KB
1	10	10	Med.
2	8	8	Med.
3	6	6	Med.
4	4	4	Med.
5	2	2	Med.
Total	30	30	
4 rounds=	120 reps	120 reps	

4 rounds of Descending Swings = 240 reps = <u>7:40 time</u>

Switch hands by performing one **Dead Clean**. Do *not* rest or break momentum while switching hands.

Descending Snatches

Set	# Reps Left	# Reps Right	Size KB
1	10	10	Med.
2	8	8	Med.
3	6	6	Med.
4	4	4	Med.
5	2	2	Med.
Total	30	30	
4 rounds=	120 reps	120 reps	

4 rounds of Descending Swings = 240 reps = <u>9:40 time</u>

Do *not* put the KB down. Switch hands using **H2H Switch** or **Half-Rotation Switch**.

Descending All 3

Snatch—Clean—Swing

Use 1 medium-size KB for all circuits.

Do not put the KB down.

No resting while switching hands or transitioning to the next exercise.

Perform one round of each: Snatch Pull, Clean Pull, and Swing Pull.

Descending Snatches

Set	# Reps Left	# Reps Right	Size KB
1	10	10	Med.
2	8	8	Med.
3	6	6	Med.
4	4	4	Med.
5	2	2	Med.
Total	30	30	Time: 2:25

Switch hands using **H2H Switch** or **Half-Rotation Switch.**

Descending Cleans

Set	# Reps Left	# Reps Right	Size KB
1	10	10	Med.
2	8	8	Med.
3	6	6	Med.
4	4	4	Med.
5	2	2	Med.
Total	30	30	Time: 1:55

Switch hands by performing one **Dead Clean.**

Descending Swings

Set	# Reps Left	# Reps Right	Size KB
1	10	10	Med.
2	8	8	Med.
3	6	6	Med.
4	4	4	Med.
5	2	2	Med.
Total	30	30	Time: 2:25

Switch hands using **H2H Switch** or **Half-Rotation Switch.**

The Basic 3

Size KB	# Reps	Exercise:
Extra Heavy	10	Russian Swing—or—Power Swing
Heavy	10	Swing Release
Medium	10	H2H Switch
	1 set = 30 reps	
	5 sets = 150 reps	Time: 5:15

Multi-Weight Cleans

Size KB	# Reps	Exercise:
Heavy	10	Clean—Right
Heavy	10	Clean—Left
Medium	10	Bottoms-up Clean—Right
Medium	10	Bottoms-up Clean—Left
	1 set = 40 reps	
	5 sets = 200 reps	Time: 9:00

Multi-Weight Snatches

Size KB	# Reps	Exercise:
Heavy	10	Snatch—Right
Heavy	10	Snatch—Left
Medium	10	Snatch—Right
Medium	10	Snatch—Left
	1 set = 40 reps	
	5 sets = 200 reps	Time: 7:30

Screaming Thrusters!

Size KB	# Reps	Exercise:
1—Medium	10	American Swing
2—Light	10	Thruster
	1 set = 40 reps	
	5 sets = 200 reps	Time: 6:00
Keep the medium KB and the pair of "light" KBs close for minimal transition time.		

Power Sprint!

Size KB	# Reps	Exercise:
1—Medium	10	Power Swing
2—Light	10	Front Squat
	1 set = 20 reps	
	5 sets = 100 reps	Time: 4:30
This is a sprint! Do *not* put the KB down. No rest! No mercy!!		

Beginners: Use medium-size KB until this workout is no longer challenging. Then graduate to the heavy KBs.

Double Sprint

Size KB	# Reps	Exercise:
2—Medium	10	Double Clean
2—Medium	10	Front Squat
	1 set = 20 reps	
	5 sets = 100 reps	Time: 4:30
Do *not* put the KB down. No rest!		

As you can see from the routines above, it doesn't take elaborate equipment or lots of time to dramatically increase your fitness level. If you want more challenging routines and the opportunity to train daily with the creator of these circuits, check out the *Busy Woman Workout* DVD series in the back of this book or on **www.tacticalathlete.com**.

V. CrossFit Kettlebell Substitution Workouts

"You can't fake performance or endurance."

—Tony Blauer

The Benchmark "Girls":

Listed below are tried-and-true CrossFit benchmark workouts with suggested kettlebell exercise substitutions. These substitutions may be necessary if you find yourself training in locations with limited equipment (i.e., no Olympic bar and weights and/or Dynamax medicine balls—no problem). The suggested KB poundage is not written in stone. Just because it's written doesn't mean you have to do it! Scale up or down to fit your conditioning and skill level.

Constantly varied, functional movement, executed at high intensity defines CrossFit. You can change the "constantly varied" portion by using the same movements with a different implement. Simply exchange kettlebells for barbells or dumbbells. You'll notice a difference. It will also decrease the risk of overly repetitive movement issues. Try performing the WODs below with kettlebells. Mix it up. The results will speak for themselves.

Elizabeth
- Double clean 135 pounds or (two 72-pound kettlebells)
- Ring dips
- 21-15-9 reps, for time

Fran
- Thrusters 95 pounds or (two 36-pound kettlebells)
- Pull-ups
- 21-15-9 reps, for time

Grace
- Clean and jerk 135 pounds (two 72-pound kettlebells)
- 30 reps for time

Note: See instructions on Long Cycle

Helen
- 400-meter run
- 1.5 poods (53 pounds) kettlebell swing x 21
- Pull-ups x 21
- 3 rounds for time

Isabel
- Snatch 135 pounds or (one-arm snatch—72-pound KB)
- 30 reps each arm for time

Jackie
- 1,000-meter row
- Thruster 45 pounds x 50 reps or (two 12-kilogram kettlebells)
- Pull-ups x 12 reps
- For time

Karen
- Wall ball 150 shots or 150 "wall ball substitute"
- For time

Note: When the going gets really tough, eliminate the squat and continue with swing-catch/push press. If the catch gets questionable, turn it into a two-arm swing release or swing.

Linda (aka "3 bars of death")
- Deadlift 1½ BW
- Bench BW or floor press two very heavy kettlebells
- Clean ¾ BW or clean two appropriate-size kettlebells
- 10/9/8/7/6/5/4/3/2/1/ rep for time

Nancy
- 400-meter run
- Overhead squat 95 pounds x 15 or use two appropriate-size kettlebells.
- 5 rounds for time

Note: Overhead squats with KBs, the arms stay vertical; they do not angle out to the sides as you would holding a bar.

Kelly
- Run 400 meters
- 30 box jump, 24-inch box
- 30 wall ball shots—20-pound ball, or wall ball substitute—36- or 26-pound kettlebell
- Rounds for time

Kettlebell Hero WOD Mods:

"High physical condition is vital to victory."

—General George Patton, U.S. Army

Hero WODs are named after CrossFitters who have given their lives in the line of duty.

Badger
In honor of Navy Chief Petty Officer Mark Carter, 27, of Virginia Beach, VA, who was killed in Iraq on December 11, 2007.

3 rounds for time:
- 30 double KB cleans and front squats (two 24 kg KBs)
- 30 pull-ups
- Run 800 meters

Daniel
Dedicated to Army Sgt 1st Class Daniel Crabtree, who was killed in Al Kut, Iraq, on Thursday, June 8, 2006.

For time:
- 50 pull-ups
- 400-meter run
- 21 KB thrusters (two 16 kg KBs)

Danny
Oakland SWAT Sergeant Daniel Sa-kai, age 35, was killed on March 21, 2009, in the line of duty along with fellow officers Sergeant Ervin Romans, Sergeant Mark Dunakin, and Officer John Hege.

AMRAP 20 min.
- 30 box jumps 24 inches
- 20 double KB push presses (two 24 kg KBs)
- 30 pull-ups

Joshie
In honor of Army Staff Sergeant Joshua Whitaker, 23, of Long Beach, CA, who was killed in Afghanistan May 15, 2007.

3 Rounds for time:
- 21 KB snatches R 24 kg
- 21 L-sit pull-ups
- 21 KB snatches L 24 kg
- 21 L-sit pull-ups
- Run 800 meters

Nate
In honor of Chief Petty Officer Nate Hardy, who was killed Sunday February 4 during combat operations in Iraq.

AMRAP 20 minutes
- 2 muscle-ups
- 4 handstand push-ups
- 8 KB swings 32 kg

Randy
In honor of Randy Simmons, 51, a 27-year LAPD veteran and SWAT team member who was killed February 6 in the line of duty. Our thoughts and prayers go out to Officer Simmons's wife and two children.

For time:
- 75 KB snatches R 24 kg
- 75 KB snatches L 24 kg

Kettlebell Rx Program Design

Tommy V

In honor of Senior Chief Petty Officer Thomas J. Valentine, 37, of Ham Lake, Minnesota, who died in a training accident in Arizona on February 13, 2008.

For time:

- 21 KB thrusters (two 16 kg KBs)
- 12 rope climbs 15 ft.
- 15 KB thrusters (two 16 kg KBs)
- 9 rope climbs 15 ft.
- 9 KB thrusters (two 16 kg KBs)
- 6 rope climbs

Hansen

Marine Staff Sgt Daniel Hansen died February 14 in Farah Province, Afghanistan, when an IED he was working on detonated.

5 rounds for time:

- 30 KB swings (24 kg)
- 30 burpees
- 30 glute-ham sit-ups

Arnie*

Los Angeles County Fire Fighter Specialist Arnaldo "Arnie" Quinones, 34, was killed in the line of duty on Sunday, August 30, 2009, during the "Station Fire." His emergency response vehicle went over the side of the road and fell 800 feet into a steep canyon during fire suppression activities protecting Camp 16 outside the City of Palmdale, CA. He is survived by his wife Lori and daughter Sophia Grace, born three weeks after his death.

For time:

Perform with one 32 kg KB

- 7 Turkish get-ups (1R/1L =1 rep)
- 50 KB swings (your choice)
- 5 overhead squats L
- 50 KB swings (your choice)
- 5 overhead squats R
- 50 KB swings (your choice)
- 7 Turkish get-ups (1R/1L = 1 rep)

*Note: Reps and sequence modified

Other CrossFit Kettlebell Benchmark WODs:

"Hard work beats talent, when talent doesn't work hard."

—**Author unknown**

Nasty Girls

3 rounds for time:

- 50 squats
- 7 muscle-ups
- 10 double cleans
- (two 32 kg kettlebells)

Filthy Fifty

For time:

- 50 box jumps 24 inches
- 50 jumping pull-ups
- 50 kettlebell swings (16 kg)
- Walking lunges, 50 steps
- 50 knees to elbows
- 50 double KB push presses
  (two 12 kg kettlebells)
- 50 back extensions
- 50 wall ball shots (16 kg)
- 50 burpees
- 50 double-unders

Sevens

Seven rounds for time:

- 7 handstand push-ups
- 7 thrusters (two 16 kg KBs)
- 7 knees to elbows
- 7 deadlifts 245/205
- 7 burpees
- 7 kettlebell swings 32 kg/24 kg
- 7 pull-ups

Heavy Fran

15, 12, 9 rep rounds for time:

- KB thruster (two 24 kg KBs)
- Weighted pull-ups 45/30 pounds

Jonesworthy

6 rounds for time:

- Air squat 80-64-50-32-16-8 reps
- KB swing 40-32-25-16-8-4 reps (24 kg KB)
- Pull-ups 20-16-12-8-4-2 reps

Conclusion

There are many kettlebell exercise variations. Master the basic lifts (virtuosity) and the principles of power generation. When training with kettlebells, use liberal amounts of common sense. Everything is scalable! Finish your sets **before** your form starts to deteriorate. **Never** go to failure! Treat each workout as a practice session and constantly try to improve your form and make each exercise effortless. You can increase the intensity and versatility of your current fitness routines by simply adding a few kettlebell exercises. It is your choice whether to pursue the simplicity of the classic kettlebell lifts or combine different styles of kettlebell training for a killer package of all-around strength and conditioning. The choices are many and the benefits are plenty.

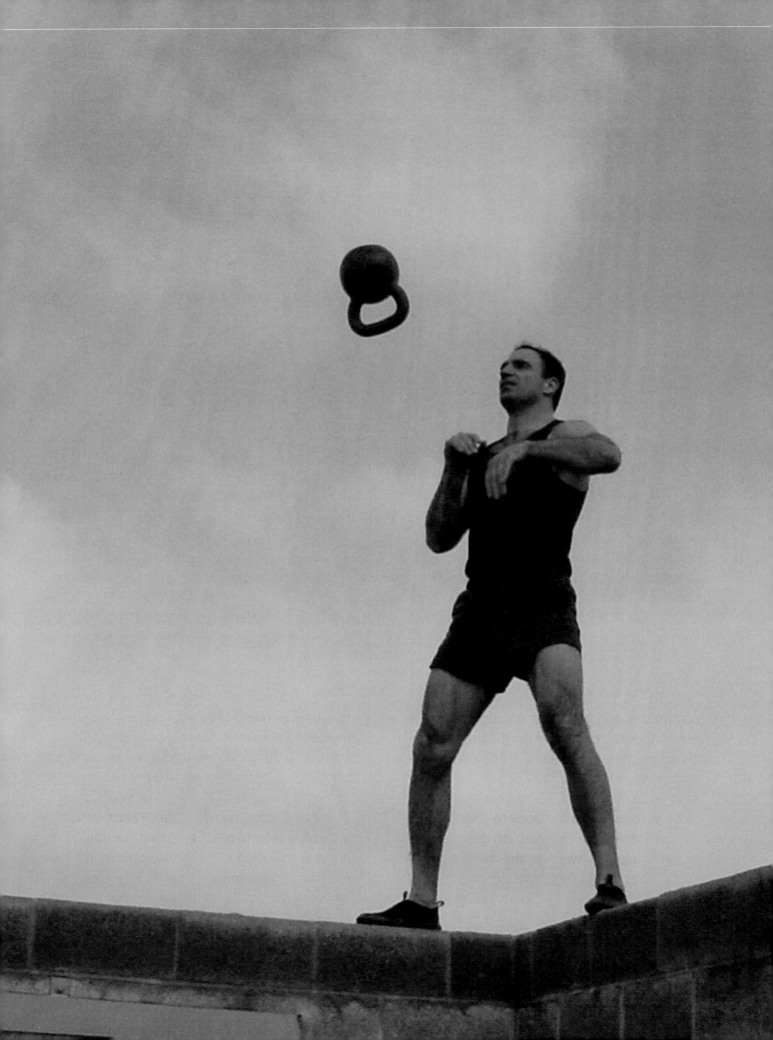

Part II

Rotational
Power Development

Most sports and life activities involve rotational movement. Athletic power is transmitted from the ground through the legs, the torso, then arms. If you want to increase overall strength that will transfer to your athletic arena, you must develop a powerful, resilient core. The core (i.e., torso) is the center that coordinates all ground-based human movements.

The term "core" usually describes the muscles surrounding the midline, or spinal column, of the body. This would include the muscles of the abs (rectus abdominus), the obliques, the transverse abdominus (TVA), and the spinal erectors. Whether you can correctly spell or pronounce these names is not as important as understanding their function. The core muscles have two competing and opposite functions: (1) to prevent undesired centerline flexion or rotation (i.e., centerline stabilization) and (2) to initiate desired centerline flexion or rotation. In other words, a solid core will allow power generated in your legs to be transferred up the body to your arms.

Let's add the muscles of the glutes and upper quad, as well as the hamstrings, hip flexors, and groin area into the core equation. The muscles of the hips and buttocks are commonly known as "the seat of power," and for good reason. They form the biggest and most powerful muscles in your body. All other mus-

cle groups become proportionally smaller and weaker from the distance they are from the center of your body. Athletes such as fighters, shot-putters, and pitchers never begin to throw a punch, shot, or baseball with the arm. The throw is initiated from the center of the body (from the hips). A powerful core is essential to transmitting maximum force.

Power is a function of speed and strength. Increasing speed of movement with the same mass lifted improves power. Increasing mass lifted and maintaining the speed of movement will increase power. The less time it takes to move a mass a certain distance, the higher the power output.

Regardless of whether you're throwing baseballs or grenades, shots or punches, swinging baseball bats or batons, or golf clubs, picking up feedbags or body-slamming bad guys, maximal rotational power and endurance is the name of the game for optimal performance.

The H2H (i.e., hand-to-hand) kettlebell drills are a unique form of training that conditions the entire body using effective multiplane, multidimensional movement patterns. These exercises will prove to be very challenging both mentally and physically and will demand your full attention. You will also discover that they are a lot of fun to practice. The best part is you only need one implement—a single kettlebell.

Benefits of H2H Kettlebell Drills

H2H kettlebell drills are a fun and effective means to build:

- Excellent centerline stabilization

- Explosive rotational power

- Hand-to-eye coordination

- High levels of cardiovascular conditioning

- Excellent lower-back endurance

- Dynamic grip strength

- Lightning-quick hand speed

H2H Training Safety

Our goal is to train, not maim others or ourselves. Safety is paramount. Please keep the following safety and performance tips in mind when you train:

1. Practice H2H drills outside, on a soft, level surface. If indoors, the preferred training surface is a clutter-free, level area, surfaced with rubber stall mats. You always want to train in an area where you can freely and safely drop your kettlebell.

2. Maintain a minimum of 5 feet of space in every direction between you, your training partner, any equipment, sleeping pets, or anything else that you wouldn't want crushed if a kettlebell accidently went flying out of your hand.

3. Follow the teaching progression in the order it is presented.

4. The difference is in the details: Carefully read each exercise description and pay close attention to the demonstrations within each photo sequence.

5. Practice with a light kettlebell, concentrating on proper form and consistency of movement.

6. Do not attempt to practice all the exercises in one session.

7. If at any point you feel that your form is beginning to deteriorate, put the KB down and choose a form of active rest. The key is to keep moving.

8. If you feel you're losing control of the kettlebell, just let it drop safely to the ground. It's not a matter of "if" you drop it, but rather "when" and how many times. Remember: "Quick feet are happy feet."

9. When in doubt, adhere to the "KILAH" principle when training: "Keep It Light and Happy."

How to Get the Most out of This Section

If you have not invested the time to master the Russian swing and one-arm swing from Part One, then you really have no business attempting any of the H2H drills in this section. I don't say that to be mean spirited, but rather for your best interest. Mastery means you have reached the autonomous stage of learning where the skill has become automatic or habitual. In other words, you should have the ability to consistently perform a skill to standard without having to consciously attend to every phase of the skill. Your balance, hip drive, back and head position, breathing, and so on must be on autopilot before practicing H2H drills. This is important for your progress and safety because it will free up your mind to concentrate on the new task at hand. Beginners have a tendency to get so focused on what they are doing with their hands that they totally forget about using their hip drive and maintaining proper back extension.

Passing the kettlebell from one hand to the other takes most people out of their comfort zone. Stress levels have a tendency to go up because nobody wants to drop their kettlebell. It makes a loud noise, draws unwanted attention, and makes you feel awkward or stupid. That's why I prefer practicing outside on the grass or sand. It's quiet and less distracting. Sand is best because it leaves less evidence of your failures!

Kettlebell selection: I would recommend for men to start with 12-kilogram kettlebells and women or teens to start with the 8–kilogram ones. The solid-cast kettlebells are more durable and easier to handle than the big hollow-cast competition-style kettlebells. Lighter is better during the initial stages of learning. However, periodically moving up one size kettlebell will keep you honest. A heavier bell pressure tests your technique and forces you to use proper mechanics. However, keep your practice sessions short and happy. Take plenty of breaks in between sets or drops. Stay as fresh as possible when training. Fatigue at the early stage of learning is counterproductive.

Keys to steady progress: Each drill builds upon the preceding drill. Master each movement, one drill at a time. If at any time you feel confused or overwhelmed, take a short break. Go back to an easier drill that you've already learned and practice it for a little while. Think about what you are doing and why. Try to develop a nice rhythm and flow to your movements. Once your head is clear and you've regained your confidence you can choose to either (a) end your training session on a positive note; or (b) recheck the photos and exercise descriptions of the drill that was giving you problems, identify where you went wrong, and then make the necessary correction. Your goal is to train like a professional!

"Amateurs practice until they get it right; Professionals train until they can't get it wrong."

– John Chapman

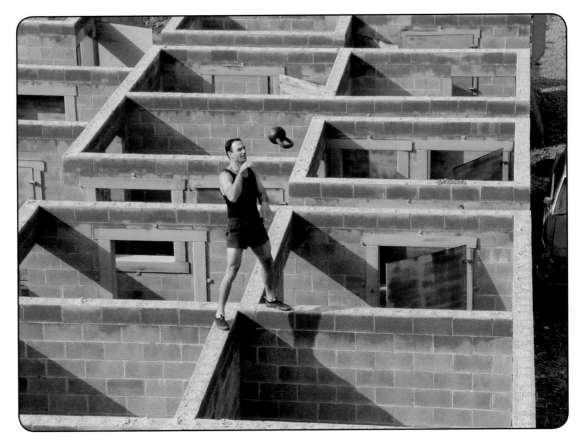

1) Around-the-Body Pass (ABP) Series

The around-the-body pass is a simple yet powerful exercise that strengthens the muscles of your hands and arms as well as all the stabilizing muscles of your core. There are two methods you will learn to pass the kettlebell around your waist. The first is the corner-to-corner method, and the second is the fingertip-to-fingertip method.

a) ABP Corner-to-Corner

The corner-to-corner method is the easiest way to get the feel for the exercise. Use it for a warm-up and to build confidence.

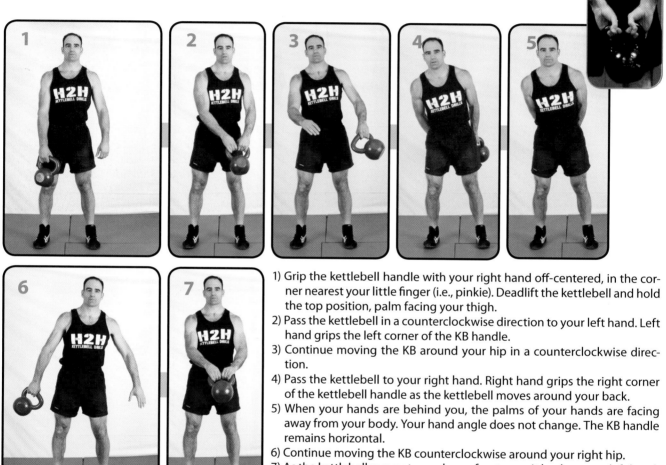

1) Grip the kettlebell handle with your right hand off-centered, in the corner nearest your little finger (i.e., pinkie). Deadlift the kettlebell and hold the top position, palm facing your thigh.
2) Pass the kettlebell in a counterclockwise direction to your left hand. Left hand grips the left corner of the KB handle.
3) Continue moving the KB around your hip in a counterclockwise direction.
4) Pass the kettlebell to your right hand. Right hand grips the right corner of the kettlebell handle as the kettlebell moves around your back.
5) When your hands are behind you, the palms of your hands are facing away from your body. Your hand angle does not change. The KB handle remains horizontal.
6) Continue moving the KB counterclockwise around your right hip.
7) As the kettlebell moves toward your front, pass it back to your left hand. This completes one full rotation. Continue passing from hand to hand for 10 reps, then change directions and repeat.

Performance Tips:

- Keep your feet firmly planted shoulder width apart.
- Look straight ahead. Do not look at your hands or the kettlebell.
- Keep your head up, chest open, and your shoulders down.
- Control the kettlebell; do not let it pull you off balance.
- Elongate your arms; "bulldogging" (i.e., bending at the elbows too much) will only lead to unnecessary stress on your elbows.
- Rhythmically shift your body weight from side to side in order to maintain balance and speed.
- Perform an equal number of reps in both directions.
- Perform for time or reps.
- Terminate before form deteriorates.

b) ABP Fingertip-to-Fingertip

This is the preferred method of passing the kettlebell. It's a more dynamic and powerful method of passing the kettlebell from hand to hand. More importantly, it puts your hand and kettlebell handle at the proper angle for all the H2H drills that follow.

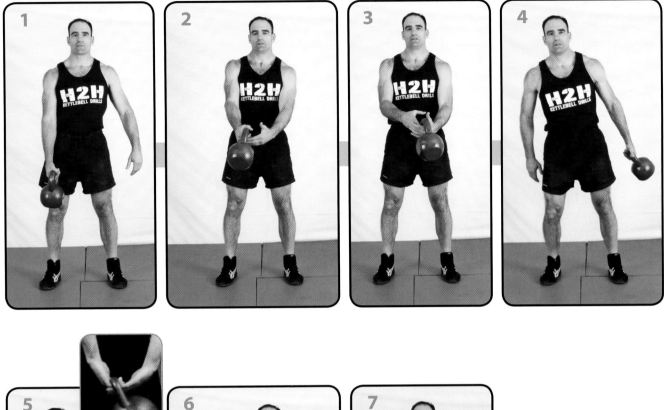

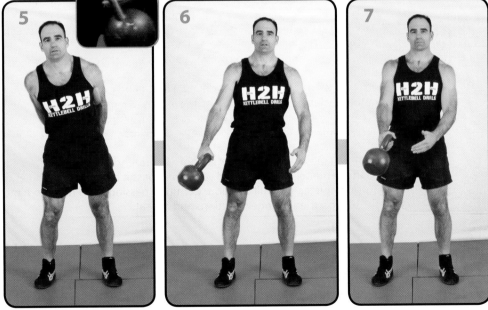

1) Grip the center of the kettlebell handle with your right hand and deadlift the kettlebell. As you reach the top position, rotate your right hand clockwise until your thumb is pointing forward, away from your body.
2) Pass the kettlebell in a counterclockwise direction toward your left hand.
3) Left hand grips the center of the KB handle.
4) Continue moving the KB around your hip in a counterclockwise direction, keeping the KB handle vertical.
5) Pass the kettlebell to your right hand behind your back, palms facing each other.
6) Continue moving the KB counterclockwise around your right hip.
7) As the kettlebell moves toward your front, pass it back to your left hand. This completes one full rotation. Continue passing from hand to hand for 10 reps, then change directions and repeat.

Changing Directions

Haphazardly attempting to change the direction of a kettlebell revolving at high speed around your torso could have the potential to cause unnecessary stress to your muscles and the connective tissue of your shoulder. To maximize safety and minimize stress:

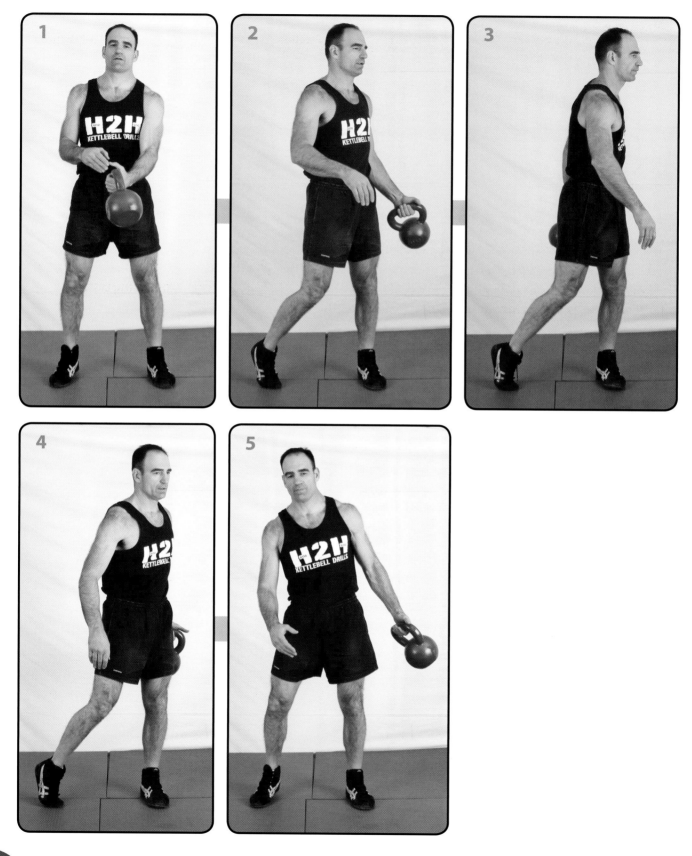

1) As your left hand receives the KB, instantly tighten all the muscles in that armpit (i.e., flexing your lats, pecs, and biceps). The best way to do this is to imagine that you have a tennis ball in your armpit and crush it. That's right, I mean really crush it! This is essential because it will activate all the protective muscles of the shoulder girdle.
2) As the kettlebell moves to the outside of your hip, shift your weight to your left foot while pivoting on the ball of your right foot.
3) Actively tighten your midsection and allow your hips and shoulders to rotate to their full range of motion. Flexing your entire core is critical to proper deceleration.
4) Reverse the direction by driving off your left foot and pivoting your hips to your right. Keep your abs and armpit tight. Initiate all movement from your hips!
5) Continue passing the kettlebell around your body in a clockwise direction for a couple of reps, then change direction.

✕ Common Problem #1:
Continually Dropping the KB

√ Corrective Action:
1. Master the "corner-to-corner" variation first.
2. Hands sweaty—Wipe them off and keep them dry. Chalk's a crutch!
3. Lack of flexibility in chest and shoulders to properly execute the "fingertip-to-fingertip" variation—practice arm-bar stretches (see pg 146)

✕ Common Problem #2:
Biceps or Elbows Sore the Next Day

√ Corrective Action:
1. Stop trying to "curl" the KB.
2. Elongate your arms and actively flex your triceps.

✕ Common Problem #3:
Do Not Feel Core Working Hard

√ Corrective Action:
1. Go faster
2. Practice switching direction every one or two rotations.
3. Try a heavier KB.

2) Figure 8 Drill

The figure 8 drill is an effective strength-endurance exercise for your core. It is an extremely versatile exercise that will be used throughout this entire section. Don't make the mistake of using a heavy KB when learning this drill. The involved muscles will fatigue quickly. Keep strict form and terminate all sets before abdominals or lower back fatigues.

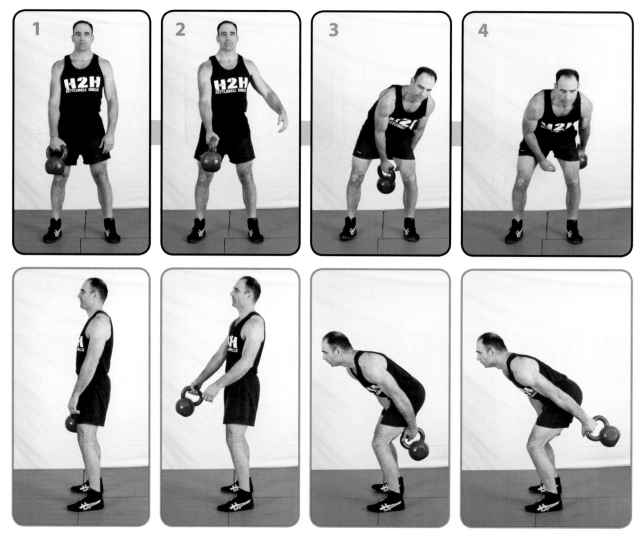

1) Grip the center of the kettlebell handle with your right hand and deadlift the kettlebell to the upright position.

2) Bump the KB off your right thigh, rotating your right hand a quarter turn in a clockwise manner (i.e., thumb is pointing away from your body). As the kettlebell reaches the top of the arc:

3) Sit back and pull the KB diagonally under the left knee. Do not turn your hand! Note: As your hips move backward, inhale through your nose as your body weight shifts to your heels. Keep your chest open, back straight, and neck neutral.

4) As the kettlebell passes from the right to left hand, shift your head position over your left foot. Note: Always pass the kettlebell from front to back, keeping your thumbs up (i.e., KB handle vertical). It's identical to the fingertip-to-fingertip pass, except the exchange happens under your thigh instead of in front of or behind your hips.

5) Once the KB is in your left hand, drive off your heels, fully extending your legs, hips, and torso to the upright position. Exhale through your teeth upon extension. This will propel the kettlebell upward, toward the front of your body. As the kettlebell reaches the top of the arc:

6) Sit back and pull the KB diagonally under the right knee. Do not turn your hand! Note: As your hips move backward, your weight shifts to your heels. Keep your chest open, back straight, and neck neutral.

7) As the kettlebell passes from the left to right hand, shift your head position over the right foot. Note: Always pass the kettlebell from front to back, keeping your thumbs up (i.e., KB handle vertical). It's identical to the fingertip-to-fingertip pass, except you transfer the KB under your thigh.

8) Once the KB is in your right hand, drive off your heels, fully extending your legs, hips, and torso to the upright position. Exhale through your teeth upon extension. This will launch the kettlebell upward, toward the front of your body. As the kettlebell reaches the top of the arc: Repeat steps 3–8 for time or reps.

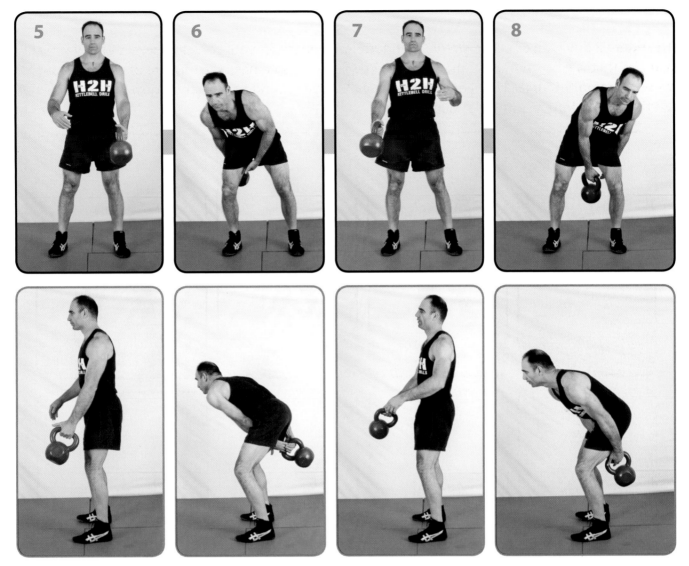

Performance Tips:

1. Slightly shift your weight from side to side when passing the kettlebell.
2. Do not look down; look straight ahead.
3. Be sure the KB handle and your thumb are pointing forward.
4. Aggressively pull the KB through your legs using the power of your lats.
5. Keep the abdominals pressurized and breathe shallowly.
6. Intensely contract all the muscles in your core.
7. Slightly shift your weight from side to side.

✕ Common Problem #1: Lower Back Fatigues Quickly

√ Corrective Action:

1. Sit back, rather than down.
2. Ensure your torso is totally upright after every hip extension.
3. Maintain intra-abdominal pressure; breathe shallowly.
4. Be sure the KB is being passed from front to back (not from the back to the front).
5. Use a lighter KB if the corrections above do not solve the problem.

✕ Common Problem #2:
Hunchback—Back and Shoulders Rounded
√ Corrective Action:

1. Sit back, chest open, weight on heels.
2. Head position neutral—look straight ahead. Do not look down or at the KB.
3. Keep the KB handle vertical and your thumb pointing forward.
4. Pass the KB directly under your knee, not your butt!
5. Review movement prep drills and corrective actions for the Russian Swing.

3) Around-the-Body–Figure 8 Combo

This combination drill is a great way to warm up and is one of the easiest and most efficient ways to change the direction of the kettlebell moving at high speed. In addition, it gives your lower back an active rest while the kettlebell travels around your body. By combining these exercises, you exponentially increase safety and your capacity to perform work. Start slow, get the movement patterns down, and then gradually increase the rate of movement.

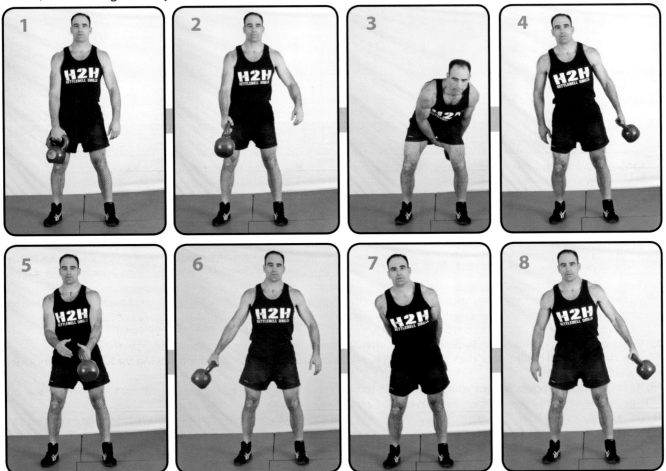

1) Grip the center of the kettlebell handle with your right hand and deadlift the kettlebell to the upright position.

2) Bump the KB off your right thigh, rotating your right hand a quarter turn in a clockwise manner (i.e., thumb is pointing away from your body). As the kettlebell reaches the top of the arc:

3) Inhale through your nose, sit back, and pull the KB diagonally under your left knee. Do not turn your hand! Note: As your hips move backward, your weight shifts to your heels. Keep your chest open, back straight, and neck neutral. As the kettlebell passes from the right to left hand, transfer your weight to your left foot. Note: Always pass the kettlebell from front to back, keeping your thumbs up (i.e., KB handle vertical). It's identical to the fingertip-to-fingertip pass, except you transfer the KB under your thigh.

4) Once the KB is in your left hand, drive off your left heel, fully extending your legs, hips, and torso to the upright position. This will launch the kettlebell upward, toward the front of your body.

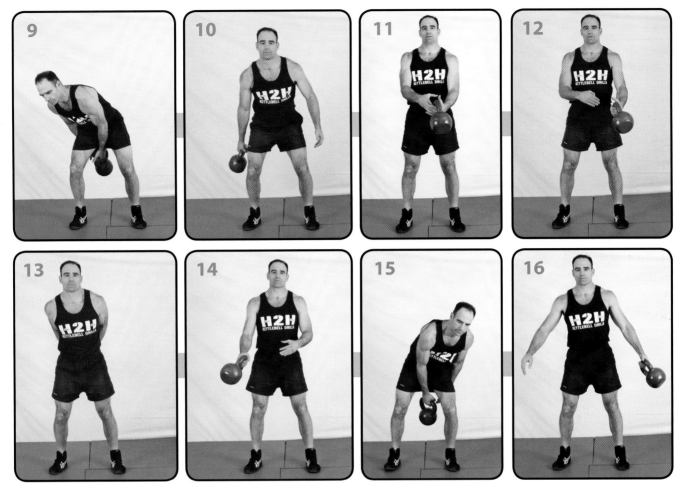

5) Perform the fingertip-to-fingertip around-the-body pass, transferring the kettlebell to your right hand.

6) Continue moving the KB around your hip in a clockwise direction, keeping the KB handle vertical.

7) Pass the kettlebell behind your back to your left hand; palms face each other.

8) Continue moving the KB counterclockwise around your right hip.

9) As the kettlebell moves toward your front, sit back and pull the KB diagonally under your right knee. Do not turn your hand! Note: As your hips move backward, your weight shifts to your heels. Keep your chest open, back straight, and neck neutral.

10) As the kettlebell passes from the left to right hand, transfer your weight to your right foot. Note: Always pass the kettlebell from front to back, keeping your thumbs up (i.e., KB handle vertical). It's identical to the fingertip-to-fingertip pass, except you transfer the KB under your thigh.

11) Once the KB is in your right hand, drive off your right heel, fully extending your legs, hips, and torso to the upright position. Exhale through your teeth upon extension. This will launch the kettlebell upward, toward the front of your body.

12) Perform the fingertip-to-fingertip around-the-body pass, transferring the kettlebell to your left hand.

13) Continue moving the KB around your hip in a counterclockwise direction, keeping the KB handle vertical.

14) Pass the kettlebell behind your back to your right hand; palms face each other. Continue moving the KB counterclockwise around your right hip.

15) As the kettlebell moves toward your front, inhale through your nose, sit back, and pull the KB diagonally under the left knee. As the kettlebell passes from the right to left hand, transfer your weight to the left foot.

16) Drive off your right heel, fully extending your legs, hips, and torso to the upright position. Exhale through your teeth upon extension. This will launch the kettlebell upward, toward the front of your body. Repeat passing the kettlebell one complete revolution around the body, then through your legs; around the body, then through your legs for time or reps. Terminate all sets before form deteriorates.

Performance Tips:

1. Talk yourself through the drill (i.e., "Around-the-body, through the legs, around the body, through the legs").
2. Always pass the kettlebell from front to back.
3. Concentrate on breathing sequence, i.e., matching the breath with the movement.
4. If you sense your shoulders rounding forward or your lower back fatiguing, then it's time to stop and rest.

4) Uppercut Series

The uppercut series is an outstanding core strength developer that creates exceptional rotational power necessary for athletic movements. The uppercut drill movement is similar to that of a fighter throwing the uppercut punch. This drill reinforces the proper sequence of generating power from the legs and hips, then transferring it through the core to extremities.

a) Uppercut (touch-and-go)

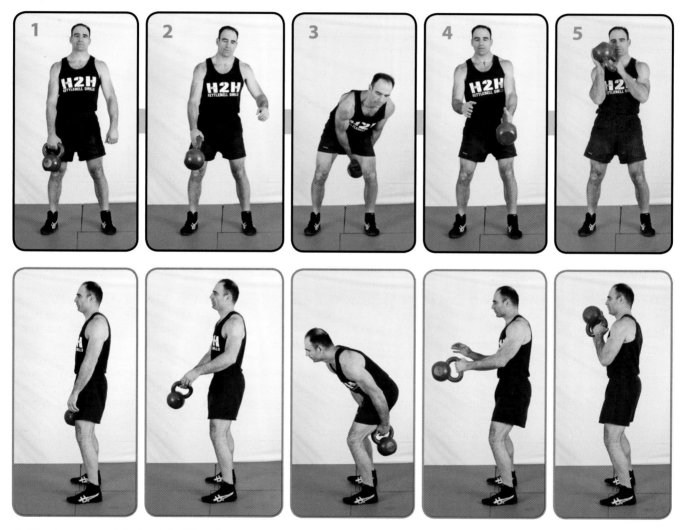

1) Grip the center of the kettlebell handle with your right hand and deadlift the kettlebell to the upright position.

2) Bump the KB off your right thigh, rotating your right hand a quarter turn in a clockwise manner (i.e., thumb is pointing away from your body). As the kettlebell reaches the top of the arc:

3) Sit back and pull the KB diagonally under your left knee. Always pass the kettlebell from front to back, keeping your thumbs up (i.e., KB handle vertical). As the kettlebell passes from the right to left hand, transfer your weight to the left foot. Note: Head is positioned directly over the left foot. Keep your chest open, back straight, and neck neutral.

4) Once the KB is in your left hand, really drive off your left foot, fully extending your legs, hips, and torso, similar to a fighter throwing an uppercut. Simultaneously, actively exhale through your teeth, keeping your left elbow tight against your side. Note: This coordinated action should "shoot" the bell like a cannon into the palm of the opposite hand.

5) As the kettlebell moves diagonally up and across your chest, quickly place the palm of your right hand on the rising bell. Use your core to decelerate and stop the kettlebell directly in front of your right shoulder. This action will load the kinetic energy in your core, similar to compressing a spring.

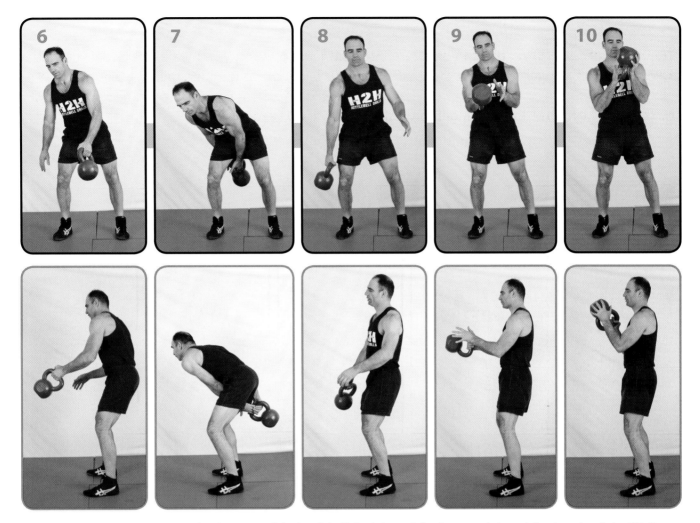

6) Recoil, immediately reversing the direction of the kettlebell. Push it straight down, and then sit back and pull the KB diagonally under your right knee. Always pass the kettlebell from front to back, keeping your thumbs up (i.e., KB handle vertical).

7) As the kettlebell passes from the left to right hand, transfer your weight to your right foot. Note: Head position is directly over the right foot. Keep your chest open, back straight, and neck neutral.

8) Once the KB is in your right hand, really drive off your right foot, fully extending your legs, hips, and torso, similar to a fighter throwing an uppercut. Simultaneously, actively exhale through your teeth, keeping your left elbow tight against your side.

9) As the kettlebell "shoots" diagonally up and across your chest, quickly place the palm of your left hand on the rising bell. Use your core to decelerate and stop the kettlebell directly in front of your left shoulder. This action will load the kinetic energy in your core similar to compressing a spring.

10) Recoil, immediately reversing the direction of the kettlebell by pushing it straight down. Repeat steps 3–10 for reps or time.

✕ Common Problem #1: Lower Back Discomfort
√ Corrective Actions:

1. Keep your chest open, shoulders back and down.
2. Power-breathe: exhale through your teeth as you uppercut, inhale through nose as you fold at the hips.
3. Ensure your torso is totally upright after every hip extension.
4. Perform fewer reps.
5. Use a lighter KB.

✕ Common Problem #2:
KB Moves Slowly; No Dynamic Power
√ Corrective Actions:

1. Be sure the handle is turned vertically when you pass it through your legs.
2. Contract your lats hard as you pull the KB through forcefully.
3. Drive off your heel and initiate explosive power from the legs, hips, and abs.
4. Keep the uppercut arm close to the ribcage.
5. Breathe!

b) Uppercut with Release
Adding the Release is a simple way to make the uppercut drill more dynamic and taxing on your core.

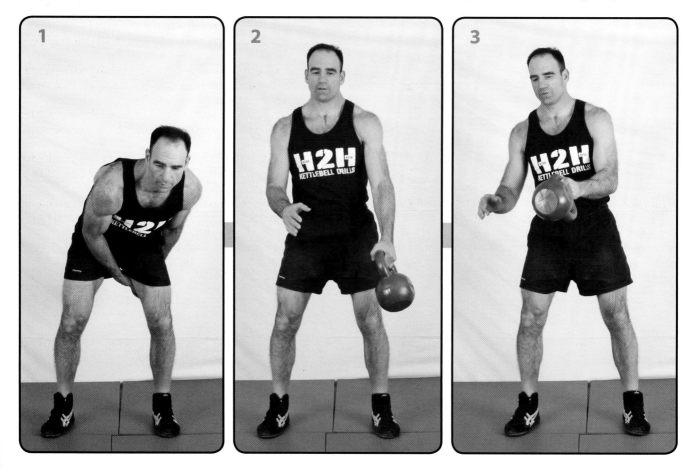

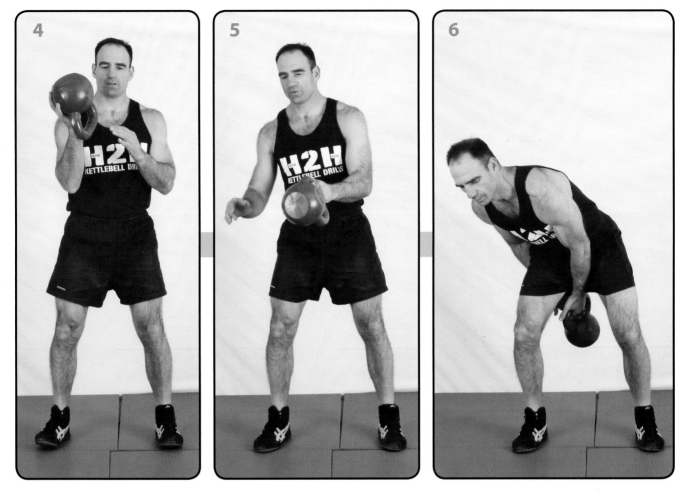

1) Grip the center of the kettlebell handle with your right hand and deadlift the kettlebell to the upright position.
   • Bump the KB off your right thigh, rotating your right hand a quarter turn in a clockwise manner (i.e., thumb is pointing away from your body). As the kettlebell reaches the top of the arc:
   • Sit back and pull the KB diagonally under the left knee. Always pass the kettlebell from front to back, keeping your thumbs up (i.e., KB handle vertical). As the kettlebell passes from the right to left hand, transfer your weight to your left foot. Note: Head is positioned directly over the left foot. Keep your chest open, back straight, and neck neutral.
2) Once the KB is in your left hand, really drive off your left foot, fully extending your legs, hips, and torso, similar to a fighter throwing an uppercut. Simultaneously, exhale actively through your teeth, keeping your left elbow tight against your side.
3) As the kettlebell "shoots" diagonally up and across the front of your chest:
4) Release the kettlebell handle from your left hand. Quickly catching the rising bell with the palm of your right hand. **Note:** Never let the KB move outside shoulder width. Use your core to decelerate and stop the kettlebell directly in front of your right shoulder. This action will load the kinetic energy in your core similar to compressing a spring.
5) Immediately reverse the direction of the kettlebell by pushing it straight down feeding the handle back to the left hand. Sit back and pull the KB diagonally under the right knee. Always pass the kettlebell from front to back, keeping your thumbs up (i.e., KB handle vertical).
6) As the kettlebell passes from the left to right hand, transfer your weight to your right foot. Note: Head position is directly over the right foot. Keep your chest open, back straight, and neck neutral. Repeat for desired time or reps.

Uppercut with Bottoms-Up Catch

The bottoms-up catch is a very challenging grip and core exercise. Be sure you have taken the time to master the bottoms-up clean on pg 196. If you have not done so, do it now.

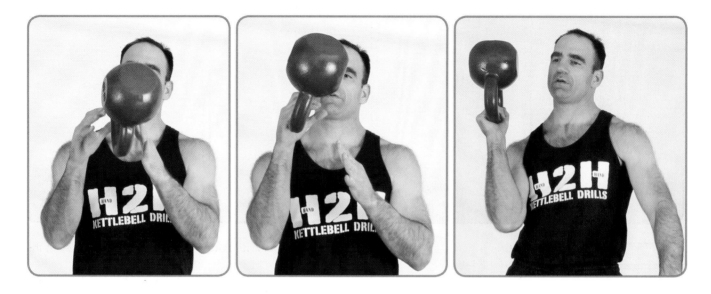

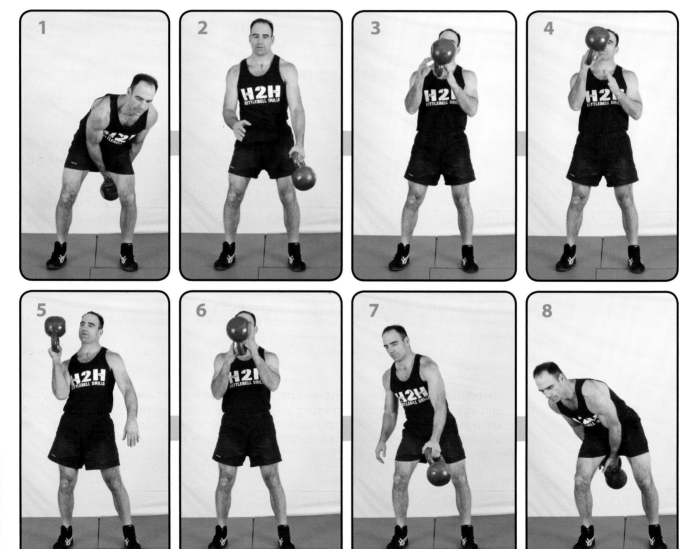

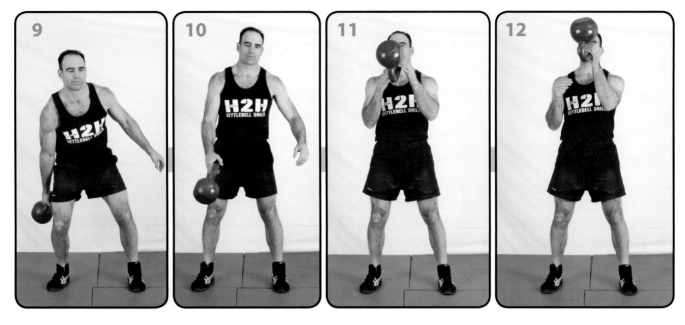

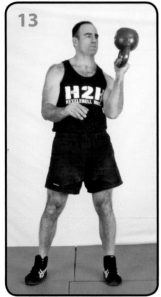

1) Grip the center of the kettlebell handle with your right hand and deadlift the kettlebell to the upright position.
   • Bump the KB off your right thigh, rotating your right hand a quarter turn in a clockwise manner (i.e., thumb is pointing away from your body). As the kettlebell reaches the top of the arc:
   • Sit back and pull the KB diagonally under your left knee and transfer your weight to your left foot as the kettlebell passes from the right to left hand. Note: Head position is directly over the left foot. Keep your chest open, back straight, and neck neutral.
2) Once the KB is in your left hand, explosively drive off your left foot. Note: The goal is to drive the kettlebell with such force that if you missed the catch, the KB would fly up and over your right shoulder.
3) As the kettlebell moves diagonally up and across your chest, release the kettlebell handle from your left hand.
4) Quickly grip the handle with your right hand.
5) Decelerate and stabilize the kettlebell by intensely gripping the handle, pulling the right elbow tightly against your torso, loading/shifting the weight to your right foot and tensing the muscles of your core.
6) Immediately reverse the direction by driving off your right foot and rotate your upper body as if you were initiating a right cross in boxing. Note: Your elbow never leaves your side. Release the kettlebell handle when your right hand starts to move away from your shoulder. Position your left hand in front of your chest.
7) Catch the KB handle at chest height, sit back, guide the KB diagonally under your left knee.
8) Transfer your weight to your right foot, as the kettlebell passes from the left to right hand. Note: Head position is directly over the right foot. Keep your chest open, back straight, and neck neutral.
9) Once the KB is in your right hand, explosively drive off your right foot.
10) Note: The goal is to drive the kettlebell with such force that if you missed the catch, the KB would fly up and over your left shoulder.
11) As the kettlebell moves diagonally up and across your chest, release the kettlebell handle from your right hand.
12) Quickly grip/catch the handle with your left hand.
13) Decelerate and stabilize the kettlebell by intensely gripping the handle, squeezing your left arm against your torso, and activating your core to prevent over-rotation. Immediately reverse the direction by driving off your left foot and rotate your upper body as if you were initiating a punch with your left hand. Repeat the sequence above for time or reps.

5) Hot Potato Drill (isolate movement)

The hot potato is a dynamic drill for strengthening the muscles of the core and upper body. This deceptively demanding exercise enhances the body's ability to absorb impact and taxes your cardio-vascular system. Start out with a light kettlebell; gradually progress with both number of reps and weight.

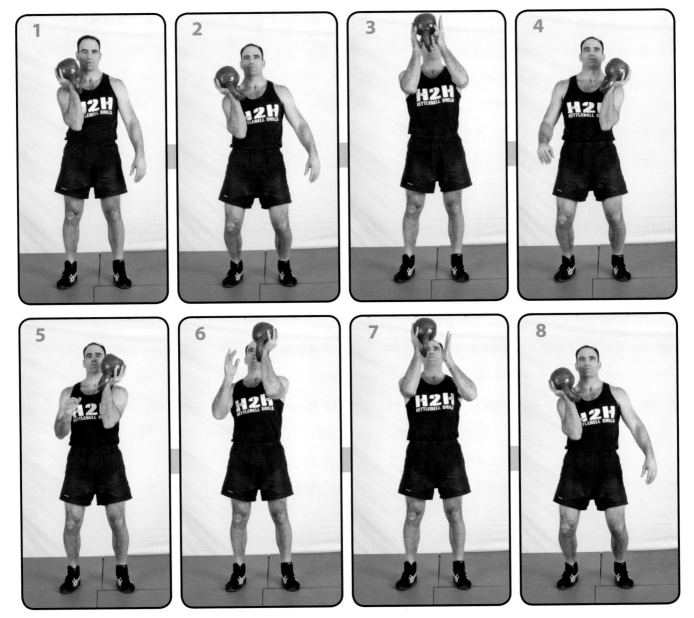

1) - Grip the center of the handle with your right hand and deadlift the kettlebell to the upright position.
   • Bump the KB off your right thigh, rotating your right hand a quarter turn in a clockwise manner (i.e., thumb is pointing away from your body). As the kettlebell reaches the top of the arc:
   • Sit back and pull the KB diagonally under the left knee and transfer your weight to your left foot.
   • Once the KB is in your left hand, explosively drive off your left foot.
   • As the kettlebell moves diagonally up and across your chest, quickly guide and catch the rising bell with the palm of your right hand, stopping the kettlebell directly in front of your right shoulder, handle down, elbow attached to your torso. From the rack position:
2) Dip straight down through your heels; allow your knees to move forward but not past your toes. Keep your hips over your heels and your torso vertical. Do not pause in this position.
3) Immediately drive through your heels with explosive hip and knee extension. This will launch the back of your arm up and off your torso, propelling the kettlebell into the air in a gentle arc. As this happens, reach up with your left hand and prepare for the catch.

4) Catch the bell with the palm of your left hand, fingers extended; handle is down, contacting the front of your forearm. Actively exhale and tighten your abs when the back of your arm contacts your torso. Note: Keep forearm vertical.
5) Dip again, straight down through your heels; allow your knees to move forward but not past your toes. Keep your hips over your heels and your torso vertical.
6) Immediately drive through your heels with explosive hip and knee extension. This will launch the back of your arm up and off your torso, propelling the kettlebell into the air in a gentle arc.
7) As this happens, reach up with your right hand to prepare for the catch.
8) Catch the bell in the palm of your right hand, fingers extended; handle is down, contacting the front of your forearm. Actively exhale and tighten your abs, when the back of your arm contacts your torso. Note: Keep forearm vertical. Repeat, passing it from hand to hand, in a rhythmic fashion for time or reps.

✕ Common Problem #1:
Wrist Strain

√ Corrective Actions:
1. Catch the kettlebell lower in the base of the palm (think palm strike).
2. Keep your wrists tight and extend your fingers as if you were palming a basketball.
3. Start out with a light kettlebell; gradually progress with both number of reps and weight.

✕ Common Problem #2:
Lower Back Discomfort

√ Corrective Actions:
1. Minimize the backward lean.
2. Tense the glutes—"pinch a coin with your cheeks."
3. Contract your core harder and keep intra-abdominal pressure high.

✕ Common Problem #3:
Using Arms and Shoulders Rather Than Core

√ Corrective Actions:
1. Press the shoulders down and press the triceps against the torso. Imagine squeezing a tennis ball in your armpit.
2. Quick, powerful, yet short hip thrust.
3. Contract the muscles of the core harder.

6) Figure 8–Uppercut–Hot Potato Combo

This is one of my favorite combination drills. It's similar to working punching combinations on a heavy bag. Initially, it may challenge your coordination, but after a few reps everything will flow more smoothly. At this point, you have already mastered the individual movements. Now it's just a matter of linking them together.

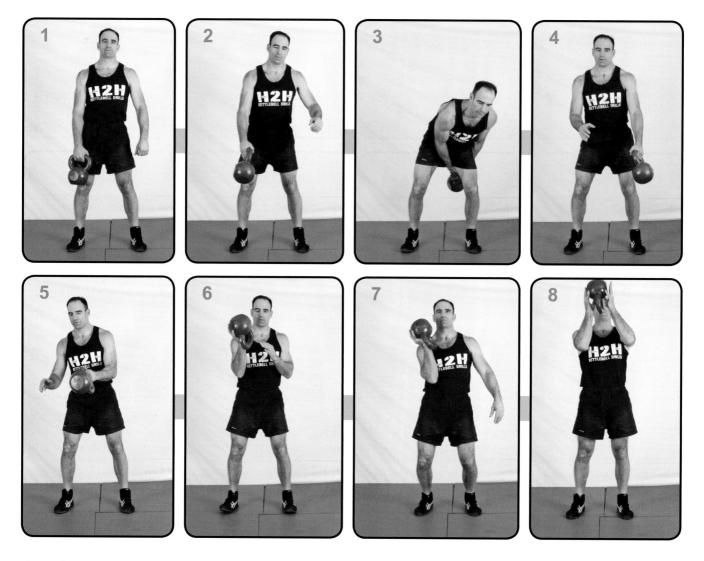

1) Grip the center of the kettlebell handle with your right hand and deadlift the kettlebell to the upright position.
2) Bump the KB off your right thigh, rotating your right hand a quarter turn in a clockwise manner (i.e., thumb is pointing away from your body). As the kettlebell reaches the top of the arc:
3) Sit back and pull the KB diagonally under your left knee. As the kettlebell passes from the right to left hand, transfer your weight to your left foot. Note: Head position is directly over the left foot. Keep your chest open, back straight, and neck neutral.
4) Once the KB is in your left hand, explosively drive off your left foot.
5) As the kettlebell moves diagonally up and across your chest:
6) Release the kettlebell handle from your left hand. Quickly guide and catch the rising bell with the palm of your right hand, stopping the kettlebell directly in front of your right shoulder, handle down, elbow attached to your torso. From this position:
7) Dip straight down through your heels; allow your knees to move forward but not past your toes. As you start to descend, keep your hips over your heels and your torso vertical.
8) Drive through you heels with explosive hip and knee extension. This will launch the back of your arm up and off your torso, propelling the kettlebell up into the air in a gentle arc. As this happens, reach up with your left hand and prepare for the catch.

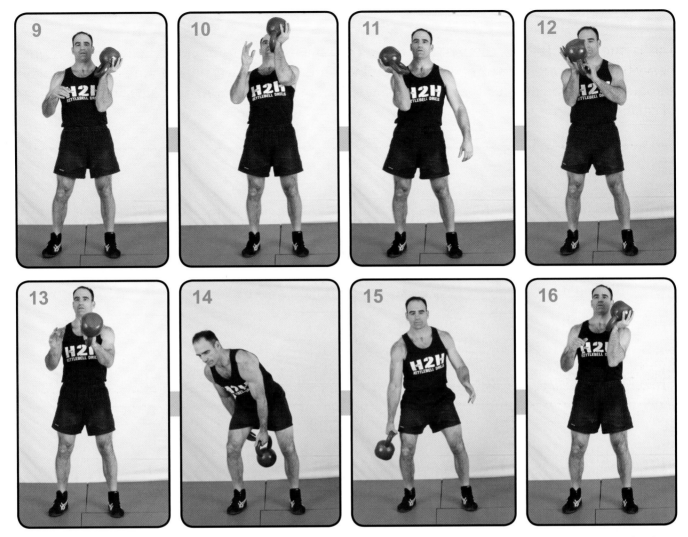

9) Catch the kettlebell with the palm of your left hand, handle down and resting on your forearm. Actively exhale and tighten your abs when the back of your arm contacts your torso. Note: Keep forearm vertical.

10) Dip straight down through your heels and then drive off your heels, launching the kettlebell up into the air in a gentle arc. As this happens, reach up with your right hand to prepare for the catch.

11) Catch the kettlebell with the palm of your right hand, handle down and resting on your forearm. Actively exhale and tighten your abs as the back of your arm contacts your torso. Note: Forearm remains vertical.

12) Dip, drive, and rotate your right shoulder as if initiating a right-handed strike. The combination of the dip, drive, and rotation will propel the kettlebell upward and out toward your centerline.

13) Grab the center of the kettlebell handle with your left hand.

14) Sit back and guide the KB diagonally under the right knee, transferring your weight over your right foot. Note: head position is over the right foot.

15) Once the KB is in your right hand, explosively drive off your right foot.

16) As the kettlebell moves diagonally up and across your chest, release the kettlebell handle from your right hand. Quickly catch the rising bell with the palm of your left hand, stopping the kettlebell directly in front of your left shoulder, handle down, elbow attached to your torso. From this position, hot-potato-pass the kettlebell to your right hand, left, then up, grab handle with your right hand, and so on. Repeat the flow for time or reps.

Training Tips:

1. Talk through each movement in simple terms
   (i.e., "though the legs, uppercut, catch, 1, 2, pass it back through").
2. Use a light kettlebell. Consistency before intensity!

7) Lunge Series

Lunges are a "must" for every athlete. They develop superior lower-body strength and stability. Reverse lunges are recommended when passing the kettlebell using the figure 8 method. Adding this one element will dramatically increase the intensity of all the previous exercises.

a) Figure 8 Lunge

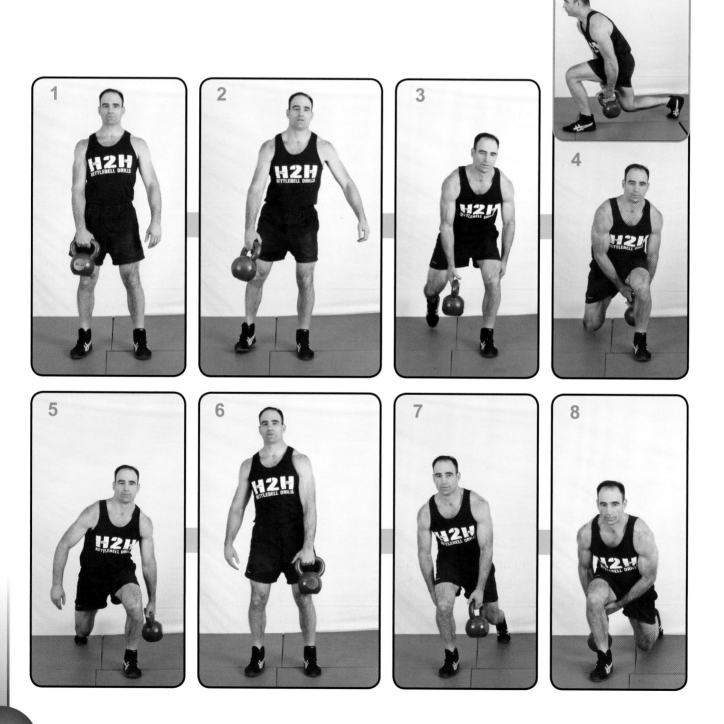

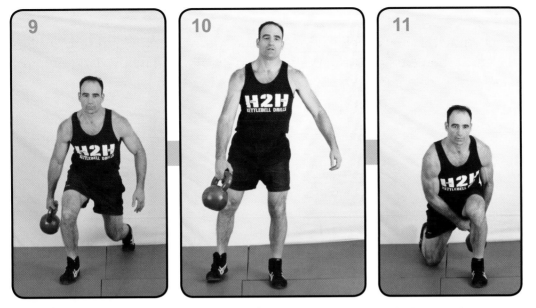

1) Grip the center of the kettlebell handle with your right hand and deadlift the kettlebell to the upright position.

2) Bump the KB off your right thigh, rotating your right hand a quarter turn in a clockwise manner (i.e., thumb is pointing away from your body). Let it bounce back into your right thigh as a kinesthetic reminder; that is the leg that will step back.

3) Step back with your right foot and pull the kettlebell back diagonally to your left.

4) Just before your right knee contacts the ground, pass the kettlebell to your left hand. Depending on the floor surface, it's your choice whether your knee touches the ground or not.

5) Keeping your left shin vertical, drive off your left heel, activating your left glute to stand up.

6) As you stand up, the kettlebell will automatically move up and around your left thigh. Allow the kettlebell to gently pendulum and lightly impact the front of your left thigh. That's the kinesthetic reminder of which leg you will step back with next.

7) Step back with your left foot and pull the kettlebell back diagonally to the right.

8) Pass the kettlebell under your right knee.

9) Keeping your right shin vertical, drive off your right heel, activating your right glute, then stand up.

10) As you stand up, the kettlebell will automatically move up and around your right thigh. Allow the kettlebell to gently pendulum and lightly impact the front of your right thigh. That's the kinesthetic reminder of which leg you will step back with next.

11) Once you're in the upright position, the kettlebell is in your right hand, in front of your right thigh. Repeat for desired time or reps.

✕ Common Problems:
Instability, Loss of Balance, Knee Strain

√ Corrective Actions:

1. Be sure your shoulders and hips are "square."
2. Keep your chest open, back straight, abs tight.
3. Be sure your toes and knees track (i.e., pointing directly forward, not in or out).
4. Step straight back, as if your feet are on railroad tracks, rather than on a tight rope.
5. Front shin remains vertical, loading the glute.
6. Look straight ahead, not down.
7. If the above tips don't solve the problem, use a lighter KB to build up strength and endurance slowly.

b) Figure 8 Lunge—Around-the-Body Pass (ABP)

By adding the around-the-body pass in between lunges you will receive an active rest, allowing you to do more reps for longer periods of time and increasing your work capacity.

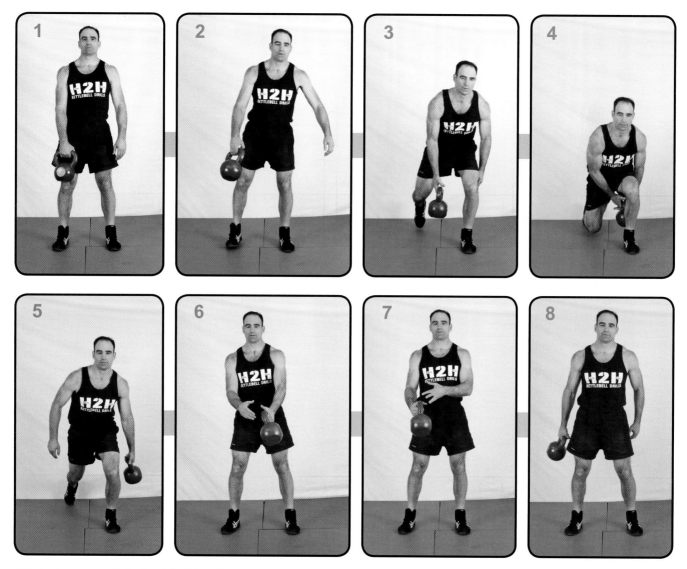

1) Grip the center of the kettlebell handle with your right hand and deadlift the kettlebell to the upright position.
2) Bump the KB off your right thigh, rotating your right hand a quarter turn in a clockwise manner (i.e., thumb is pointing away from your body). Let it bounce back into your right thigh as a kinesthetic reminder; that is the leg that will step back.
3) Step back with your right foot and pull the kettlebell back diagonally to your left.
4) Just before your right knee contacts the ground, pass the kettlebell to your left hand. Depending on the floor surface, it's your choice whether your knee touches the ground or not.
5) Keep your left shin vertical, drive off your left heel (i.e., activating your left glute), and stand up.
6) As you stand up, the kettlebell will automatically move up and around your left thigh. Continue moving the kettlebell in a clockwise direction.
7) Perform the fingertip-to-fingertip around-the-body pass, transferring the kettlebell to your right hand.
8) Continue moving the KB around your right leg in a clockwise direction.

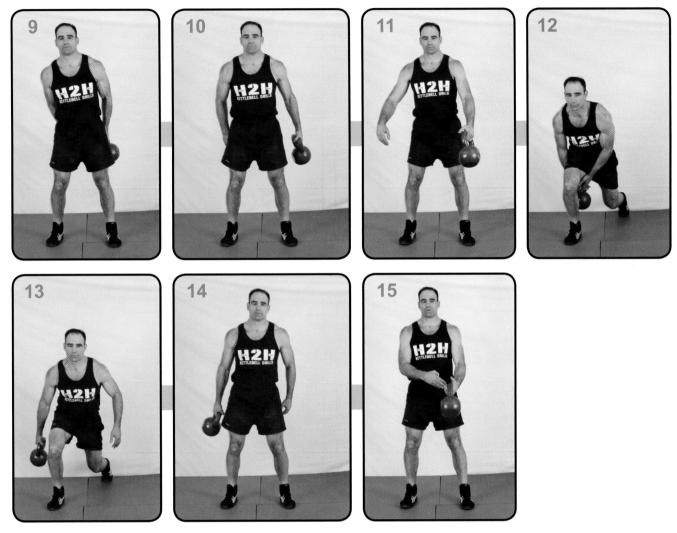

9) Pass the kettlebell to your left hand, behind your back, palms facing each other.

10) Continue moving the KB clockwise around your left leg.

11) As soon as the KB is 45 degrees off your left leg:

12) Simultaneously step back with your left foot and pull the kettlebell back diagonally to the right, passing the kettlebell under your right knee.

13) Keeping your right shin near vertical, drive off your right heel, activating your right glute, and stand up.

14) As you stand up, the kettlebell will automatically move up and around your right thigh. Continue moving the kettlebell in a counterclockwise direction.

15) Perform the fingertip-to-fingertip around-the-body pass transferring the kettlebell to your left hand. Continue passing the kettlebell around the body, reverse lunge, around-the-body, reverse lunge, alternating. Repeat for desired time or reps.

c) Figure 8 Lunge–Uppercut

Grab a light kettlebell and have fun practicing this combination. This is a particularly demanding exercise. The key to success is to powerfully load your outside glute, driving off the heel of your front foot.

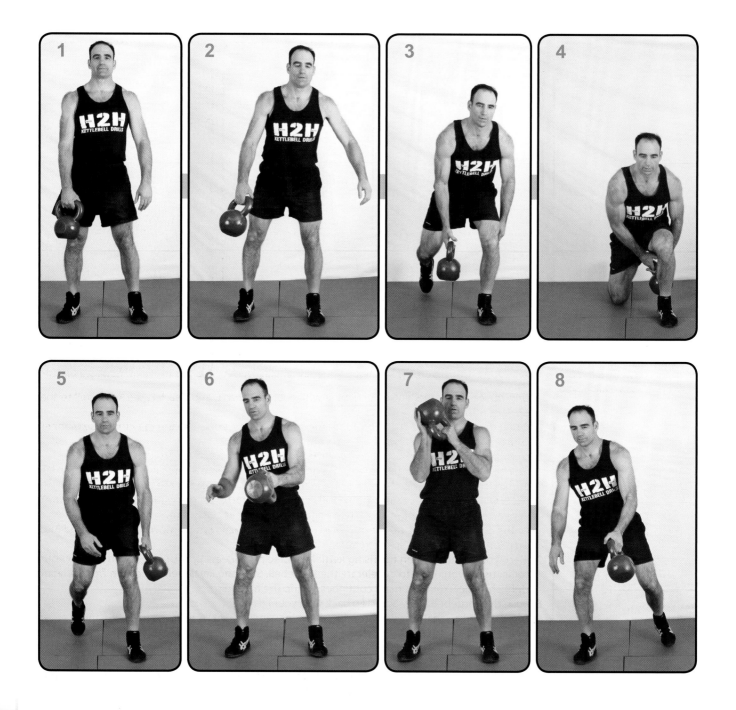

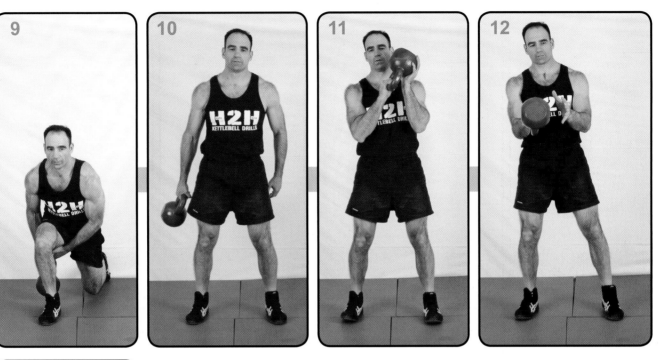

1) Grip the center of the kettlebell handle with your right hand and deadlift the kettlebell to the upright position.
2) Bump the KB off your right thigh, rotating your right hand a quarter turn in a clockwise manner (i.e., thumb is pointing away from your body).
3) Step back with your right foot and pull the kettlebell back diagonally to your left.
4) Just before your right knee contacts the ground, pass the kettlebell to your left hand. Depending on the floor surface, it's your choice whether your knee touches the ground or not.
5) Keeping your left shin vertical, powerfully drive off your left heel (i.e., activating your left glute), actively exhale through your teeth to engage your core, and stand up.
6) As the kettlebell moves up diagonally in front of your chest, quickly move your right hand into position to decelerate the rising bell.
7) Place your right hand on the rising kettlebell, bracing/squeezing your upper arm against your torso, using your core to decelerate the kettlebell. Stop the kettlebell directly in front of your right shoulder. Your left hand continues to grip the handle.
8) Push the kettlebell away and step back with your left foot.
9) Pull the KB diagonally under your right knee, passing the kettlebell to your right hand. As you pull, you should feel a strong contraction in your left lat and across your midsection. Note: Always pass the kettlebell from front to back while maintaining the thumbs-up position (i.e., KB handle vertical).
10) Keeping your right shin vertical, powerfully drive off your right heel (i.e., activating your right glute), actively exhale through your teeth to engage your core, and stand up.
11) As the kettlebell moves up diagonally in front of your chest, quickly move your left hand into position to decelerate the rising bell. Brace and squeeze your upper left arm against your torso and use your core to decelerate the kettlebell, stopping the kettlebell directly in front of your left shoulder. Right hand continues to grip the handle.
12) Push the kettlebell away with your left hand.
13) Pass the kettlebell underneath your left leg. Repeat the movements for time or reps. Note: If you're getting smoked too fast, add the around-body-pass as a form of active rest, or practice more sets of lower reps.

e) Figure 8 Lunge–Uppercut Release

Focus on the fundamentals and efficiency of movement. The release makes this drill more dynamic and forces you to generate more speed/power from your hips and core.

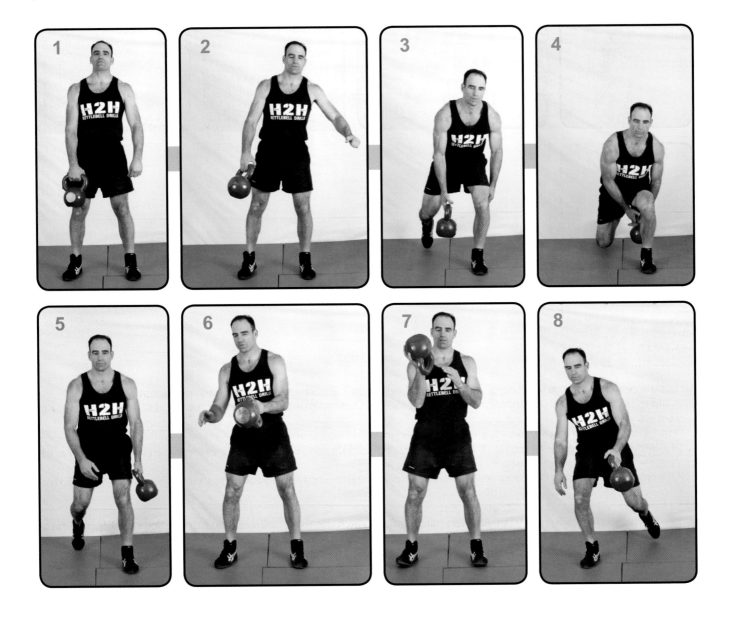

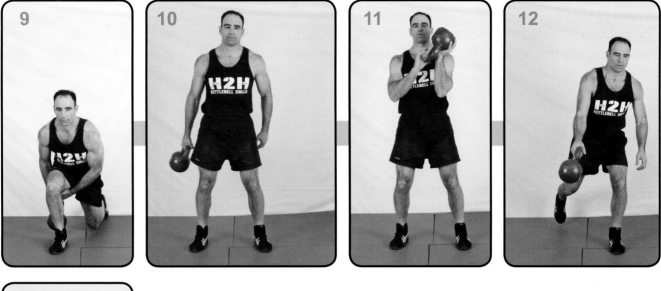

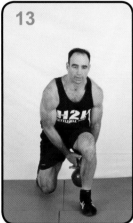

1) Grip the center of the kettlebell handle with your right hand and deadlift the kettlebell to the upright position.

2) Bump the KB off your right thigh, rotating your right hand a quarter turn in a clockwise manner (i.e., thumb is pointing away from your body).

3) Step back with your right foot and pull the kettlebell back diagonally to your left.

4) Just before your right knee contacts the ground, pass the kettlebell to your left hand. Depending on the floor surface, it's your choice whether your knee touches the ground or not.

5) Keeping your left shin vertical, powerfully drive off your left heel (i.e., activating your left glute), actively exhale through your teeth to engage your core, and stand up.

6) As the kettlebell moves diagonally up and across your chest:

7) Release the kettlebell handle from your left hand. Quickly catch the rising bell with the palm of your right hand. Brace/squeeze your upper arm against your torso and use your core to decelerate the kettlebell. Stop the kettlebell directly in front of your right shoulder. Note: Do not let the KB move outside shoulder width.

8) Dip and drive the kettlebell up and out toward your centerline. Reach out with your left hand, catch the handle, and step back with your left foot.

9) Guide the KB diagonally under your right knee, passing the kettlebell to your right hand. As you pull, you should feel a strong contraction in your left lat and across your midsection. Note: Always pass the kettlebell from front to back and maintain the thumbs-up position (i.e., KB handle vertical).

10) Keeping your right shin vertical, powerfully drive off your right heel (i.e., activating your right glute), actively exhale through your teeth to engage your core, and stand up.

11) As the kettlebell moves up diagonally in front of your chest, release the kettlebell handle from your right hand. Quickly catch the rising bell with the palm of your left hand. Brace/squeeze your upper arm against your torso and use your core to decelerate the kettlebell. Stop the kettlebell directly in front of your left shoulder. Note: Do not let the KB drift past shoulder width.

12) Dip and drive the kettlebell up and out toward your centerline. Reach out with your right hand, catch the handle, and step back with your right foot.

13) Guide the KB diagonally under the left knee and continue, repeating the movements for time or reps. Note: If this drill is smoking you too fast, add the around-body-pass as a form of active rest or practice more sets of lower reps.

g) Figure 8 Lunge–Uppercut–Hot Potato Combo

This is one of the most demanding combination drills. Initially, it may challenge your coordination, but after a few reps everything will flow more smoothly. It's just a matter of practice.

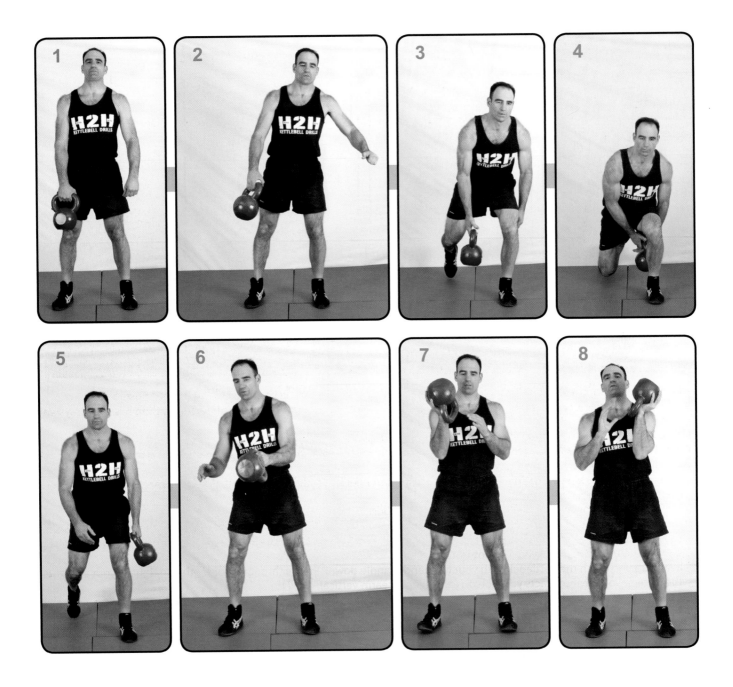

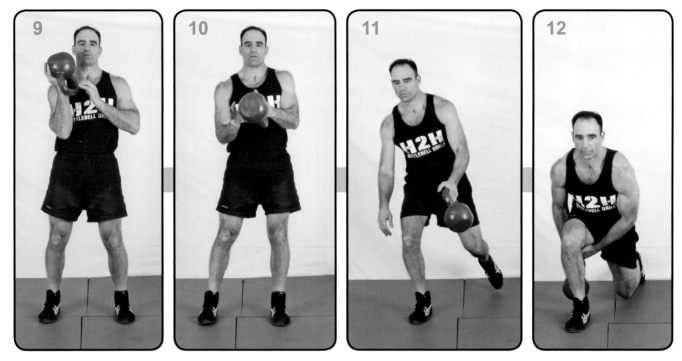

1) Grip the center of the kettlebell handle with your right hand and deadlift the kettlebell to the upright position.
2) Bump the KB off your right thigh, rotating your right hand a quarter turn in a clockwise manner (i.e., thumb is pointing away from your body).
3) Step back with your right foot and pull the kettlebell back diagonally to your left.
4) Just before your right knee contacts the ground, pass the kettlebell to your left hand. Depending on the floor surface, it's your choice whether your knee touches the ground or not.
5) Keeping your left shin vertical, powerfully drive off your left heel (i.e., activating your left glute), actively exhale through your teeth to engage your core, and stand up.
6) As the kettlebell moves diagonally up and across your chest:
7) Release the kettlebell handle from your left hand. Quickly catch the rising bell with the palm of your right hand. Brace/squeeze your upper arm against your torso and use your core to decelerate the kettlebell. Dip and drive the kettlebell up and over toward your left hand (i.e., hot-potato).
8) Reach up and catch the kettlebell with your left hand (handle down). Exhale through your teeth and tighten your abs when the back of your arm contacts your torso. Note: Keep forearm vertical.
9) Repeat: Dip and drive the kettlebell back up toward your left hand (i.e., hot-potato). As the kettlebell ascends to its maximum height, reach up with your right hand to catch and guide it back to the rack position.
10) Dip and drive the kettlebell up and out toward your centerline. Reach out with your left hand and:
11) Catch/grip the kettlebell handle while stepping back with your left foot.
12) Guide the KB diagonally under your right knee, passing the kettlebell to your right hand. Repeat the movements for time or reps. Terminate all sets before your form deteriorates.

h) Figure 8 Lunge–Uppercut–Bottoms-Up Catch Combo

This combination drill will tax everything from your hips to grip . . . enjoy!

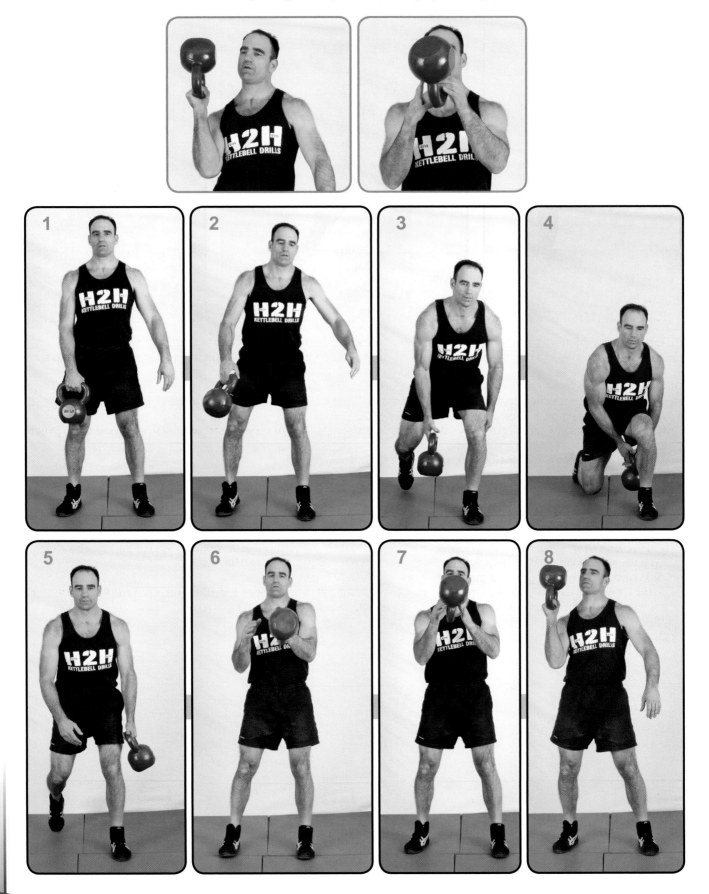

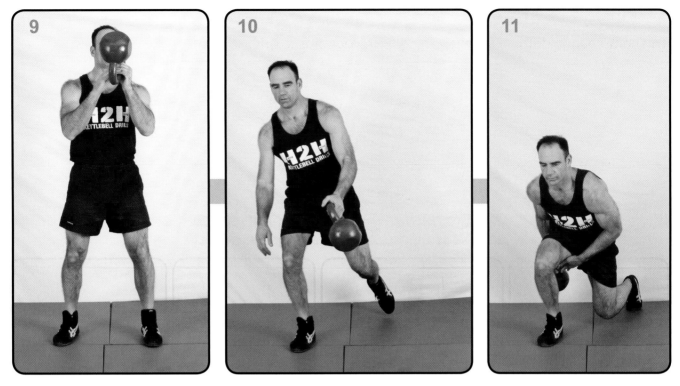

1) Grip the center of the kettlebell handle with your right hand and deadlift the kettlebell to the upright position.

2) Bump the KB off your right thigh, rotating your right hand a quarter turn in a clockwise manner (i.e., thumb is pointing away from your body).

3) Step back with your right foot and pull the kettlebell back diagonally to your left.

4) Just before your right knee contacts the ground, pass the kettlebell to your left hand. Depending on the floor surface, it's your choice whether your knee touches the ground or not.

5) Keeping your left shin vertical, powerfully drive off your left heel (i.e., activating your left glute), actively exhale through your teeth to engage your core, and stand up.

6) As the kettlebell moves diagonally up and across your chest:

7) Release the kettlebell handle from your left hand.

8) Quickly grip the handle with your right hand. Decelerate and stabilize the kettlebell by intensely gripping the handle, pulling your right elbow tightly against your torso, loading/shifting the weight to your right foot, and tensing the muscles of your core.

9) Slightly dip, drive, and rotate your right shoulder, as if initiating a punch. This movement will propel the kettlebell upward and out toward your centerline. As your right hand begins to move away from your shoulder, release the kettlebell handle with your right hand. Immediately reach out with your left hand and grasp the KB handle.

10) Step back with your left foot and guide the KB diagonally between your legs.

11) Just before your left knee touches the ground, pass the kettlebell to your right hand. (Depending on the floor surface, it's your choice whether your knee contacts the ground or not.) Repeat for desired time or reps.

H2H Program Design

In the beginning, I recommend two H2H training sessions a week. Pick a few skills and just focus on becoming more skillful. Have fun and use it as a form of active recovery. Your conditioning levels will automatically improve just by practicing your skills. Keep the weight light and strive to make all your movements as smooth, efficient, and effortless as possible.

If you're a person who needs more structure, then consider circuit training. It's a more systematic way to increase your conditioning levels without the risk of overtraining. The only thing you will need in addition to your kettlebell is an interval timer (i.e., watch, ring timer, gym boss, etc.). Each circuit consists of three elements. Familiarize yourself and practice each element individually. Follow the principles outlined below and use it for dynamic warm-ups, active recovery, or a challenging total-body workout.

"It doesn't matter what you know, if you can't make it flow."

—Jeff Martone

H2H Circuits

Regardless of your fitness level or kettlebell lifting experience, it's highly recommended that everyone start out at the beginner level. Please keep in mind there is a learning curve to overcome. This is especially true as the drills begin to link together. Progress slowly, allowing your body to adapt to new demands and routines. This is the key for preventing overuse injuries.

There are three levels of H2H circuit programming. The beginner circuit is six weeks long. This is the place to start when implementing newly learned drills. The intermediate and advanced circuits are each seven weeks long. As you progress through the levels, your work periods gradually increase while rest periods decrease.

The general "rule of thumb" is to complete a circuit three times (three separate training sessions) at a particular level before progressing to the next level. In other words, if you find yourself "waiting" for your rest interval to end, then it's time to move to the next level.

Please note: This is just a guide. Stay at each level for a minimum of three training sessions. It doesn't matter if you stay at a given phase for three days or three weeks. The key is consistency and determination. Stay the course!

You can't develop work capacity without work. The key, whether you're working at high intensity or low intensity, is to continue moving. This builds work capacity and mental toughness. There's an old saying "If you can't run anymore—jog. If you can't jog anymore—walk. If you can't walk anymore—crawl." Likewise, when fatigued at any point during the circuits, substitute an easier drill.

The key to the effectiveness of this training is to stay in constant motion. If on the second or third rounds you find that you're having problems performing a KB drill safely, put the kettlebell down and continue on with one of the following body weight exercises until your time is up:

Element #1:
Jumping jacks, jogging in place, shadow boxing

Element #2:
Burpees, Hindu push-ups or upward/downward dog

Element #3:
Body weight squat, body weight lunge, box step-ups

Listed below are three samples of possible elements choices for your H2H circuits.

Sample H2H Circuit
Element #1: Around-the-Body Pass
Element #2: Hot Potato Drill
Element #3: Figure 8 Drill

Sample H2H Circuit
Element #1: Around-the-Body Pass, Figure 8 Combo
Element #2: Figure 8 with Lunge
Element #3: Upper Cut Drill

Sample H2H Circuit
Element #1: Two Hand Swing and Release
Element #2: Figure 8 Lunge, Uppercut Release
Element #3: Around-the-Body Pass, Figure 8 Combo

No fluff, no frills – just practice the drills!

Beginner Circuit

Interval Training Phase:

Week One:

Element 1: 30 seconds work / 30 seconds rest interval

Element 2: 30 seconds work / 30 seconds rest interval

Element 3: 30 seconds work / 30 seconds rest interval

Repeat this circuit three times (3 rounds).

Total Time: 9 minutes

Week Two:

Element 1: 30 seconds work / 15 seconds rest interval

Element 2: 30 seconds work / 15 seconds rest interval

Element 3: 30 seconds work / 15 seconds rest interval

Repeat this circuit three times (3 rounds).

Total Time: 6 minutes, 45 seconds

Circuit Training Phase:
(no rest in between elements, rest interval between rounds)

Week Three:

Element 1: 30 seconds of work / 0 seconds of rest interval

Element 2: 30 seconds of work / 0 seconds of rest interval

Element 3: 30 seconds of work / 45 seconds of rest interval

Repeat this circuit three times (3 rounds).

Total Time: 6 minutes, 45 seconds

Week Four:

Element 1: 30 seconds of work / 0 seconds of rest interval

Element 2: 30 seconds of work / 0 seconds of rest interval

Element 3: 30 seconds of work / 30 seconds of rest interval

Repeat this circuit three times (3 rounds).

Total Time: 6 minutes

Week Five:

Element 1: 30 seconds of work / 0 seconds of rest interval

Element 2: 30 seconds of work / 0 seconds of rest interval

Element 3: 30 seconds of work / 15 seconds of rest interval

Repeat this circuit three times (3 rounds).

Total Time: 5 minutes, 15 seconds

Intermediate Circuit

Interval Training Phase:

Week One:

Element 1: 1 minute work / 45 seconds rest interval

Element 2: 1 minute work / 45 seconds rest interval

Element 3: 1 minute work / 45 seconds rest interval

Repeat this circuit three times (3 rounds).

Total Time: 15 minutes, 45 seconds

Week Two:

Element 1: 1 minute work / 30 seconds rest interval

Element 2: 1 minute work / 30 seconds rest interval

Element 3: 1 minute work / 30 seconds rest interval

Repeat this circuit three times (3 rounds).

Total Time: 13 minutes, 30 seconds

Week Three:

Element 1: 1 minute work / 15 seconds rest interval

Element 2: 1 minute work / 15 seconds rest interval

Element 3: 1 minute work / 15 seconds rest interval

Repeat this circuit three times (3 rounds)

Total Time: 11 minutes, 15 seconds

Circuit Training Phase:
(no rest in between elements, rest interval between rounds)

Week Four:

Element 1: 1 minute work / 0 seconds of rest interval

Element 2: 1 minute work / 0 seconds of rest interval

Element 3: 1 minute work / 45 seconds of rest interval

Repeat this circuit three times (3 rounds).

Total Time: 11 minutes, 15 seconds

Week Five:

Element 1: 1 minute work / 0 seconds of rest interval

Element 2: 1 minute work / 0 seconds of rest interval

Element 3: 1 minute work / 30 seconds of rest interval

Repeat this circuit three times (3 rounds).

Total Time: 10 minutes, 30 seconds

Week Six:

Element 1: 1 minute work / 0 seconds of rest interval

Element 2: 1 minute work / 0 seconds of rest interval

Element 3: 1 minute work / 15 seconds of rest interval

Repeat this circuit three times (3 rounds).

Total Time: 9 minutes, 45 seconds

Non-Stop, Free-Flow Phase:
(no rest in between elements or rounds)

Week Seven:

Element 1: 1 minute work / 0 seconds of rest interval

Element 2: 1 minute work / 0 seconds of rest interval

Element 3: 1 minute work / 0 seconds of rest interval

Repeat this circuit three times (3 rounds).

Total Time: 9 minutes

H2H Program Design

Advanced Circuit

Interval Training Phase:

Week One:

Element 1: 2 minute work / 45 seconds rest interval

Element 2: 2 minute work / 45 seconds rest interval

Element 3: 2 minute work / 45 seconds rest interval

Repeat this circuit three times (3 rounds).

Total Time: 24 minutes, 45 seconds

Week Two:

Element 1: 2 minute work / 30 seconds rest interval

Element 2: 2 minute work / 30 seconds rest interval

Element 3: 2 minute work / 30 seconds rest interval

Repeat this circuit three times (3 rounds).

Total Time: 22 minutes, 30 seconds

Week Three:

Element 1: 2 minute work / 15 seconds rest interval

Element 2: 2 minute work / 15 seconds rest interval

Element 3: 2 minute work / 15 seconds rest interval

Repeat this circuit three times (3 rounds)

Total Time: 20 minutes, 15 seconds

Circuit Training Phase:
(no rest in between elements, rest interval between rounds)

Week Four:

Element 1: 2 minute work / 0 seconds of rest interval

Element 2: 2 minute work / 0 seconds of rest interval

Element 3: 2 minute work / 45 seconds of rest interval

Repeat this circuit three times (3 rounds).

Total Time: 20 minutes, 15 seconds

Week Five:

Element 1: 2 minute work / 0 seconds of rest interval

Element 2: 2 minute work / 0 seconds of rest interval

Element 3: 2 minute work / 30 seconds of rest interval

Repeat this circuit three times (3 rounds).

Total Time: 19 minutes, 30 seconds

Week Six:

Element 1: 2 minute work / 0 seconds of rest interval

Element 2: 2 minute work / 0 seconds of rest interval

Element 3: 2 minute work / 15 seconds of rest interval

Repeat this circuit three times (3 rounds).

Total Time: 18 minutes, 45 seconds

Non-Stop, Free-Flow Phase:
(no rest in between elements or rounds)

Week Seven:

Element 1: 2 minute work / 0 seconds of rest interval

Element 2: 2 minute work / 0 seconds of rest interval

Element 3: 2 minute work / 0 seconds of rest interval

Repeat this circuit three times (3 rounds).

Total Time: 18 minutes

Note: The circuit-training format is extremely flexible. It doesn't have to be limited to H2H Drills only. You can add any variety of swings, cleans, or snatches into the mix. For more information on H2H Drills and Circuits, check us out online at www.tacticalathlete.com.

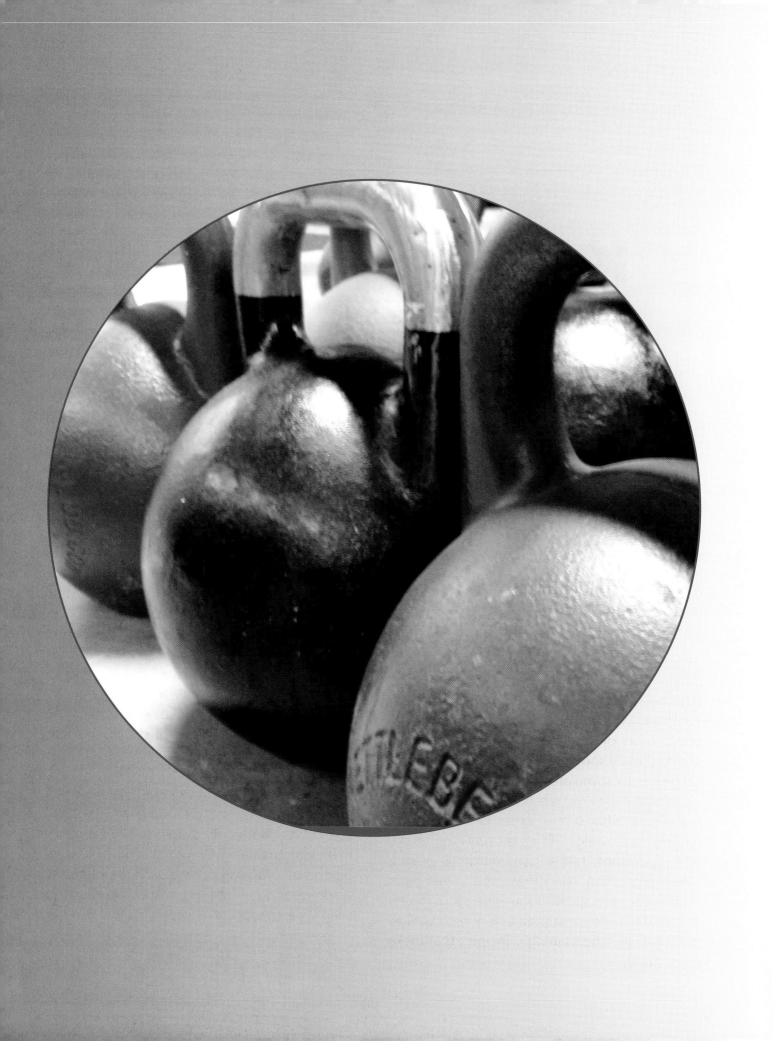

Part III

Introduction to Kettlebell Sport

"Physical fitness develops not only speed, energy, and agility to move faster, but it also develops the endurance to maintain that speed for longer durations. With endurance, we not only outpace the enemy but maintain a higher tempo longer than he can."

— Warfighting, USMC

A book on kettlebell training would not be complete without addressing the Russian national sport of kettlebell lifting (aka kettlebell sport, girevoy sport, or GS). The purpose of this section is to stimulate awareness of kettlebell sport and the many benefits of practicing sport technique. What distinguishes kettlebell sport among other weightlifting sports is that maximal repetitions, rather than maximal weight, determine who becomes the champion. Throughout this section, you will be introduced to current world-champions, honored coaches of Russia, and the training principles that make them great.

"Methods are many, principles are few. Methods always change, principles never do."

—Anonymous

The following information is by no means an exhaustive treatise or definitive guide to the sport of kettlebell lifting, nor is it intended to get you to the rank of master of sport. Rather, it's a primer designed to elucidate the type of performance you can achieve by correctly understanding and applying the principles and scientific training methods of kettlebell sport. The results speak for themselves.

I sincerely hope the following information will inspire, motivate, and challenge you to study the classic kettlebell exercises and practice them with greater virtuosity. Who knows? Maybe one day you will compete on the platform, work toward the rank of master of sport, or even set a new world record!

The Short of Kettlebell Sport

Listed below is a synopsis of the competitive exercises and events of kettlebell sport. For more detailed information, see the complete IKSFA ranking tables located at the end of this chapter.

- Classified as a cyclical sport, composed of competitive exercises that last for up to 10 minutes.

- Competition kettlebells have standard dimensions: height 280 mm, body diameter 210 mm, handle diameter 35 mm, handle length 115 mm.

- Competition kettlebells are color-coded 16 kg (yellow), 24 kg (green), 32 kg (red).

- Athletes compete according to sex, age, and weight category.

- One judge is assigned to each athlete to ensure correct technique and all rules are followed. The judge keeps score and his decision is final.

The Classic Kettlebell Exercises

- **Jerk:** two kettlebells are cleaned once to the chest (i.e., rack position), then jerked as many times overhead as possible. The finish position must have knees and elbows in full lockout.

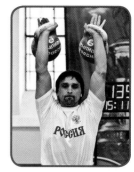

Sergey Rachinsky,

IKSFA President, HMS (Honored Master of Sport), MSWC (Master of Sport World Class), Honored Coach of Russia, 9-time World Champion, 12-time Champion of Russia, and father of the Kettlebell Sport Relay event.

Photo courtesy of IKSFA

- **Snatch:** a single kettlebell is swung between your legs and up to the overhead position in one uninterrupted movement, finishing with the arm fully extended overhead. Only one hand switch is permitted.

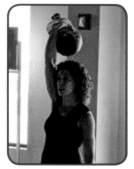

Lorna Kleidman,

2-Time World Champion, 3-Time Int'l Master of Sport, Master of Sport (20 kg Snatch for MSWC IKSFA/IKFF ranking—176 reps. 92 Right and 84 Left.)

- **Long Cycle:** one exercise preformed in three steps: clean two kettlebells to chest, Jerk them to the overhead position, then allow the kettlebells to drop into the back-swing position and repeat this cycle for reps.

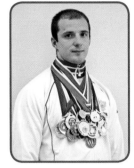

Denis Vasiliev,

Master of Sport World Class, 2-time World Champion, 3-time Champion of Europe, 3-time Champion of Russia. Long Cycle record holder: 84 reps (World Record in 80 kg weight class).

Photo courtesy of IKSFA

Traditional Events

- **Biathlon:** combination of two events jerk and snatch. Competitors jerk two kettlebells overhead for as many reps as possible (AMRAP) in 10 minutes, followed by a 30-minute rest period, then 10 minutes of snatches: AMRAP in 5 minutes with one hand, then AMRAP in 5 minutes the other hand, only one hand switch is permitted.

- **Long Cycle:** stand-alone event; AMRAP for 10 minutes.

Special Events

- **Marathon:** One-arm jerk, AMRAP in 1 hour. Multiple hand switches are permitted. Set ends when time expires or kettlebell is placed on the ground.

Jad Marinovic,

founder of Kettlebell Athletica, achieved a total of 546 jerks with 16 kg without putting the Kettlebell down, setting a new record.

Australia's 1st International Girevoy Sport Marathon champion Jad Marinovic, wins the highest title in the 1-hour kettlebell marathon discipline at the Italian Girevoy Sport Federation Marathon Championships in Milan, Italy, on the 12/06/2011. Eight months later, Jad competed in a half-marathon and achieved 523 jerks with a 16 kg kettlebell in 30 minutes.

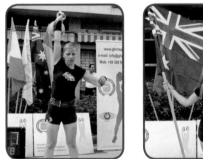
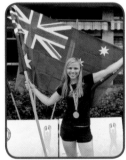

Photos courtesy of Jad

- **Relay:** Sergey Rachinsky is the father of relays in kettlebell sport. The relay was first included in the 2002 Championships and Cups of Russia. Relays are either classic jerk or long cycle (2 kettlebells). There are seven weight categories, and consists of seven competitors per team and a 3-minute all-out sprint (fastest pace possible). The team with the most repetitions wins.

Not Fully Convinced

Truth is stranger than fiction. If you told me two years ago that I would be joyfully competing in kettlebell sport today, I would have laughed out loud and thought you were on drugs. Up until a few of months ago, I have never really had the desire to compete in kettlebell sport. I know that may sound odd coming from one of the "pioneers" of the modern-day kettlebell movement in the United States, but it's the truth.

I supported the sport and served as a judge in some of the very first American GS competitions. Even my wife enjoyed competing and became the 2004 Florida State Champion in both snatch and long cycle. I was happy for her and everyone else who competed. However, I had absolutely no interest in competing. I was very content to train with kettlebells to improve my general physical preparation (GPP) and the performance of my job skills (i.e., combatives, marksmanship, and small-unit tactics). From what I observed at that time, the risk/benefit ratio of doing kettlebell sport seemed a bit off.

I strived to keep an open mind to new training methods and follow the "always a student, sometimes an instructor" philosophy. At that time in America, the information regarding kettlebell sport was limited and slightly outdated. Later in 2006, I had an opportunity to train with a former GS world champion. I wanted to broaden my knowledge, understanding, and skill base. As a result of this training, my snatch technique became more efficient; I learned the importance of tempo/pacing and bought a set of competition kettlebells. On the down side, the training stimulated more questions than answers and my brief experience on the platform only confirmed my suspicions that this had to be the most miserable sport in existence. At that time, I couldn't figure out what was more painful, performing timed sets or watching others perform timed sets.

This GS training experience was reminiscent of my mid-eighties boxing experience at the Natick Boxing Club. I'd show up, do a quick warm-up, put the gloves on, spar, punch the heavy bag, jump rope, shadow box, go home, and repeat. The coaches gave minimal training advice and explanations. As the weeks turned into months, my skill did improve, but only out of shear will and determination. It was a slow and frustrating learning process. I didn't know any different, so I just kept moving forward. Knowing what I know now, I could have avoided a fair amount of punishment and character building if I'd had different coaches.

It wasn't until fifteen years later, when I was training with boxing coach Steve Bacarri, that my eyes were opened to a more excellent way. I learned more about the technical aspects of boxing in a few days with Steve than I did in two years at my old club. When I expressed this to Steve, he said:

"If boxing was about just being tough, then we could just get in the ring and take turns hitting each other with a two-by-four."

The Litmus Test for a Training Program

Listed below are five criteria for testing a sound, proper, and successful training program.

1. Training must be valid, producing the desired result.
2. Training must be relevant, pertinent.
3. Training must be effective, prepared, and available for service.
4. Training must be efficient, performing or functioning in the best possible manner with the least waste of time and effort.
5. Training must support the personal growth of the athlete.

I can honestly say that I'm not emotionally attached to one method of training or training implement. If something increases my performance and lowers my chance of injury, I keep it. Otherwise I get rid of it. It's that simple.

Based on my experience and the limited the kettlebell sport training I had been exposed to up to that point seemed to fail the "litmus test" in just about every aspect. It appeared like a good way to dislocate a shoulder or injure the lower back, and it didn't seem relevant to my personal or professional goals. The entire concept of the sport didn't make sense to me, nor could I see any practical application or transfer of skills to other sports or professions.

As I mentioned earlier, a comedian once said there were only three things you needed to do to be a successful boxer:

1. Train everyday
2. Get a good nickname, and
3. Train everyday

At that point, this was my translation of what it took to be a successful kettlebell lifter:

1. Crush yourself everyday
2. Get a Russian accent, and
3. Crush yourself everyday

Five Years Later

On June 25, 2011, I competed in my first competition, the New York Open Kettlebell Championship. I chose the long cycle event, a 10-minute event where you continuously clean and jerk two 24 kg kettlebells. I had three goals: (1) have fun, (2) stay on the platform for the entire 10 minutes, and (3) perform seventy repetitions (Rank I) without sacrificing form.

By God's grace I actually achieved all my goals, plus an extra three reps! When I made the decision to compete, it was less than three weeks prior to the event and I had never attempted a continuous ten-minute set with the 24 kg bells before, only with the 16s. Did I achieve my goals because of my athletic prowess? Not hardly. I was blessed with excellent coaches and friends who inspired me to sharpen my technique and follow through to the logical conclusion of my training.

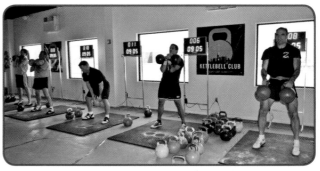

Photo by Nazo, courtesy of IKSFA

Long Cycle Event,
New York Open Kettlebell Championship.

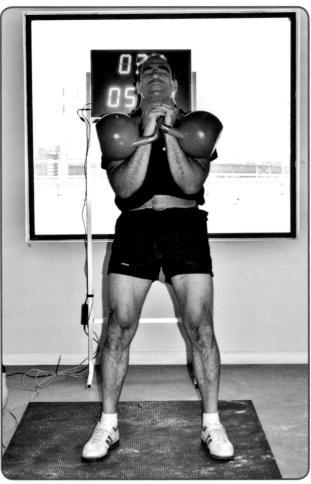

Photo by Nazo, courtesy of IKSFA

Halfway point!
Q: Resting, sleeping, or praying?
A: All of the above!

John Wild Buckley
Congratulating Jeff for achieving Rank 1 at
New York Open Kettlebell Championships.

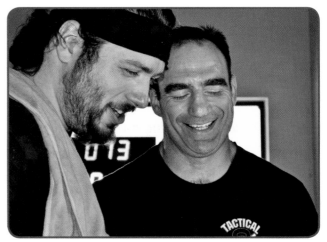

Photo by Nazo, courtesy of IKSFA

So what changed in five years?

The short answer: Two trips to St. Petersburg, Russia, where I trained with current GS World Champions and Honored Coaches of Russia; that's what changed it all!

Attitude of Gratitude

Before moving on, I need to give credit to the people who are responsible for adding this chapter in my life and this book.

Tom Corrigan and Mikhail Marshak are first and foremost. Their passion for the sport, training tips, and insight has proven invaluable. Thank you for introducing me to the IKSFA and encouraging me to attend their first training camp in St. Petersburg, Russia.

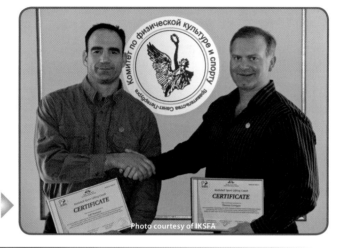

Photo courtesy of IKSFA

Tom Corrigan and Jeff Martone, graduation ceremony St. Petersburg, Russia.

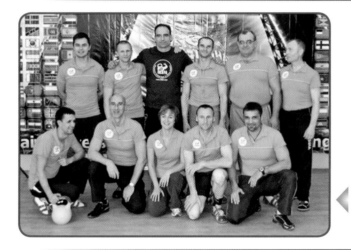

A very special thanks to Aleksandr Khasin, IKSFA CEO, "the man behind the scenes," for creating a world-class organization of true professionals. Thank you for giving me permission to use information from the IKSFA manual, photos, and addition resources.

Top Row:
A. Zhernakav, S Rudnev, J. martone, V. Andreychuk, S. Mishin, V. Tiknov
Bottom Row:
A. Semenov, A. Khasin, O. Nikifor, S. Merkulin, S. Rachinsky

I would like to personally thank all my friends, athletes, and coaches within the IKSFA for being a constant source of inspiration.

Thank you Nazo for taking awesome photos!

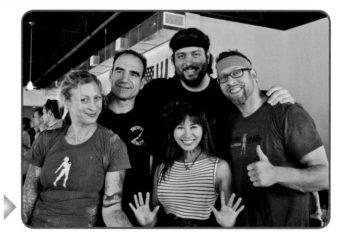

Juliet, Jeff, John, Nazo, Jason

History of Kettlebell Sport

The information below is a glimpse into the rich history of kettlebell lifting. It should give you the big picture of how the sport began and developed over the years.

Kettlebell Lifting B.S. (Before Sport)

Throughout the history, within every culture, strength has always been held in high esteem. In ancient times, the Russians were constantly defended against foreign invasions of the Mongols, Turks, and others. For any culture to survive and thrive, physical strength, power, and endurance are essential to support martial skills. For centuries Russian folk festivals and national holidays consisted of exciting events and tournaments. Fist fighting, wrestling, and lifting weights (i.e., logs, stones, millstones, bags of grain, anvils, etc.) were the favorite entertainment for the ordinary people of the working class. Even traditional Russian folk dancing was designed to build incredible strength endurance and cardiovascular conditioning.

- Girya is the Russian word for "kettlebell."

- Before competitions existed, a kettlebell was simply a weight with a handle used on scales to measures grain. The standard weight of grain was a pood, the equivalent of 16 kg.

The original girya, or kettlebell.

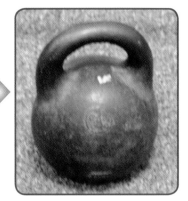

- Gireviks are athletes who lift kettlebells.

- The handle made it easy to lift and carry around the marketplace and flour mills. Wherever weights were commonplace, some kind of competition and display of strength were to be expected.

- If scale weights were unavailable, kettlebells were improvised by forge-welding handles onto cannon balls for general physical conditioning.

- Competitions were held not only among rural strongmen, but in the army and navy as well.

- Kettlebell lifting was used as assistance exercises to develop strength and endurance for the competitive sports of wrestling, boxing, and fencing.

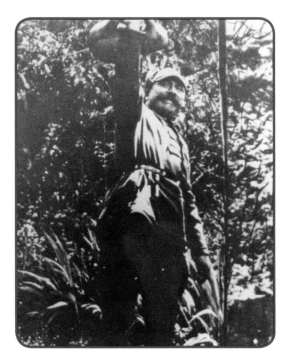

- Traveling circus shows toured the countryside with strongmen, performing complex strength routines and challenges and juggling kettlebells.

- By the 1900s most physical culturists and strongmen from around the world trained with kettlebells.

- After World War II, Russia was in need of strong hands and backs to restore their economy and protect their homeland.

- The kettlebell was the most accessible and low-cost means for developing strength and endurance, especially in rural areas.

- Weightlifting became one of the most prestigious and popular sports in the international arena. Many famous Russian weightlifters of those years got started by lifting kettlebells.

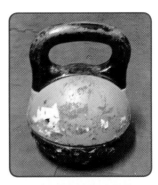

1950 era adjustable kettlebell. Internal weights allowed the kettlebell to weigh 16, 24, or 32 kg.

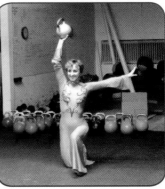

Oksana Nikifor - Power Juggling 2x World Champion 11x Champion of Russia

Kettlebell Sport: Fast Facts
The following information traces the development of modern kettlebell sport.

- Birth date: August 10, 1885; St. Petersburg, Russia.

- Founder: Physician V. Kraevski.

- Girevoy sport is the national weightlifting sport of Russia.

- 1897: Nationwide weightlifting championships began.

- 1948: The "first" official All-Union kettlebell competition. From this point forward, kettlebell lifting went from GPP to SPP (special physical preparation), becoming a sport all its own.

- 1962: Kettlebell rules and weight classes were established (i.e., 60, 70, 80, 90+ kg). Competition was a triathlon consisting of the press, jerk, and snatch; no time limits.

- 1974: Kettlebell sport is officially declared the ethnic sport of Russia.

- 1977: Snatch technique changed to what we see today.

- 1984: Kettlebell press removed from competition.

- 1985: First Championship of the USSR, introduction of prestigious title Master of Sport.

- 1989: Ten-minute time limits established. Long cycle became an event (Zaytcev).

- 1989: Power juggling was developed to promote kettlebell sport and entertain spectators with artistic display of strength and skill.

- 1998: Rachinsky introduced the relay event: five competitors per team, five weight categories, three-minute sprint each, traditional jerk, short jerk.

- 2009: Modified weight classes to 60, 65, 70, 75, 80, 90+ kg.

- 2010: Weight classes changed to international standard: 63, 68, 73, 78, 85, 95, 105, 105+.

- Professional kettlebell lifters refer to themselves as "sportsmen."

Historical Significance

Edmund Burke (1729–1797) said, "Those who don't know history are destined to repeat it."

I will close with an interesting insight straight from the former USSR. In 1981, an official commission enforced mandatory kettlebell training for the masses, relying on kettlebells as "an effective yet simple tool to increase productivity and decrease health care costs." It makes perfect sense from a health and productivity standpoint.

There's a staggering price to be paid for softness. Our nation's exploding obesity rates and the staggering health care and disability costs are alarming. However, what's more alarming is a quote from one of the most decorated and distinguished military leaders this nation has ever produced:

"Our country won't go on forever. If we stay soft as we are now, there won't be any AMERICA because some foreign soldiery will invade us and take our women and breed a hardier race!"—Lt. Gen. Lewis B. "Chesty" Puller, USMC

—**Lt. Gen. Lewis B. "Chesty" Puller, USMC**

Ouch!!

Benefits of Learning Sport Technique

"Weightlifting is physics, mathematics and biomechanics."

—**Louie Simmons, Westside Barbell Club**

The above statement is equally true if you insert the word kettlebell for weight. The Russians have a tremendous amount of science behind their sports (i.e., kettlebell lifting, power lifting, Olympic lifting, etc.). It's not about just lifting weights. It's about producing observable, measurable, repeatable results. There are different approaches to training based on different training goals. However, the notion that there are two distinct styles of kettlebell lifting (hard vs. soft) has more to do with a marketing strategy to create brand loyalty than it does with physics, mathematics, and biomechanics.

Regardless of your political orientation or motivation to train with kettlebells, please consider exploring the benefits of using sport technique and training methods for the following reasons:

1. Kettlebell sport is classified as a cyclical sport with competitive exercises lasting up to ten minutes. Athletes experience the same physiological benefits of other cyclical sports, such as rowing, biking, cross-country skiing, and long-distance running, without having to leave a four-foot-square platform.
2. Sport technique doesn't tear up your hands.
3. Economy of movement—no wasted energy, body doesn't break down under high volume and/or load.
4. Training with competition kettlebells provides maximum comfort while performing maximum number of reps.

5. Builds tremendous grip endurance and finger strength.
6. Anatomical breathing coordinates breathing with movement for greater endurance and rhythmic power under load.
7. Strengthens the abdominal muscles, trunk extensors, and muscles surrounding the hips, knees, and ankles.
8. Increases work capacity.
9. Increases shoulder flexibility and stability.

"The physiological basis of training comprises progressive functional and structural changes that occur in the body under the influence of repetitive training with gradually increased training load. These changes represent the basis of general progress and increase of work capacity of the body. GS athlete typically has harmoniously developed all organs and muscle groups with significant hypertrophy of extensors of the back, lower limbs and arms. Also, considerable changes are observed in the development of muscular-skeletal apparatus, cardio-vascular and respiratory system."

(Odintsov)

Extraordinary Endurance

"If you always put limits on everything you do, physical or anything else, it will spread into your work and into your life. There are no limits. There are only plateaus, and you must not stay there, you must go beyond them."

—Bruce Lee

CrossFit builds an excellent foundation of GPP.
Kettlebell sport training consists of both GPP and SPP. The goal of SPP in Kettlebell Sport is to form optimal technique (virtuosity) and special endurance in the classic kettlebell lifts (i.e., snatch, jerk, long cycle).

Endurance, the ability to resist fatigue and the ability to effectively recover during and after activity, is a determining physical factor in kettlebell sport. Endurance is typically characterized by either the number of possible exercise repetitions until failure, or by the time one can maintain a prescribed pace of lifts or a posture. Listed below are some amazing feats of endurance from one of my coaches.

Champion of the Guinness Book of Records

1. Jerk Kettlebell, 24 kg, 12 hours, 5,555 times.
2. Squat Barbell, 225 lb, 180 times.
3. Squat Barbell, 225 lb, 212 times.
4. Jerk Kettlebell OALC, 24 kg, 1 hour, 915 times.
5. Squat Barbell, 176 lb, 1 hour, 520 times.

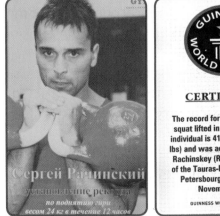

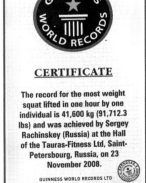

CERTIFICATE

The record for the most weight squat lifted in one hour by one individual is 41,600 kg (91,712.3 lbs) and was achieved by Sergey Rachinskey (Russia) at the Hall of the Tauras-Fitness Ltd, Saint-Petersbourg, Russia, on 23 November 2008.

GUINNESS WORLD RECORDS LTD

Switch from Sprint to Endurance Mode

It is important to understand that strength endurance is not a determining factor in kettlebell sport. In other words, performing competition lifts at a fast tempo of 30+ reps per minute for 1–3 minutes is purely a function of strength endurance (aka speed strength). This means that the main energy source comes from glycogen stored in the muscles and liver, which quickly produces oxygen debt, causing athletes to terminate sets prematurely.

On the other hand, the main energy source to complete 10 minutes of continuous lifting comes from the oxidative capability of slow twitch (red) muscle fibers. That's why it is critical to establish the right pace/tempo and breathing cycles that facilitate a steady supply of oxygen, allowing for sufficient recovery between repetitions. Stop and think about this for a couple of seconds.

In Olympic weightlifting, the main work is done by fast low-endurance (white) muscle fibers. It's a 6-second sport. In kettlebell lifting, the main work is done by both slow and high-endurance (red) muscle fibers. It's a 10-minute sport dominated by high oxidative activity. The first 3 minutes is glycolic. The last 7 minutes oxidative. This concept is the key that unlocks the "why" behind the methods used in kettlebell sport.

For example, this is why:

- Kettlebell sport is classified as a cyclical sport.
- Coaches speak in terms of number of reps per minute (rpm).
- Coaches emphasize the importance of proper breathing: "breathe, breathe, always breathe."
- It's important to develop special flexibility to allow your structure to take the load and your muscles to completely relax and recover in between reps.
- Kettlebell sport technique is so efficient yet looks a bit "odd" to the casual observer.
- It takes two to four years to become a master of sport. I liken it to earning rank in BJJ; there are no shortcuts!
- The only way to expedite the process is to find a qualified coach.

If you were in the market for a coach, you would be wise to consider the following standards:

"A prospective instructor must meet all three criteria before they can coach for me. They must be a:
1. World-class practitioner
2. World-class teacher
3. World-class person
If one of these elements is missing, I'll look for someone else."

—George Ryan, creator of CrossFit Striking, LAPD SWAT officer

A Coach's Coach:

Coach Rudnev prepared: approx. 200 CMS (Candidate Master of Sport), 35 MS (Master of Sport), 6 MSWC (Master of Sport World Class), 1 HMS (Honored Master of Sport), and me.

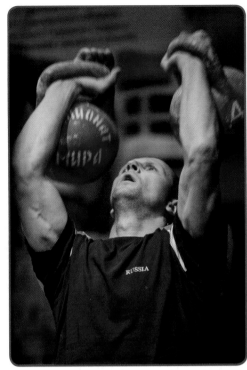

Sergey Rudnev,
HMS (Honored Master of Sport), MSWC (Master of Sport World Class), Honored Coach of Russia, 5-time World Champion, 5-time Champion of Russia; professor of Department of Physical Education and Sport, Girevoy Sport Specialization, Far-East Military Institute; trainer of the Russian National Team 2008–present.

Transferable Skills

Without a doubt, endurance is an important attribute for many athletes, especially fighters. Kettlebell sport technique and training protocols have proven to build elite levels of endurance to enhance performance of combat sports. As a matter of fact, that was one of the original purposes of lifting kettlebells in the first place.

What's not so obvious is that kettlebell sport technique develops an entire host of transferable skills:

1. Double knee bend is similar and complimentary to the movements of Olympic weightlifting.

2. Double knee bend and extension mimics how wrestlers pick up their opponents (your hips get under their hips, then simultaneous extension of knee, hips, back, and neck).

3. Movement of the hips and deflecting torso (i.e., leaning backward) similar technique to stone lifting, keg lifting, and other strongman/odd object lifts.

4. The connection of the elbow to the hip in the rack position and the extension of the hips during one-arm jerks mimic how a fighter would throw a shovel punch and an uppercut in boxing.

5. Rack position reinforces defensive position and ability to relax under pressure.

6. Hip movement during acceleration pull reinforces the principle that power originates from hips, moves through core, then out through a relaxed arm.

7. Asymmetrical load and continuous work develops core and respiratory endurance.

8. How to breathe properly and continuously with weight on chest (i.e., breathing under pressure) and during repeated efforts is essential for optimum performance transfers in striking and grappling sports.

9. Efficient clean and snatch technique reduces the chance of injury to wrists, elbow, shoulder.

Points to Ponder:

Watch the videos of the top champions and you will see different techniques, but all the variations are still based upon the principles of optimal use of energy. Kettlebell sport lifters' techniques are based upon their body type and size, limb length, injury history, and their own personal strengths and weaknesses. Smaller lifters bend their knees more to jerk than heavier ones do, and they also either squat more and/or lean over more when they load up to clean or snatch. Lifters with strong lower backs snatch and clean much differently than other lifters who rely on their leg and hip strength more.

Through years, even decades, of training and millions of reps, each champion has found technique variations that work for him or her personally. Beginning lifters should try to learn the general way to do the lifts and then modify them (hopefully under the guidance of an experience coach) according to their body. Imitating a champion with a completely different body structure is not the best way to go. Don't try and lift like a Clydesdale if you're an Arabian!

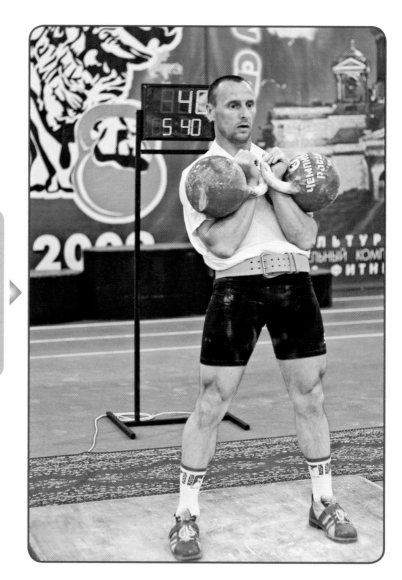

Sergey Merkulin,
MSWC, 15-time Champion of Russia,15-time World Champion, 5-time Champion of Europe. Multiple times record holder in long cycle, jerk, and biathlon.
Best results: Jerk—122;
Snatch—85 + 85;
Long Cycle—78; (current world record in 70 kg weight category)

In Closing

By nature, CrossFitters love to compete in everything—Olympic weightlifting, power lifting, triathlons, biking, running, paddle boarding, and so on. Why not give kettlebell sport a try?

You don't have to be an athlete to start, but you have to start to be an athlete. If you are in search of a new sport, I would highly recommend trying your hand at kettlebell sport. You have nothing to lose and everything to gain. Even if you have no desire to compete, the application of kettlebell sport principles and virtuosity will prove to be an invaluable tool for increasing your work capacity and performance over broad domains.

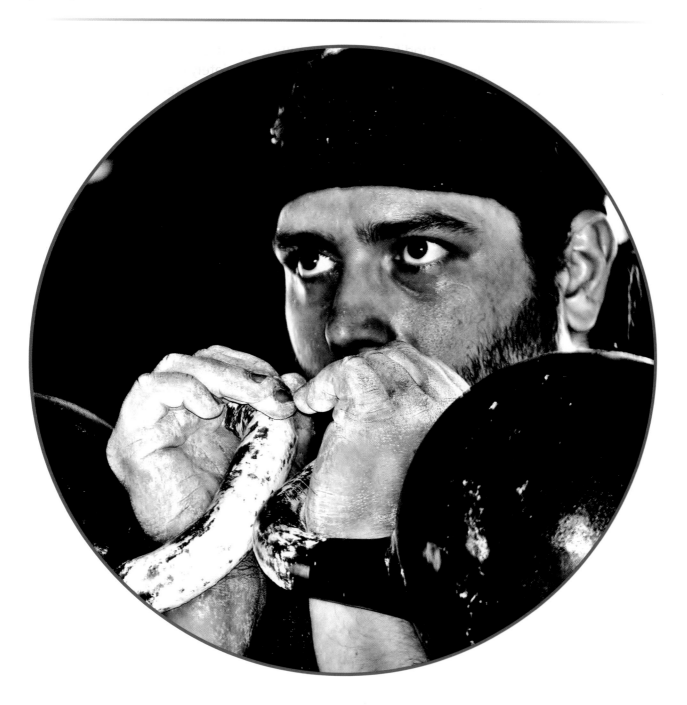

IKSFA INTERNATIONAL RANKING TABLE

Biathlon = jerk + snatch

Men's Biathlon: every lift in Jerk is 1 point and every lift in Snatch is 0.5 points. The snatch score is calculated as the sum of total lifts made with both hands, divided by 2. For example: 35 lifts were done in Jerk and the snatch = 24 lifts with right hand and 40 with left hand. The total count of points = 35 + (24 +40)/ 2 = 35 +64/2 = 35 +32 = 77 points.

Women's Biathlon: every jerk with one hand is 0.5 points and every snatch with one hand is 0.5 points. In the jerk and snatch, total number of points = sum of total lifts done by both hands, divided by 2. Example: Jerk - 35 +30 lifts were done with both right and left hand. Snatch - 24 right hand and 40 left hand. The total count for the event = (35 +30)/2 + (24 +40)/2 = 65/2 +64/2 = 32.5 +32 = 64.5 points.

Men's Long Cycle: every lift =1 point.

Women's Long Cycle: every lift by each hand = 1 point. The total number of points is determined by the amount of lifts performed by each hand.

Men's Jerk: every lift =1 point.

Women's Jerk: every lift =1 point. The total number of points is determined by the amount of lifts performed by each hand.

Snatch - Men and Women: every lift = 1 point. The total number of points is determined by the amount of lifts performed by each hand.

CMS = Candidate Master of Sport

MS = Master of Sport

MSIC = Master of Sport International Class

Men's Biathlon

Weight Categories (kg)	60	64	69	75	82	90	100	100+	KB weight	
MSIC	130	145	157	168	178	185	190	193	32kg	Ranks
MS	80	95	108	119	129	136	141	145		in category
CMS	50	62	73	83	92	96	101	105		HIGH MASTERY OF SPORT
CMS	100	120	135	148	159	168	177	185	24kg	Ranks
1	70	85	98	109	117	124	130	135		in category
2	50	62	74	84	91	98	103	107		SPORTING
3	29	39	49	58	65	72	77	80		PERFECTION
1	125	136	146	155	164	172	178	182	16kg	Ranks
2	85	93	100	106	112	118	124	130		in category
3	56	63	70	76	82	87	91	94		GPP
1	149	160	170	179	187	194	200	205	12kg	Ranks
2	106	115	122	129	136	143	149	153		in category
3	63	70	75	80	85	90	95	100		HEALTH

Men's Snatch

Weight Categories (kg)	60	64	69	75	82	90	100	100+	KB weight	
MSIC	126	140	154	166	174	182	188	192	32kg	Ranks
MS	80	94	106	116	126	134	140	144		in category
CMS	48	58	68	76	84	92	98	102		HIGH MASTERY OF SPORT
CMS	120	130	140	150	160	168	176	182	24kg	Ranks
1	80	90	98	106	114	120	126	130		in category
2	52	62	70	78	86	94	100	104		SPORTING
3	28	38	46	54	62	70	76	80		PERFECTION
1	134	146	156	164	172	180	189	190	16kg	Ranks
2	98	106	114	120	126	132	138	142		in category
3	66	74	80	86	90	94	98	100		GPP
1	150	160	168	176	184	190	196	200	12kg	Ranks
2	116	126	134	142	148	154	160	164		in category
3	78	86	92	98	104	110	116	120		HEALTH

Men's Long Cycle

Weight Categories (kg)	60	64	69	75	82	90	100	100+	KB weight	
MSIC	41	51	59	66	71	74	77	79	32kg	Ranks
MS	30	38	45	50	54	58	60	63		in category
CMS	20	29	36	42	46	51	53	55		HIGH MASTERY OF SPORT
CMS	50	58	65	72	78	83	87	90	24kg	Ranks
1	37	44	50	55	60	67	69	72		in category
2	27	32	37	41	45	49	53	56		SPORTING
3	17	21	25	29	33	37	40	42		PERFECTION
1	49	53	57	61	65	69	72	74	16kg	Ranks
2	38	42	45	48	51	54	57	59		in category
3	27	30	33	36	39	42	45	47		GPP
1	57	63	68	72	75	78	81	83	12kg	Ranks
2	48	52	55	58	61	64	67	69		in category
3	40	44	47	50	53	56	59	61		HEALTH

Men's Age to 18 Biathlon

Weight Categories (kg)	56	60	64	69	75	82	82+	KB weight	
CMS	80	100	120	135	148	159	164	24kg	Ranks
1	55	70	85	98	109	117	121		in category
2	38	50	62	74	84	91	95		SPORTING
3	19	29	39	49	58	65	69		PERFECTION
1	112	125	136	146	155	164	169	16kg	Ranks
2	75	85	93	100	106	112	116		in category
3	48	56	63	70	76	82	85		GPP
1	137	149	160	170	179	187	192	12kg	Ranks
2	98	106	115	122	129	136	141		in category
3	57	63	70	75	80	85	88		HEALTH

Men's Jerk

Weight Categories (kg)	60	64	69	75	82	90	100	100+	KB weight	
MSIC	90	100	109	117	124	130	135	138	32kg	Ranks
MS	60	71	81	90	97	103	108	112		in category
CMS	36	46	56	66	74	80	86	90		HIGH MASTERY OF SPORT
CMS	77	89	100	110	119	127	134	140	24kg	Ranks
1	59	69	78	86	94	101	107	112		in category
2	42	50	58	65	72	78	83	88		SPORTING
3	27	34	40	45	50	55	59	62		PERFECTION
1	85	92	98	103	108	113	117	120	16kg	Ranks
2	63	68	73	78	83	87	91	94		in category
3	47	51	55	59	63	67	70	72		GPP
1	106	112	117	122	127	131	135	139	12kg	Ranks
2	82	89	95	100	105	109	113	116		in category
3	57	63	68	73	78	82	86	89		HEALTH

Men's Age to 18 Long Cycle

Weight Categories (kg)	56	60	64	69	75	82	82+	KB weight	
CMS	41	50	58	65	72	78	81	24kg	Ranks
1	30	37	44	50	55	60	65		in category
2	21	27	32	37	41	45	47		SPORTING
3	13	17	21	25	29	33	35		PERFECTION
1	44	49	53	57	61	65	67	16kg	Ranks
2	34	38	42	45	48	51	53		in category
3	24	27	30	33	36	39	41		GPP
1	51	57	63	68	72	75	77	12kg	Ranks
2	43	48	52	55	58	61	63		in category
3	36	40	44	47	50	53	55		HEALTH

Men's Age to 18 Jerk

Weight Categories (kg)	56	60	64	69	75	82	82+	KB Weight	
CMS	65	77	89	100	110	119	124	24kg	Ranks
1	49	59	69	78	86	94	98		in category
2	34	42	50	58	65	72	76		SPORTING
3	20	27	34	40	45	50	53		PERFECTION
1	77	85	92	98	103	108	111	16kg	Ranks
2	57	63	68	73	78	83	85		in category
3	42	47	51	55	59	63	65		GPP
1	99	106	112	117	122	127	129	12kg	Ranks
2	74	82	89	95	100	105	107		in category
3	51	57	63	68	73	78	80		HEALTH

Men's Age to 18 Snatch

Weight Categories (kg)	56	60	64	69	75	82	82+	KB Weight	
CMS	110	120	130	140	150	160	166	24kg	Ranks
1	70	80	90	98	106	114	118		in category
2	42	52	62	70	78	86	90		SPORTING
3	18	28	38	46	54	62	68		PERFECTION
1	122	134	146	156	164	172	176	16kg	Ranks
2	88	98	106	114	120	126	130		in category
3	58	66	74	80	86	90	92		GPP
1	140	150	160	168	176	184	188	12kg	Ranks
2	106	116	126	134	142	148	152		in category
3	70	78	86	92	98	104	108		HEALTH

Men's Age to 16 Biathlon

Weight Categories (kg)	52	56	60	64	69	75	75+	KB Weight	
1	98	112	125	136	146	155	160	16kg	Ranks
2	63	75	85	93	100	106	110		in category
3	38	48	56	63	70	76	80		GPP
1	124	137	149	160	170	179	185	12kg	Ranks
2	86	98	106	115	122	129	134		in category
3	51	57	63	70	75	80	83		HEALTH

Men's Age to 16 Long Cycle

Weight Categories (kg)	52	56	60	64	69	75	75+	KB Weight	
1	39	44	49	53	57	61	63	16kg	Ranks
2	29	34	38	42	45	48	50		in category
3	20	24	27	30	33	36	38		GPP
1	44	51	57	63	68	72	44	12kg	Ranks
2	37	43	48	52	55	58	60		in category
3	31	36	40	44	47	50	52		HEALTH

Men's Age to 16 Jerk

Weight Categories (kg)	52	56	60	64	69	75	75+	KB Weight	
1	68	77	85	92	98	103	106	16kg	Ranks
2	50	57	63	68	73	78	81		in category
3	36	42	47	51	55	59	61		GPP
1	88	99	106	112	117	122	125	12kg	Ranks
2	65	74	82	89	95	100	103		in category
3	45	51	57	63	68	73	45		HEALTH

Men's Age to 16 Snatch

Weight Categories (kg)	52	56	60	64	69	75	75+	KB Weight	
1	110	122	134	146	156	164	168	16kg	Ranks
2	78	88	98	106	114	120	124		in category
3	50	58	66	74	80	86	88		GPP
1	128	140	150	160	168	176	180	12kg	Ranks
2	96	106	116	126	134	142	146		in category
3	62	70	78	86	92	98	102		HEALTH

Men's Age to 14 Biathlon

Weight Categories (kg)	48	52	56	60	64	69	69+	KB Weight	
1	110	124	137	149	160	170	177	12kg	Ranks
2	76	86	98	106	115	122	127		in category
3	45	51	57	63	70	75	78		HEALTH

Men's Age to 14 Long Cycle

Weight Categories (kg)	48	52	56	60	64	69	69+	KB Weight	
1	37	44	51	57	63	68	70	12kg	Ranks
2	31	37	43	48	52	55	57		in category
3	26	31	36	40	44	47	49		HEALTH

Men's Age to 14 Jerk

Weight Categories (kg)	48	52	56	60	64	69	69+	KB Weight	
1	75	88	99	106	112	117	120	12kg	Ranks
2	55	65	74	82	89	95	98		in category
3	38	45	51	57	63	68	71		HEALTH

Men's Age to 14 Snatch

Weight Categories (kg)	48	52	56	60	64	69	69+	KB Weight	
1	116	128	140	150	160	168	172	12kg	Ranks
2	84	96	106	116	126	134	140		in category
3	54	62	70	78	86	92	96		HEALTH

Women's Biathlon

Weight Categories (kg)	50	54	59	65	72	72+	KB Weight	
MSIC	136	144	152	160	166	170	20kg	Ranks
MS	108	120	126	134	140	144		in category
CMS	90	98	104	110	116	120		HIGH MASTERY OF SPORT
CMS	134	142	150	158	164	168	16kg	Ranks
1	106	118	124	132	138	142		in category
2	88	96	104	108	114	118		SPORTING
3	62	68	74	80	84	88		PERFECTION
1	126	136	144	150	156	160	12kg	Ranks
2	102	110	116	122	126	130		in category
3	84	92	98	64	84	104		GPP
1	146	154	162	170	176	180	8kg	Ranks
2	120	128	134	140	146	150		in category
3	96	102	108	114	118	122		HEALTH

Women's Snatch

Weight Categories (kg)	50	54	59	65	72	72+	KB Weight	
MSIC	140	154	166	176	184	190	20kg	Ranks
MS	100	12	124	134	142	148		in category
CMS	58	70	80	88	96	102		HIGH MASTERY OF SPORT
CMS	130	144	156	166	174	180	16kg	Ranks
1	92	104	114	124	132	138		in category
2	70	78	86	92	98	102		SPORTING
3	52	60	66	72	78	82		PERFECTION
1	118	132	144	154	162	168	12kg	Ranks
2	94	102	110	122	126	128		in category
3	68	74	80	84	88	90		GPP
1	144	158	170	182	192	200	8kg	Ranks
2	112	122	130	138	144	148		in category
3	88	94	60	80	94	98		HEALTH

Women's Long Cycle

Weight Categories (kg)	50	54	59	65	72	72+	KB Weight	
MSIC	96	104	112	120	126	130	24kg	Ranks
MS	76	84	90	96	102	108		in category
MS	92	100	106	112	118	122	20kg	HIGH
CMS	58	64	70	74	78	82	24kg	MASTERY
CMS	70	78	84	90	96	100	20kg	OF SPORT
1	80	88	98	106	114	120	16kg	Ranks
2	62	70	78	84	90	94		in category
3	46	52	58	62	66	70		SPORTING PERFECTION
1	108	114	118	122	126	130	12kg	Ranks
2	82	86	90	94	98	100		in category
3	56	60	64	68	72	74		GPP
1	122	126	130	134	138	140	8kg	Ranks
2	104	108	112	116	120	122		in category
3	84	88	92	96	100	102		HEALTH

Women's Age to 18 Biathlon

Weight Categories (kg)	47	50	54	59	65	65+	KB Weight	
CMS	124	134	142	150	158	162	16kg	Ranks
1	96	106	118	124	132	136		in category
2	78	88	96	104	108	112		SPORTING
3	54	62	68	74	80	82		PERFECTION
1	116	126	136	144	150	154	12kg	Ranks
2	94	102	110	116	122	124		in category
3	74	84	92	98	64	74		GPP
1	136	146	154	162	170	150	8kg	Ranks
2	112	120	128	134	140	144		in category
3	88	96	102	108	114	116		HEALTH

Women's Age to 18 Long Cycle

Weight Categories (kg)	47	50	54	59	65	65+	KB Weight	
1	72	80	88	98	106	110	16kg	Ranks
2	54	62	70	78	84	88		in category
3	40	46	52	58	62	64		SPORTING PERFFECTION
1	102	108	114	118	122	124	12kg	Ranks
2	76	82	86	90	94	96		in category
3	52	56	60	64	68	70		GPP
1	118	122	126	130	134	136	8kg	Ranks
2	100	104	108	112	116	118		in category
3	80	84	88	92	96	98		HEALTH

Women's Jerk

Weight Categories (kg)	50	54	59	65	72	72+	KB Weight	
MSIC	144	158	170	180	188	194	20kg	Ranks
MS	118	128	138	148	158	166		in category
CMS	96	108	118	126	134	140		HIGH MASTERY OF SPORT
CMS	134	148	160	170	178	186	16kg	Ranks
1	112	122	132	140	148	154		in category
2	92	100	108	114	120	124		SPORTING
3	74	80	86	92	96	100		PERFECTION
1	134	146	156	166	174	180	12kg	Ranks
2	106	114	122	128	134	138		in category
3	82	86	90	94	98	100		GPP
1	156	168	180	190	198	204	8kg	Ranks
2	122	130	136	142	148	152		in category
3	90	94	98	102	106	108		HEALTH

Women's Age to 18 Jerk

Weight Categories (kg)	47	50	54	59	65	65+	KB Weight	
CMS	120	134	148	160	170	174	16kg	Ranks
1	100	112	122	132	140	144		in category
2	84	92	100	108	114	118		SPORTING
3	68	74	80	86	92	94		PERFECTION
1	122	134	146	156	166	170	12kg	Ranks
2	98	106	114	122	128	132		in category
3	78	82	86	90	94	96		GPP
1	144	156	168	180	190	194	8kg	Ranks
2	114	122	130	136	142	146		in category
3	86	90	94	98	102	104		HEALTH

Women's Age to 18 Snatch

Weight Categories (kg)	47	50	54	59	65	65+	KB Weight	Ranks
CMS	116	130	144	156	166	170	16kg	Ranks
1	80	92	104	114	124	128		in category
2	62	70	78	86	92	96		SPORTING
3	44	52	60	66	72	76		PERFECTION
1	104	118	132	144	154	160	12kg	Ranks
2	84	94	102	110	122	124		in category
3	60	68	74	80	84	86		GPP
1	128	144	158	170	182	188	8kg	Ranks
2	102	112	122	130	138	142		in category
3	80	88	94	60	80	88		HEALTH

Women's Age to 16 Biathlon

Weight Categories (kg)	44	47	50	54	59	59+	KB Weight	Ranks
1	106	116	126	136	144	148	12kg	Ranks
2	86	94	102	110	116	120		in category
3	64	74	84	92	98	102		GPP
1	126	136	146	154	162	128	8kg	Ranks
2	104	112	120	128	134	138		in category
3	80	88	96	102	108	112		HEALTH

Women's Age to 16 Long Cycle

Weight Categories (kg)	44	47	50	54	59	59+	KB Weight	Ranks
1	96	102	108	114	118	120	12kg	Ranks
2	68	76	82	86	90	92		in category
3	46	52	56	60	64	66		GPP
1	112	118	122	126	130	132	8kg	Ranks
2	94	100	104	108	112	114		in category
3	76	80	84	88	92	94		HEALTH

Women's Age to 16 Jerk

Weight Categories (kg)	44	47	50	54	59	59+	KB Weight	Ranks
1	108	122	134	146	156	162	12kg	Ranks
2	90	98	106	114	122	124		in category
3	74	78	82	86	90	92		GPP
1	130	144	156	168	180	186	8kg	Ranks
2	106	114	122	130	136	140		in category
3	82	86	90	94	98	100		HEALTH

Women's Age to 16 Snatch

Weight Categories (kg)	44	47	50	54	59	59+	KB Weight	Ranks
1	88	104	118	132	144	150	12kg	Ranks
2	72	84	94	102	110	118		in category
3	52	60	68	74	80	82		GPP
1	112	128	144	158	170	178	8kg	Ranks
2	90	102	112	122	130	134		in category
3	70	80	88	94	60	70		HEALTH

Women's Age to 14 Biathlon

Weight Categories (kg)	41	44	47	50	54	54+	KB Weight	Ranks
1	114	126	136	146	154	164	8kg	Ranks
2	94	104	112	120	128	132		in category
3	72	80	88	96	102	106		HEALTH

Women's Age to 14 Long Cycle

Weight Categories (kg)	41	44	47	50	54	54+	KB Weight	Ranks
1	106	112	118	122	126	128	8kg	Ranks
2	88	94	100	104	108	110		in category
3	72	76	80	84	88	90		HEALTH

Women's Age to 14 Jerk

Weight Categories (kg)	41	44	47	50	54	54+	KB Weight	Ranks
1	114	130	144	156	168	176	8kg	Ranks
2	96	106	114	122	130	134		in category
3	78	82	86	90	94	96		HEALTH

Women's Age to 14 Snatch

Weight Categories (kg)	41	44	47	50	54	54+	KB Weight	Ranks
1	96	112	128	144	158	166	8kg	Ranks
2	76	90	102	112	122	126		in category
3	60	70	80	88	94	98		HEALTH

Division information:

Weight Class – Refer to the rankings above.

Female Divisions:
· Amateur Adult (8 kg, 12 kg, and 16 kg k-bell) – any age
· Professional Adult (20 kg and 24 kg bell) – any age
· Juniors (8 kg k-bell) – up to 14 years
· Juniors (8 kg or 12 kg k-bell) – up to 16 years
· Juniors(8 kg, 12 kg, or 16 kg k-bell) – up to 18 years
· Masters (12 kg bell) – 40 +
· Seniors (8 kg bell) – 55+

Male Divisions:

· Amateur Adult(12 kg or 16 kg k-bell) – any age
· Professional Adult (24 kg or 32 kg k- bell) – any age
· Juniors (12 kg k-bell) – up to 14 years
· Juniors (12 kg or 16 kg k-bell) – up to 16 years
· Junior (12 kg, 16 kg or 24 kg k-bell) – up to 18 years
· Masters (16 kg bell) – 40 +
· Seniors (12 kg bell) – 55+